Fundamentals of
Hair and Scalp Dermoscopy

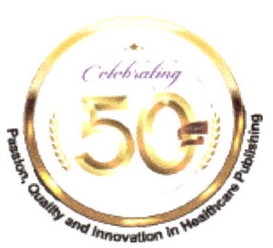

Fundamentals of Hair and Scalp Dermoscopy

Editor

Isabella Doche MD PhD
Department of Dermatology
University of São Paulo Medical School
São Paulo, Brazil

Co-editors

Patricia Damasco MD
Department of Dermatology
Hospital Regional da Asa Norte
Brasília, DF, Brazil

Giselle Martins MD
Department of Dermatology
Santa Casa de Misericórdia of Porto Alegre
Federal University of Health Sciences of Porto Alegre
Porto Alegre, RS, Brazil

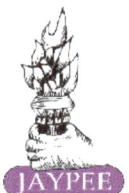

JAYPEE BROTHERS MEDICAL PUBLISHERS
The Health Sciences Publisher
New Delhi | London | Panama

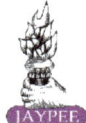 **Jaypee Brothers Medical Publishers (P) Ltd**

Headquarters
Jaypee Brothers Medical Publishers (P) Ltd
4838/24, Ansari Road, Daryaganj
New Delhi 110 002, India
Phone: +91-11-43574357
Fax: +91-11-43574314
Email: jaypee@jaypeebrothers.com

Overseas Offices

J.P. Medical Ltd
83 Victoria Street, London
SW1H 0HW (UK)
Phone: +44 20 3170 8910
Fax: +44 (0)20 3008 6180
Email: info@jpmedpub.com

Jaypee-Highlights Medical Publishers Inc
City of Knowledge, Bld. 235, 2nd Floor
Clayton, Panama City, Panama
Phone: +1 507-301-0496
Fax: +1 507-301-0499
Email: cservice@jphmedical.com

Jaypee Brothers Medical Publishers (P) Ltd
Bhotahity, Kathmandu, Nepal
Phone: +977-9741283608
Email: kathmandu@jaypeebrothers.com

Website: www.jaypeebrothers.com
Website: www.jaypeedigital.com

© 2019, Jaypee Brothers Medical Publishers

The views and opinions expressed in this book are solely those of the original contributor(s)/author(s) and do not necessarily represent those of editor(s) of the book.

All rights reserved. No part of this publication may be reproduced, stored or transmitted in any form or by any means, electronic, mechanical, photocopying, recording or otherwise, without the prior permission in writing of the publishers.

All brand names and product names used in this book are trade names, service marks, trademarks or registered trademarks of their respective owners. The publisher is not associated with any product or vendor mentioned in this book.

Medical knowledge and practice change constantly. This book is designed to provide accurate, authoritative information about the subject matter in question. However, readers are advised to check the most current information available on procedures included and check information from the manufacturer of each product to be administered, to verify the recommended dose, formula, method and duration of administration, adverse effects and contraindications. It is the responsibility of the practitioner to take all appropriate safety precautions. Neither the publisher nor the author(s)/editor(s) assume any liability for any injury and/or damage to persons or property arising from or related to use of material in this book.

This book is sold on the understanding that the publisher is not engaged in providing professional medical services. If such advice or services are required, the services of a competent medical professional should be sought.

Every effort has been made where necessary to contact holders of copyright to obtain permission to reproduce copyright material. If any have been inadvertently overlooked, the publisher will be pleased to make the necessary arrangements at the first opportunity. The **CD/DVD-ROM** (if any) provided in the sealed envelope with this book is complimentary and free of cost. **Not meant for sale**.

Inquiries for bulk sales may be solicited at: jaypee@jaypeebrothers.com

Fundamentals of Hair and Scalp Dermoscopy

First Edition: **2019**

ISBN 978-93-5270-561-0

Printed at

Contributors

Alessandra Anzai MD
Division of Dermatology
Hospital das Clínicas
University of São Paulo Medical School
São Paulo, Brazil

Amy McMichael MD
Chair, Department of Dermatology
Wake Forest University School of Medicine
Winston-Salem, North Carolina, USA

Antonella Tosti MD
Department of Dermatology and Cutaneous Surgery
University of Miami Miller School of Medicine
Miami, Florida, USA

Cyro Festa Neto MD PhD
Chair, Department of Dermatology
University of São Paulo Medical School
São Paulo, Brazil

Daniel Asz-Sigall MD
Onco Dermatology Clinic
National Autonomous University of Mexico
Ciudad de Mexico, CDMX, Mexico

Emilie Jane Fowler BS
Department of Dermatology and Cutaneous Surgery
University of Miami Miller School of Medicine
Miami, Florida, USA

Giselle Martins MD
Department of Dermatology
Santa Casa de Misericórdia of Porto Alegre
Federal University of Health Sciences of Porto Alegre
Porto Alegre, RS, Brazil

Iris Zalaudek MD
Chair, Dermatology Clinic
Hospital Maggiore, University of Trieste
Trieste, TS, Italy

Isabella Doche MD PhD
Department of Dermatology
University of São Paulo Medical School
São Paulo, Brazil

Jade Cury Martins MD PhD
Department of Dermatology
University of São Paulo Medical School and ICESP
São Paulo, Brazil

José Antonio Sanches MD PhD
Chair, Department of Dermatology
University of São Paulo Medical School
São Paulo, Brazil

Laura N Uwakwe MD
Department of Dermatology
Wake Forest University School of Medicine
Winston-Salem, North Carolina, USA

Lidia Rudnicka MD PhD
Department of Dermatology
Medical University of Warsaw
Warszawa, Poland

Maria Abril Martínez-Velasco MD
Onco Dermatology Clinic
National Autonomous University of Mexico
Ciudad de Mexico, CDMX, Mexico

Maria Cecília da Matta Rivitti Machado MD
Division of Dermatology
Hospital das Clínicas
University of São Paulo Medical School
São Paulo, Brazil

Maria de Fátima Maklouf Amorim Ruiz MD
Department of Dermatology
Escola Paulista de Medicina
Federal University of São Paulo
São Paulo, Brazil

Maria K Hordinsky MD
Chair, Department of Dermatology
University of Minnesota Medical School
Minneapolis, Minnesota, USA

Marina Lino Vieira MD
Division of Dermatology
Hospital das Clínicas
University of São Paulo Medical School
São Paulo, Brazil

Marta Kurzeja MD PhD
Private Practice
Warsaw, Poland

Maximilian Uranitsch MD
Department of Dermatology and Venereology
Medical University of Graz
Graz, Austria

Neusa Yuriko Sakai Valente MD PhD
Division of Dermatology
Hospital das Clínicas
University of São Paulo Medical School
São Paulo, Brazil

Norma Elizabeth Vázquez-Herrera MD
Department of Dermatology
Tecnologico de Monterrey
Monterrey, Nuevo León, Mexico

Patricia Damasco MD
Department of Dermatology
Hospital Regional da Asa Norte
Brasília, DF, Brazil

Ricardo Romiti MD PhD
Division of Dermatology
Hospital das Clínicas
University of São Paulo Medical School
São Paulo, Brazil

Roberta Giuffrida MD
Department of Clinical and Experimental Medicine
Section of Dermatology
University of Messina
Messina, ME, Italy

Roberto Arenas MD
Micology Section
"Dr Manuel Gea González" General Hospital
Ciudad de Mexico, CDMX, Mexico

Valeria Petri MD PhD
Department of Dermatology
Federal University of São Paulo
São Paulo, Brazil

Zilda Najjar Prado de Oliveira MD PhD
Division of Dermatology
Hospital das Clínicas
University of São Paulo Medical School
São Paulo, Brazil

Preface

The idea of making a book on hair and scalp dermoscopy arose partly because of an increased need to teach more about this noninvasive and practical tool in daily practice. Hair dermoscopy or trichoscopy not only allows a more accurate diagnosis, but also enhance treatment and follow-up in many cases of hair diseases. In this book, we tried to gather the most updated findings and features in the main hair and scalp disorders, and to discuss some tips and pearls we have learned in the last years practicing the examination, although there is so much to learn and discover in this amazing field.

The second reason was based on the inspiring mentors that not only thought me a lot about this technique, but also about perseverance, enthusiasm and altruism. I hope this book inspires the readers to make new discoveries and also share their experiences in this fascinating field of hair diseases.

Isabella Doche

Acknowledgments

I would like to acknowledge my friends, colleagues and professors from the University of São Paulo, for the friendship and fully support.

My sincere gratitude to Dr Damasco and Dr Martins, for having accepted my invitation to co-edit this project, and to my colleagues and all book contributors who encouraged and helped me in this journey, especially Dr Maria K Hordinsky, Dr Antonella Tosti and Dr Lidia Rudnicka, for being great mentors and leaders in the field of hair diseases.

Last but not least, I thank my family for the tireless support and God, who always give me strength to keep moving forward.

Contents

Chapter 1. **Normal Scalp** 1
Patricia Damasco, Giselle Martins, Isabella Doche

Chapter 2. **Devices for Hair and Scalp Dermoscopy** 5
Giselle Martins, Patricia Damasco, Isabella Doche

Chapter 3. **Trichoscopy Patterns and Tips to Enhance Your Exam** 8
Isabella Doche, Giselle Martins, Patricia Damasco

Chapter 4. **Nonscarring Alopecias** 33

    4.1 **Androgenetic Alopecia or Male-Pattern Hair Loss** 33
Patricia Damasco, Giselle Martins, Isabella Doche

    4.2 **Female-Pattern Hair Loss** 37
Giselle Martins, Patricia Damasco, Isabella Doche

    4.3 **Senescent or Senile Alopecia** 40
Isabella Doche

    4.4 **Telogen Effluvium** 42
Patricia Damasco, Giselle Martins, Isabella Doche

    4.5 **Alopecia Areata** 44
Isabella Doche, Maria K Hordinsky

    4.6 **Alopecia Areata Incognito** 49
Emilie Jane Fowler, Antonella Tosti

    4.7 **Trichotillomania** 51
Lidia Rudnicka

    4.8 **Dissecting Cellulitis (Initial Stage)** 53
Isabella Doche

    4.9 **Chemotherapy-induced Alopecia** 56
Giselle Martins, Patricia Damasco, Isabella Doche

    4.10 **Radiotherapy-induced Alopecia** 59
Giselle Martins, Patricia Damasco, Isabella Doche

    4.11 **Traction Alopecia (Initial Stage)** 62
Patricia Damasco, Giselle Martins, Isabella Doche

    4.12 **Pressure-induced Alopecia** 65
Isabella Doche

Chapter 5 **Scarring Alopecias** 67

    5.1 **Lichen Planopilaris** 68
Isabella Doche

    5.2 **Frontal Fibrosing Alopecia** 74
Isabella Doche

5.3 **Fibrosing Alopecia in a Pattern Distribution** 80
Giselle Martins, Patricia Damasco, Isabella Doche

5.4 **Discoid Lupus Erythematosus** 84
Patricia Damasco, Giselle Martins, Isabella Doche

5.5 **Traction Alopecia (Late Stage)** 88
Patricia Damasco, Giselle Martins, Isabella Doche

5.6 **Central Centrifugal Cicatricial Alopecia** 91
Laura N Uwakwe, Amy McMichael, Patricia Damasco, Isabella Doche

5.7 **Pseudopelade of Brocq** 93
Isabella Doche

5.8 **Alopecia Mucinosa and Folliculotropic Mycosis Fungoides** 95
Lidia Rudnicka

5.9 **Keratosis Follicularis Spinulosa Decalvans** 97
Isabella Doche

5.10 **Folliculitis Decalvans** 100
Giselle Martins, Patricia Damasco, Isabella Doche

5.11 **Dissecting Cellulitis (Late Stage)** 104
Isabella Doche

5.12 **Acne Keloidalis Nuchae** 106
Maria Cecília da Matta Rivitti Machado, Isabella Doche

5.13 **Erosive Pustular Dermatosis of the Scalp** 108
Giselle Martins, Patricia Damasco, Isabella Doche

Chapter 6. Inflammatory Scalp Disorders 111

6.1 **Seborrheic Dermatitis/Pityriasis Amiantacea** 111
Isabella Doche

6.2 **Psoriasis** 114
Ricardo Romiti, Alessandra Anzai

6.3 **Contact Dermatitis** 117
Emilie Jane Fowler, Antonella Tosti

6.4 **Rosacea-like Dermatosis** 119
Giselle Martins, Patricia Damasco, Isabella Doche

Chapter 7. Systemic Diseases 121

7.1 **Systemic Lupus Erythematosus** 121
Patricia Damasco, Giselle Martins, Isabella Doche

7.2 **Dermatomyositis** 124
Isabella Doche, Maria K Hordinsky

7.3 **Scleroderma** 127
Ricardo Romiti, Alessandra Anzai

7.4 **Sarcoidosis** 130
Isabella Doche

7.5 **Amyloidosis** 132
Giselle Martins, Patricia Damasco, Isabella Doche

Chapter 8. Infections and Infestations 133

8.1 **Localized Infectious Diseases** 133
Daniel Asz-Sigall, Maria Abril Martínez-Velasco, Norma Elizabeth Vásquez-Herrera, Roberto Arenas, Antonella Tosti

8.2 Systemic Infectious Diseases 138
Maria de Fátima Maklouf Amorim Ruiz, Valeria Petri, Isabella Doche

Chapter 9 Alopecia During Childhood 141

9.1 Aplasia Cutis Congenita 141
Giselle Martins, Patricia Damasco, Isabella Doche

9.2 Congenital Triangular Alopecia 144
Giselle Martins, Patricia Damasco, Isabella Doche

9.3 Loose Anagen Syndrome 146
Giselle Martins, Patricia Damasco, Isabella Doche

9.4 Short Anagen Syndrome 148
Giselle Martins, Patricia Damasco, Isabella Doche

Chapter 10. Genetic Skin Diseases 150

10.1 Ichthyosis 150
Marina Lino Vieira, Maria Cecilia da Matta Rivitti Machado, Zilda Najjar Prado de Oliveira, Isabella Doche

10.2 Ectodermal Dysplasia 152
Marina Lino Vieira, Maria Cecilia da Matta Rivitti Machado, Zilda Najjar Prado de Oliveira, Isabella Doche

10.3 Congenital Epidermolysis Bullosa 154
Zilda Najjar Prado de Oliveira, Maria Cecilia da Matta Rivitti Machado, Marina Lino Vieira, Isabella Doche

Chapter 11. Autoimmune Bullous Disorders 156
Marta Kurzeja

Chapter 12. Hair Shaft Disorders 163

12.1 Monilethrix 163
Giselle Martins, Patricia Damasco, Isabella Doche, Neusa Yuriko Sakai Valente

12.2 Pili Torti 166
Giselle Martins, Patricia Damasco, Isabella Doche

12.3 Pili Annulati 169
Giselle Martins, Patricia Damasco, Isabella Doche

12.4 Trichorrhexis Invaginata 171
Giselle Martins, Patricia Damasco, Isabella Doche

12.5 Woolly Hair 173
Giselle Martins, Patricia Damasco, Isabella Doche

12.6 Pili Trianguli et Canaliculi 175
Neusa Yuriko Sakai Valente, Isabella Doche

12.7 Trichothiodystrophy 178
Neusa Yuriko Sakai Valente, Isabella Doche

12.8 Silvery Hair Syndromes 180
Neusa Yuriko Sakai Valente, Isabella Doche

12.9 Trichorrhexis Nodosa 183
Patricia Damasco, Giselle Martins, Isabella Doche

12.10 Bubble Hair 186
Patricia Damasco, Giselle Martins, Isabella Doche

12.11 Trichoptilosis 187
Patricia Damasco, Giselle Martins, Isabella Doche

12.12 Trichonodosis 189
Patricia Damasco, Giselle Martins, Isabella Doche

Chapter 13.	**Eyebrows and Eyelashes Disorders**	**190**
	Patricia Damasco, Giselle Martins, Isabella Doche	
Chapter 14.	**Cosmetic Hair Products**	**199**
	14.1 Camouflage 199	
	Patricia Damasco, Giselle Martins, Isabella Doche	
	14.2 Extensions 201	
	Patricia Damasco, Giselle Martins, Isabella Doche	
	14.3 Micropigmentation and Tattoo 203	
	Patricia Damasco, Giselle Martins, Isabella Doche	
	14.4 Dry Shampoos, Hair Sprays, and Others 206	
	Patricia Damasco, Giselle Martins, Isabella Doche	
	14.5 Hair Matting 208	
	Patricia Damasco, Giselle Martins, Isabella Doche	
Chapter 15.	**Nonmelanocytic Scalp Tumors**	**210**
	Jade Cury Martins, José Antonio Sanches, Cyro Festa Neto	
Chapter 16.	**Melanocytic Scalp Tumors**	**224**
	Melanoma 224	
	Maximilian Uranitsch, Roberta Giuffrida, Iris Zalaudek	
	Benign Tumors 226	
	Maximilian Uranitsch, Roberta Giuffrida, Iris Zalaudek	
Chapter 17.	**Pearls and Pitfalls**	**231**
	Isabella Doche, Giselle Martins, Patricia Damasco	
Index		*243*

CHAPTER 1

Normal Scalp

Patricia Damasco, Giselle Martins, Isabella Doche

INTRODUCTION

Dermoscopy of hair and scalp or trichoscopy is a useful technique that can help clinicians to better detect hair and scalp disorders. With this technique, it is possible to measure and compare the hair shaft thickness in different scalp areas, to evaluate hair shaft abnormalities and to assess perifollicular and interfollicular patterns. Only few studies on normal scalp have been published, focusing mainly on hair shafts, hair follicle openings, and vascular patterns.

Normal hair shafts are uniform in thickness, shape, and color with continuous, interrupted, fragmented, or absent medulla. About 20% of human scalp hairs can be thin and up to 10% are vellus hairs. An increased proportion of thin hairs is characteristic of androgenetic alopecia.

For classification purposes, the hair can be divided into three main groups according to their racial origin: (1) Caucasian, (2) African, and (3) Asian. These groups differ mainly in their appearance, geometry, mechanical properties and water content.

NORMAL CAUCASIAN SCALP

On the scalp, there are evenly spaced groups of few hair shafts coming out of the same follicular ostium. In healthy individuals, two to three hairs emerge from one follicular unit (average: 2.6). Less than 5% of all follicular units consist of follicular units with four or more hairs. In the temporal area, up to 40% of the follicular units can have one hair (Figs. 1.1A to D). In the frontal region, single follicular units should be less than 35% and in the occipital area, less than 30%. The number of single follicular units increases with aging and some hair disorders.

There are marked differences in hair shaft structure among different ethnic groups. The shape of the hair shaft is partly formed by the shape of the hair follicle (Figs. 1.2 and 1.3). Caucasian hair is described as having intermediate thickness, between African and Asian hairs. The cross-sectional diameter ranges from 0.04 mm (in blond-haired people) to 0.09 mm (in dark-haired individuals). Some trichoscopic features, such as empty follicular openings and yellow dots are occasionally seen in healthy individuals.

The appearance of cutaneous microvessels may vary in type, arrangement, and number. Normal scalp vessels include thin arborizing vessels, found usually in the occipital and temporal areas, and interfollicular simple red loops, mainly observed in the frontal scalp (Figs. 1.4 and 1.5).

NORMAL AFRICAN SCALP

African descents have a large variability in their hair shaft diameter, ranging from 0.06 mm to 0.1 mm. Shafts are asymmetrical, with an elliptical or oval cross-sectional shape with a curved bulb, giving the African hair a curly and frizzy appearance. Because the hairs exit the epidermis

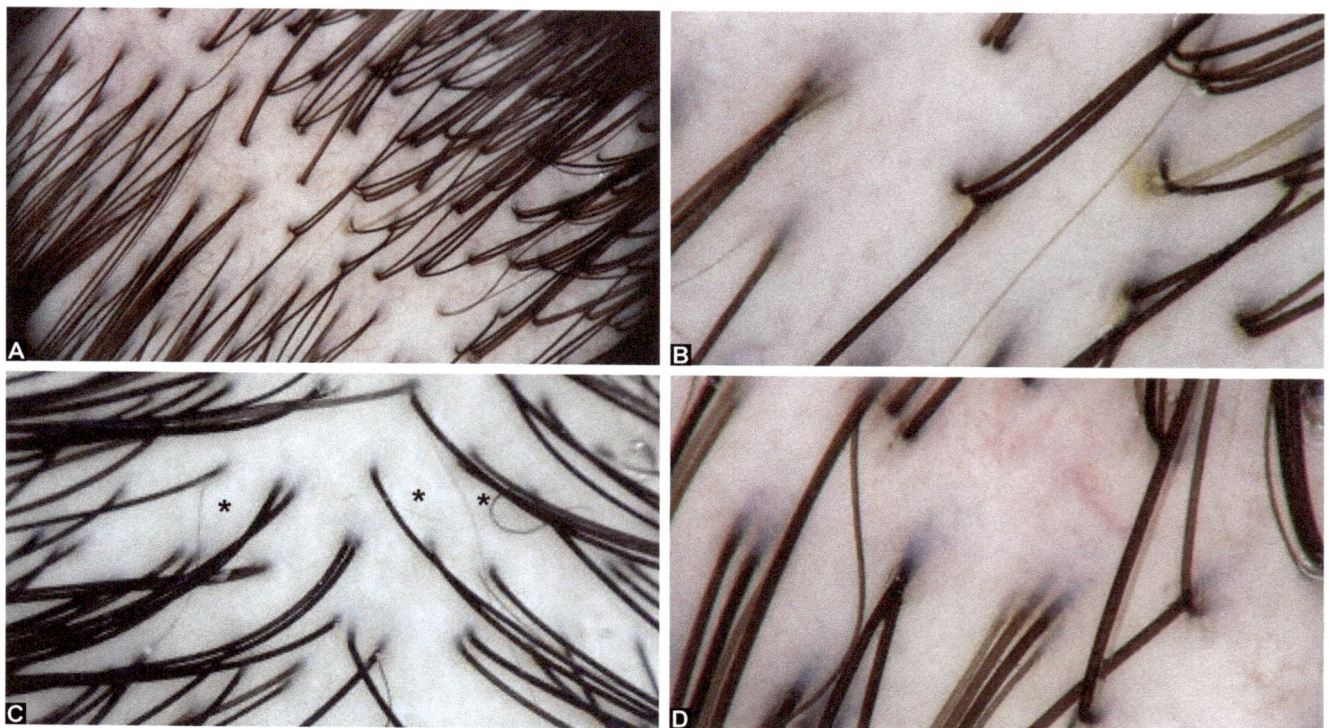

Figs. 1.1A to D: Normal Caucasian vertex scalp. (A) Normal hair shafts are uniform in thickness, shape, and color. Most follicular units are composed of two to three hairs. (B) Thin hairs may account for up to 20% of the total number of hairs. (C) Note the presence of less than 10% of vellus hairs. These are hairs that are nonmedullated, poorly pigmented, short (less than 3 cm), and fine (less than 0.03 mm)(*). (D) Follicular units with four or more hairs are rare and account for less than 5% of all follicular units.

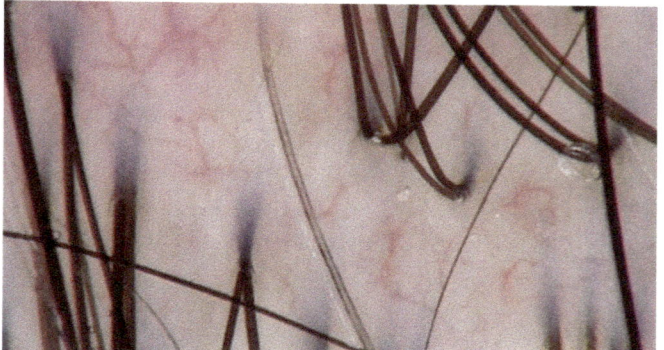

Fig. 1.2: Normal Caucasian occipital scalp. Note a blond hair with no medulla.

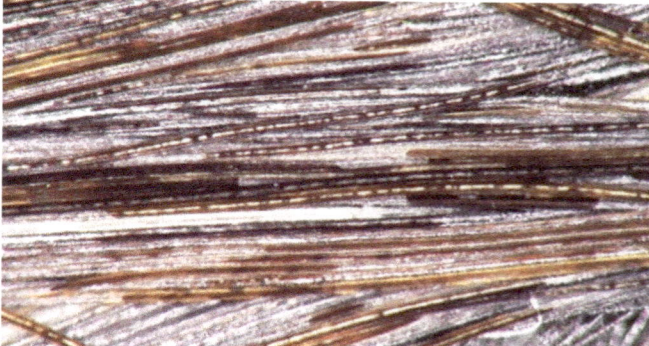

Fig. 1.3: Normal Caucasian hair shaft. Note the interrupted and fragmented medulla. Interrupted medulla may be differentiated from pili annulati. In normal subjects, the medulla covers less than 50% of the interior of the hair shaft. In pili annulati, it covers 50–100%.

Normal Scalp

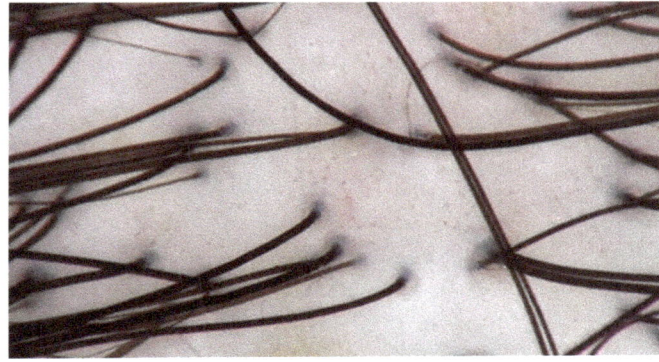

Fig. 1.4: Normal Caucasian vertex scalp. Interfollicular simple red loops. They are best viewed at 50X or higher magnifications with the camera probe angled tangentially.

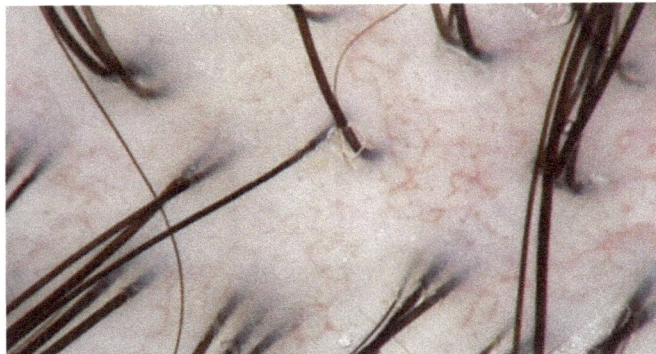

Fig. 1.5: Normal Caucasian temporal scalp. Thin arborizing vessels are best viewed at 20X or higher magnifications.

> **Take-Home Message**
> - Normal Caucasian hair shafts are uniform in thickness, shape, and color with continuous, interrupted, fragmented, or absent medulla.
> - Most follicular units consist of two to three hairs.
> - Normal scalp vessels include thin arborizing vessels (usually found in occipital and temporal areas) and interfollicular simple red loops (mainly in the frontal scalp).

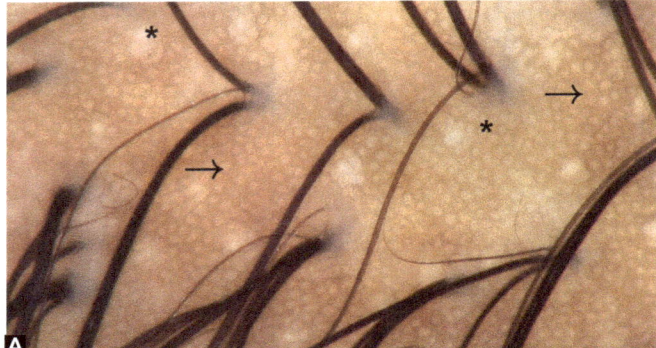

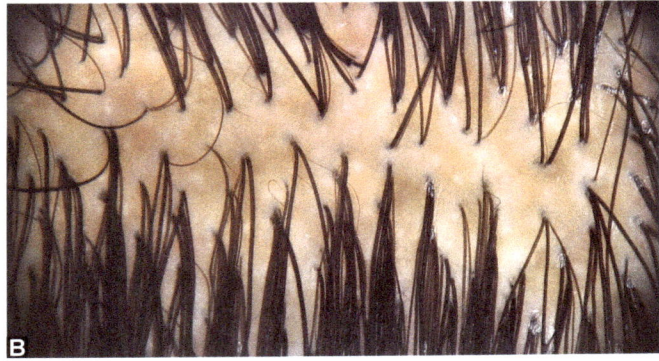

Figs. 1.6A and B: Normal African vertex scalp. (A) Honeycomb-pigmented network (→) and pinpoint white dots(*). (B) Most follicular units consist of one or two vellus hairs and between two to four terminal hairs.

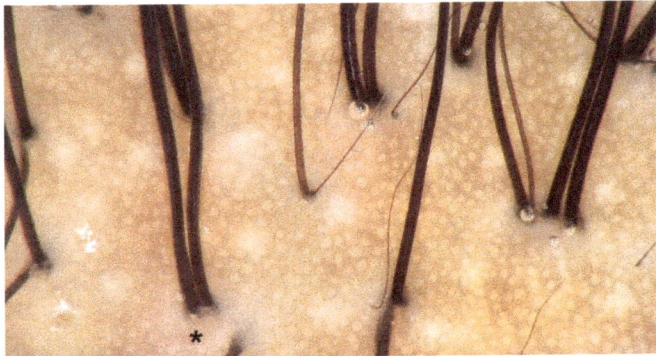

Fig. 1.7: Normal African scalp can show a mild erythema due to excessive traction(*). Also note few vellus and short regrowing hairs.

at an oblique angle to the skin, this population has a higher prevalence of certain diseases, such as pseudofolliculitis barbae and acne keloidalis nuchae. African hairs have less tensile strength, less moisture, and tend to break more easily during combing or manipulation.

On trichoscopic examination, small pinpoint white dots regularly distributed on the scalp which correspond to follicular and eccrine sweat gland duct openings, and honeycomb-pigmented network can be observed (Figs. 1.6A and B). Scalp color varies from light brown to black. Usually vessels cannot be visualized. However, perifollicular and interfollicular erythema can sometimes be seen (Fig. 1.7). Hair density is significantly lower than in Caucasian patients but the hair diameter is larger. Each follicular unit contains one or two vellus hairs and two to four terminal hairs. Hair shafts show a coarser and curlier texture with irregular torsions (Fig. 1.8). The scalp frequently presents scales and residues of products used for hair styling and moisturizing the scalp.

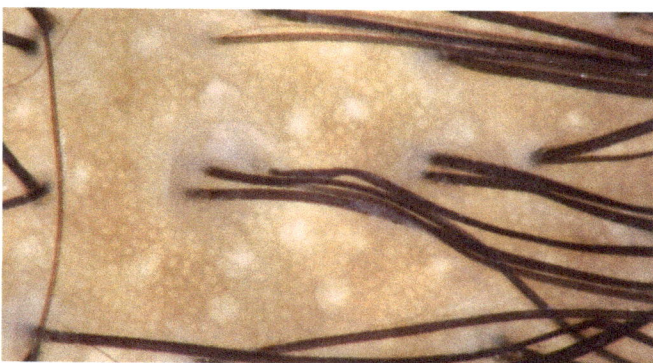

Fig. 1.8: Normal African hair shafts have a flattened shape and some irregular torsions.

> **Take-Home Message**
> - African hair follicles are asymmetrical, with an elliptical or oval cross-sectional shape.
> - Most follicular units consist of two hairs.
> - Pinpoint white dots and honeycomb-pigmented network can usually be seen.

NORMAL ASIAN SCALP

Asians have round-shaped and straight hair shafts with a relatively large diameter, ranging from 0.08 mm to 0.12 mm and a higher thin-hair ratio (12.9%) (Fig. 1.9). Hair cuticle layers are more numerous, compact, and thicker compared to Caucasian hairs. These differences are important in determining increased resistance to chemical procedures, ultraviolet radiation, and mechanical trauma. Trichoscopic features are similar to those of Caucasians; however, the frequencies of the pigment patterns are different because of the contrast effect of the skin and hair color.

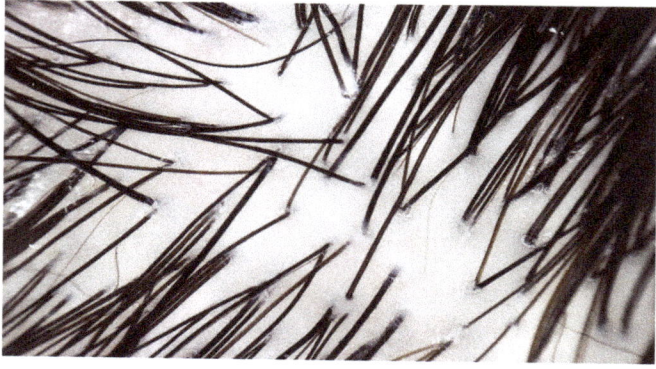

Fig. 1.9: Normal Asian vertex scalp. Hair shafts are uniform in thickness, shape, and color, similar to Caucasian hairs. Few vellus hairs can be present.

> **Take-Home Message**
> - Normal Asian hair shafts have a round shape with a larger diameter.
> - Hair cuticle layers are more numerous, compact, and thicker.
> - Higher thin-hair ratio compared to Caucasian subjects.
> - Trichoscopic features are similar to those of Caucasians.

SUGGESTED READING

1. Abraham LS, Pineiro-Maceira J, Duque-Estrada B, et al. Pinpoint white dots in the scalp: dermoscopic and histopathologic correlation. J Am Acad Dermatol. 2010;63(4):721-2.
2. Franbourg A, Hallegot P, Baltenneck F, et al. Current research on ethnic hair. J Am Acad Dermatol. 2003;48(6 Suppl):S115-9.
3. Inui S. Trichoscopy in Asian patients. In: Rudnicka L, Olszewska M, Rakowska A (Eds). Atlas of Trichoscopy: Dermoscopy in Hair and Scalp Disease. Berlin: Springer; 2012. pp. 433-8.
4. Kim BJ, Na JI, Park WS, et al. Hair cuticle differences between Asian and Caucasian females. Int J Dermatol. 2006;45(12):1435-7.
5. Kim JE, Lee JH, Choi KH, et al. Phototrichogram analysis of normal scalp hair characteristics with aging. Eur J Dermatol. 2013;23(6);849-56.
6. Lacarrubba F, Micali G, Tosti A. Scalp dermoscopy or trichoscopy. Curr Probl Dermatol. 2015;47:21-32.
7. Lawson CN, Hollinger J, Sethi S, et al. Updates in the understanding and treatments of skin and hair disorders in women of color. Int J Womens Dermatol. 2017;3(1 Suppl):S21-37.
8. Lindsay SF, Tosti A. Ethnic hair disorders. Curr Probl Dermatol. 2015;47:139-49.
9. Miteva M, Tosti A. Hair and scalp dermatoscopy. J Am Acad Dermatol. 2012;67(5):1040-8.
10. Rakowska A. Trichoscopy (hair and scalp videodermoscopy) in the healthy female. Method standardization and norms for measurable parameters. J Dermatol Case Rep. 2009;5(1):14-9.
11. Rodney IJ, Onwudiwe OC, Callender VD, et al. Hair and scalp disorders in ethnic populations. J Drugs Dermatol. 2013;12(4):420-7.
12. Rudnicka L, Olszewska M, Rakowska A, et al. Trichoscopy update 2011. J Dermatol Case Rep. 2011;5(4):82-8.
13. Rudnicka L, Rakowska A, Kurzeja M, et al. Hair shafts in trichoscopy. Clues for diagnosis of hair and scalp diseases. Dermaltol Clin. 2013;31(4):695-708.
14. Rudnicka L, Rakowska A, Olszewska M. Trichoscopy. How it may help the clinician. Dermatol Clin. 2013;31(1):29-41.
15. Sperling LC. Hair density in African-Americans. Arch Dermatol. 1999;135(6):656-8.
16. Takahashi T, Havashi R, Okamoto M, et al. Morphology and properties of Asian and Caucasian hair. J Cosmet Sci. 2006;57(4):327-38.
17. Tanus A, Oliveira CC, Villarreal DJ, et al. Black women's hair: the main scalp dermatoses and aesthetic practices in women of African ethnicity. An Bras Dermatol. 2015;90(4):450-65.

CHAPTER 2

Devices for Hair and Scalp Dermoscopy

Giselle Martins, Patricia Damasco, Isabella Doche

INTRODUCTION

Trichoscopy or hair dermoscopy is a noninvasive and practical tool to examine hair and scalp disorders. Dermoscopy can also be useful for some hair shaft disorders and for the examination of hair roots obtained from pull test.

DERMOSCOPES

The dermoscope consists of a lense of 10X or above magnification, with nonpolarized or polarized lights (Table 2.1). Dermoscopy can be perfomed using polarized (noncontact) or nonpolarized (contact) light in handheld or videodermoscope devices (digital epiluminescence).

Table 2.1: Handheld dermoscopes*.

Devices/Characteristics	DL200 HR DermLite®	DL200 Hybrid DermLite®	DL3N DermLite®	DL4 DermLite®	Heine Delta 20T®
Polarization	Polarized	Polarized and nonpolarized	Polarized and nonpolarized	Polarized and nonpolarized	Polarized and nonpolarized
Optics	10X/21 white polarized LEDs	10X/21 white LEDs (15 polarized, 6 nonpolarized)	10X/18 white LEDs (12 polarized, 6 nonpolarized), 10 orange polarized LEDs	10X/18 white LEDs (12 polarized, 6 nonpolarized), 6 orange polarized LEDs	10X/6-white polarized LEDs (LEDs-High Quality)
Infection control	IceCap	IceCap	–	IceCap	Detachable and autoclavable contact plates
Battery	Rechargeable/USB	Rechargeable/USB	Rechargeable	Rechargeable/USB	Rechargeable/USB
Camera compatibility	Yes	Yes	Yes	Yes	Yes
Smartphone/Tablet compatibility	Yes	Yes	Yes	Yes	No
Prices	$	$	$$	$$	$$
Comments	Contact and noncontact dermoscopy	Contact and noncontact dermoscopy	Contact and noncontact dermoscopy	Contact and noncontact dermoscopy	Contact dermoscopy only

*Prices ranged from $ (less than $1,000), $$ ($1,000–10,000) to $$$ (above $10,000).

Fundamentals of Hair and Scalp Dermoscopy

Table 2.2: Smartphone/Tablet compatibility and digital dermoscopes*.

Devices/ Characteristics	Heine iC 1®	FotoFinder handyscope®	FotoFinder®	MoleMax HD®	Vidix®	Dino-Lite Edge® AM7515MZT
Polarization	Polarized and nonpolarized	Polarized and nonpolarized	Polarized and nonpolarized	Polarized and nonpolarized	Polarized and nonpolarized	Adjustable polarization
Optics	15X optical magnification (40X digital)/4 LEDs	20X/6 white nonpolarized LEDs and 6 polarized	20X–70X optical magnification /6 white LEDs	20X–100X optical magnification	7X–100X optical magnification /18 white LEDS	20X–220X/8-white polarized
Infection control	No	No	No	No	No	Interchangeable front cap
Battery	Rechargeable/ USB	Rechargeable/ USB	Computer	Computer	Computer	USB
Camera compatibility	No	No	Medicam 1000: 140X magnification	Yes	Resolution of 5 million pixels (2560 × 1920) wireless camera	5.0 MP camera (2592 × 1944 resolution)
Smartphone/ Tablet compatibility	Smartphone 12 MP image quality	Yes	No	No	Camera 18 MP	Yes (WF-10 or USB OTG cable)
Prices	$	$	$$$	$$$	$$$	$$
Comments	Contact dermoscopy only	Contact and noncontact dermoscopy	Contact and noncontact dermoscopy	Contact and noncontact dermoscopy, true HDMI transfer data, two monitors, LCD on camera	Contact and noncontact dermoscopy, two monitors, dual circular LED illuminator	Contact and noncontact dermoscopy
Devices						

*Prices ranged from $ (less than $1,000), $$ ($1,000–10,000) to $$$ (above $10,000).
(MP: Megapixel; USB: Universal serial bus; OTG: On-the-go; HDMI: High-definition multimedia interface; LCD: Liquid crystal display; LED: Light emiting diode)
Note: We thank all the companies for device specifications and images.

Digital dermoscopes can be attached to variable softwares and reach magnifications ranging from 20X to 1000X. They can store images for further comparison and follow-up. Nowadays, smartphone/tablet compatibility devices also allow one to store and compare images (Table 2.2). However, it may be difficult to track the same areas in each patient's visit.

Nonpolarized or contact dermoscopy demands the use of a liquid medium in order to eliminate skin surface reflections. For immersion fluid, prefer the use of alcohol or spring thermal water sprays, because the gel can get stuck on the lenses producing artifacts and pseudonodes.

Hair dermoscopy can be done using nonpolarized or polarized lights. In general, polarized dermoscopy allows better visualization of scales, casts, and scarring alopecias. Scales should always be examined with dry dermoscopy. However, polarized or low-pressure contact dermoscopy should be preferred for vascular patterns.

There is no ideal device to perform the examination, although some specific characteristics may be taken into consideration before deciding which one to use.

> **Take-Home Message**
> - Hair dermoscopy can be performed with polarized (noncontact) or nonpolarized (contact) dermoscopy.
> - Digital dermoscopy allows higher magnifications and better quality images besides image storage for further follow-up.
> - Polarized dermoscopy allows better visualization of scales, casts, and scarring alopecias.
> - Polarized or low-pressure contact dermoscopy should be preferred for vascular patterns.
> - Nonpolarized dermoscopy demands immersion fluids like alcohol or spring water spray.
> - Always start scalp dermoscopy with dry dermoscopy to assess scales and casts.

SUGGESTED READING

1. Benvenuto-Andrade C, Dusza SW, Agero AL, et al. Differences between polarized light dermoscopy and immersion contact dermoscopy for the evaluation of skin lesions. Arch Dermatol. 2007;143(3):329-38.
2. Dhurat R, Saraogi P. Hair evaluation methods: merits and demerits. Int J Trichology. 2009;1(2):108-19.
3. Gewirtzman AJ, Saurat JH, Braun RP. Na evaluation of dermoscopy fluids and application techniques. Br J Dermatol. 2003;149(1):59-63.
4. Karadag Köse Ö, Güleç AT. Clinical evaluation of alopecias using a handheld dermatoscope. J Am Acad Dermatol. 2012;67(2):206-14.
5. Lacarrubba F, Micali G, Tosti A. Scalp dermoscopy or trichoscopy. Curr Probl Dermatol. 2015;47:21-32.
6. Miteva M, Tosti A. Hair and scalp dermoscopy. J Am Acad Dermatol. 2012;67(5):1040-8.
7. Nikam VV, Mehta HH. A nonrandomized study of trichoscopy patterns using nonpolarized (contat) and polarized (noncontact) dermoscopy in hair and shaft disorders. Int J Trichol. 2014;6(2):54-62.
8. Rakowska A. Trichoscopy (hair and scalp videodermoscopy) in the healthy female. Method standardization and norms for measurable parameters. J Dermatol Case Rep. 2009;3(1):14-9.
9. Rogers NE. Scoping scalp disorders: practical use of a novel dermatoscope to diagnose hair and scalp conditions. J Drugs Dermatol. 2013;12(3):283-90.
10. Ross EK, Vincenzi C, Tosti A. Videodermoscopy in the evaluation of hair and scalp disorders. J Am Acad Dermatol. 2006;55(5):799-806.
11. Rudnicka L, Olszewska M, Rakowska A, et al. Trichoscopy: a new method for diagnosing hair loss. J Drugs Dermatol. 2008;7(7):651-4.
12. Rudnicka L, Rakowska A, Olszewska M. Trichoscopy: how it may help the clinician. Dermatol Clin. 2013;31(1):29-41.
13. Silverberg NB, Silverberg JI, Wong ML. Trichoscopy using a handheld dermoscope: na in-office technique to diagnose genetic disease of the hair. Arch Dermatol. 2009;14(5):600-1.
14. Tasli L, Oguz O. The role of various immersion liquids at digital dermoscopy in structural analysis. Indian J Dermatol Venereol Leprol. 2011;77(1):110.
15. Tonćić RJ, Lipozenćić J, Pastar Z. Videodermoscopy in the evaluation of hair and scalp disorders. Acta Dermatovenereol Croat. 2007;15(2):116-8.
16. Verzì AE, Lacarrubba F, Micali G. Use of low-cost videomicroscopy versus standard videodermatoscopy in trichoscopy: a controlled, blinded noninferiority trial. Skin Appendage Disord. 2016;1(4):172-4.

CHAPTER 3

Trichoscopy Patterns and Tips to Enhance Your Exam

Isabella Doche, Giselle Martins, Patricia Damasco

INTRODUCTION

Hair dermoscopy, also known as trichoscopy, is a noninvasive and practical tool for the diagnosis and follow-up of many hair shafts and scalp disorders. There are several devices with magnification ranging from 10X (manual dermoscope) to 1000X (videodermoscope) and both polarized (noncontact) and nonpolarized (contact) modes can be used to perform the examination.

TRICHOSCOPY PATTERNS

The identification of normal versus abnormal trichoscopic patterns is fundamental to understand the findings and the processes going on in the hair and scalp.

Hair and scalp patterns that should be analyzed (Box 3.1):
1. Follicular
2. Interfollicular
3. Hair shafts
4. Hair roots

Box 3.1 Follicular hair and scalp patterns.

- Follicular patterns
  - Follicular openings
  - Pinpoint white dots
  - Red dots
  - Target blue-gray dots
  - Peripilar sign (brown dots)
  - Exogen substances
  - Yellow dots
  - Black dots
  - Gray-white halos
  - Keratotic plugs
  - Peripilar scale

Follicular Patterns

Follicular Openings (Figs. 3.1A and B)

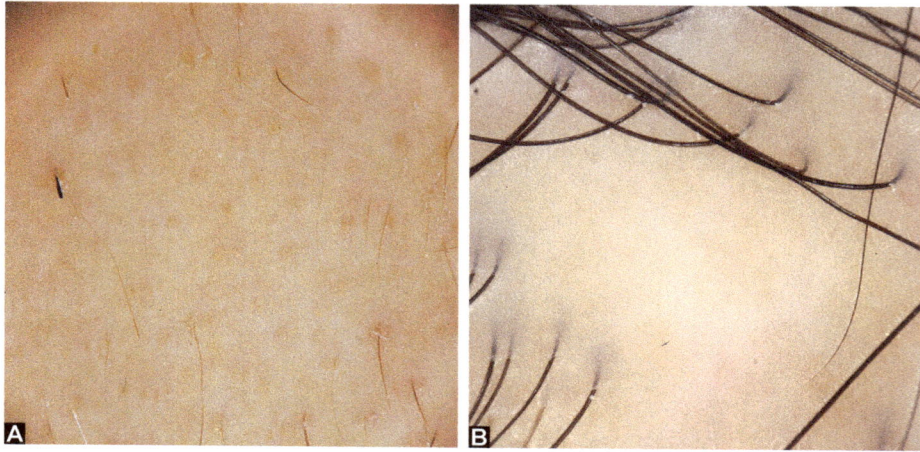

Figs. 3.1A and B: (A) Note the presence of follicular openings. Empty follicles are represented by multiple yellow dots in a patient with alopecia areata. (B) Note the whitish scarring area. No follicular openings can be seen in this patient with frontal fibrosing alopecia.

Trichoscopy Patterns and Tips to Enhance Your Exam

Take-Home Message
The presence of follicular openings is the most important criterion to distinguish nonscarring from scarring alopecia.

Yellow Dots (Figs. 3.2A and B)

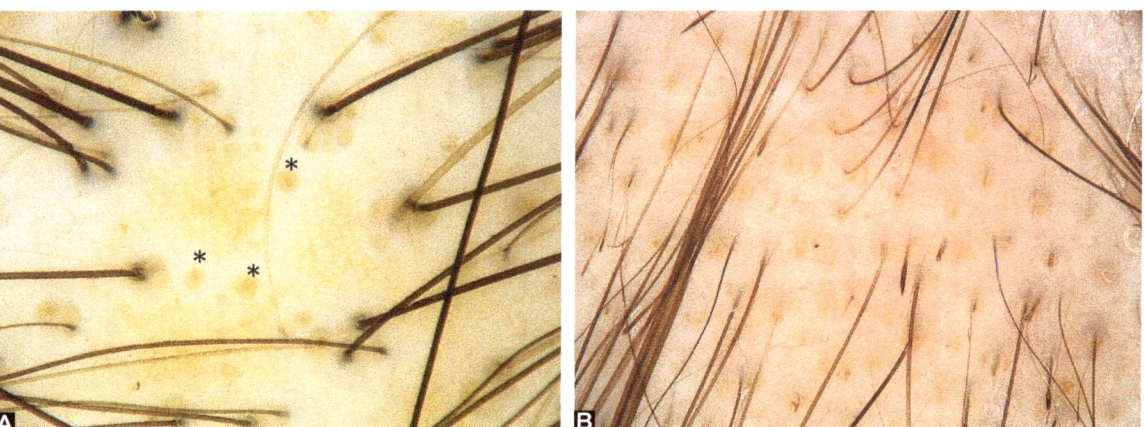

Figs. 3.2A and B: (A) Yellow dots (*) filled with sebum and keratotic materials in a patient with severe androgenetic alopecia. (B) Multiple yellow dots, some surrounding miniaturized, dystrophic, and small broken hairs in a patient with alopecia areata.
Source: (B) Division of Dermatology, Hospital das Clínicas, University of São Paulo Medical School.

Take-Home Message
- Yellow dots are small round structures filled with sebum and rests of keratinocytes.
- Yellow dots correspond to follicles with intense miniaturization and can be completely empty or contain residues of hair.
- Multiple regularly distributed yellow dots are more common in alopecia areata and few irregularly distributed yellow dots in long-lasting androgenetic alopecia.
- Many causes of temporary and chronic nonscarring alopecias can cause yellow dots.
- These structures are not seen in high skin phototypes.

Pinpoint White Dots (Figs. 3.3A and B)

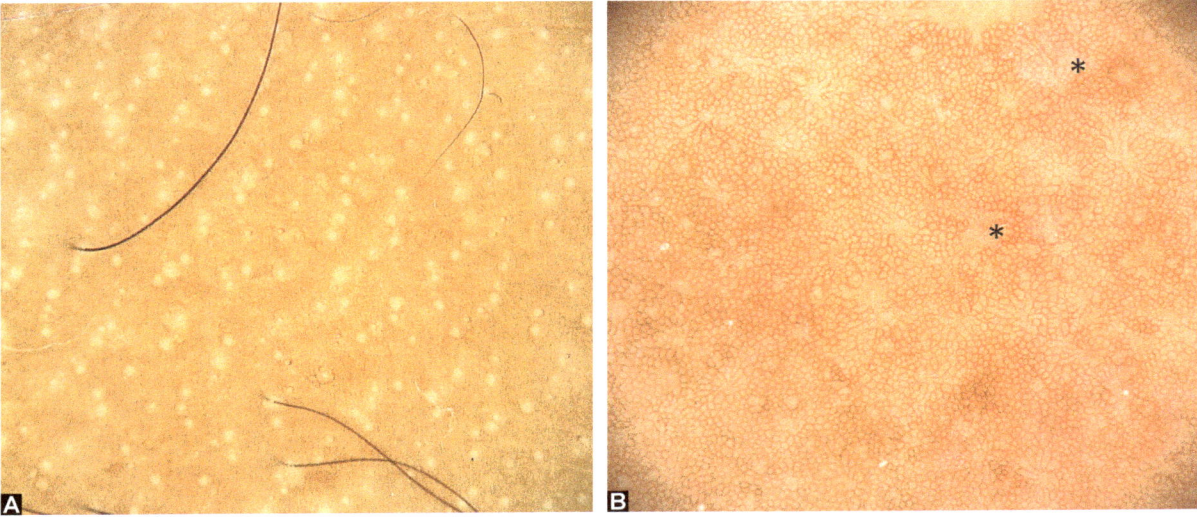

Figs. 3.3A and B: (A) Note small white dots (pinpoints) regularly distributed in a patient with early stage of traction alopecia. (B) Irregular distribution of pinpoints white dots in a patient with late stage of traction alopecia. Note white fibrotic areas (*) with no follicular openings, a sign of a scarring process.

> **Take-Home Message**
> - Pinpoint white dots are very small round structures that correspond to follicular and sweat gland openings.
> - Pinpoint dots are a normal finding in black scalps.
> - Absence or irregular distribution of pinpoint white dots can be a sign of a scarring process.

Black Dots (Figs. 3.4A and B)

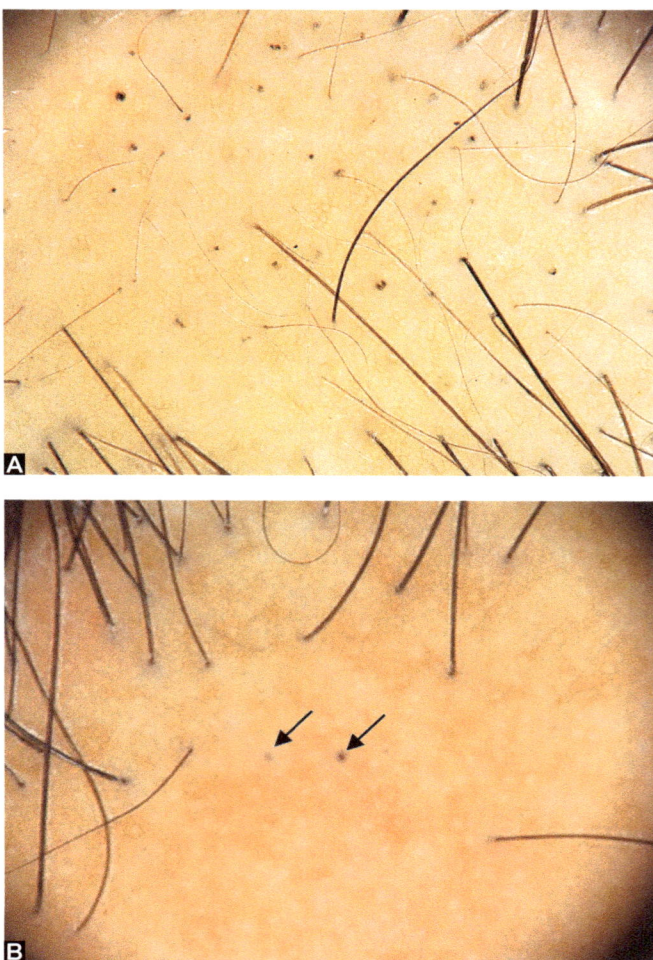

Figs. 3.4A and B: (A) Multiple black dots in a patient with alopecia areata. (B) Few black dots (→) can be noted in a patient with frontal fibrosing alopecia.
Source: Division of Dermatology, Hospital das Clínicas, University of São Paulo Medical School.

> **Take-Home Message**
> - Black dots, also known as "cadaverized hairs," correspond to hairs fractured in the level of the follicle emergence.
> - Multiple black dots usually indicate active alopecia areata.
> - Scarring alopecias can show few isolated black dots.
> - Black dots can also be seen in trichotillomania, tinea capitis, dissecting cellulitis, and more rarely in chronic alopecia areata, monilethrix, traction alopecia, chemotherapy-induced alopecia, and aplasia cutis congenita.

Trichoscopy Patterns and Tips to Enhance Your Exam

Red Dots (Figs. 3.5A to C)

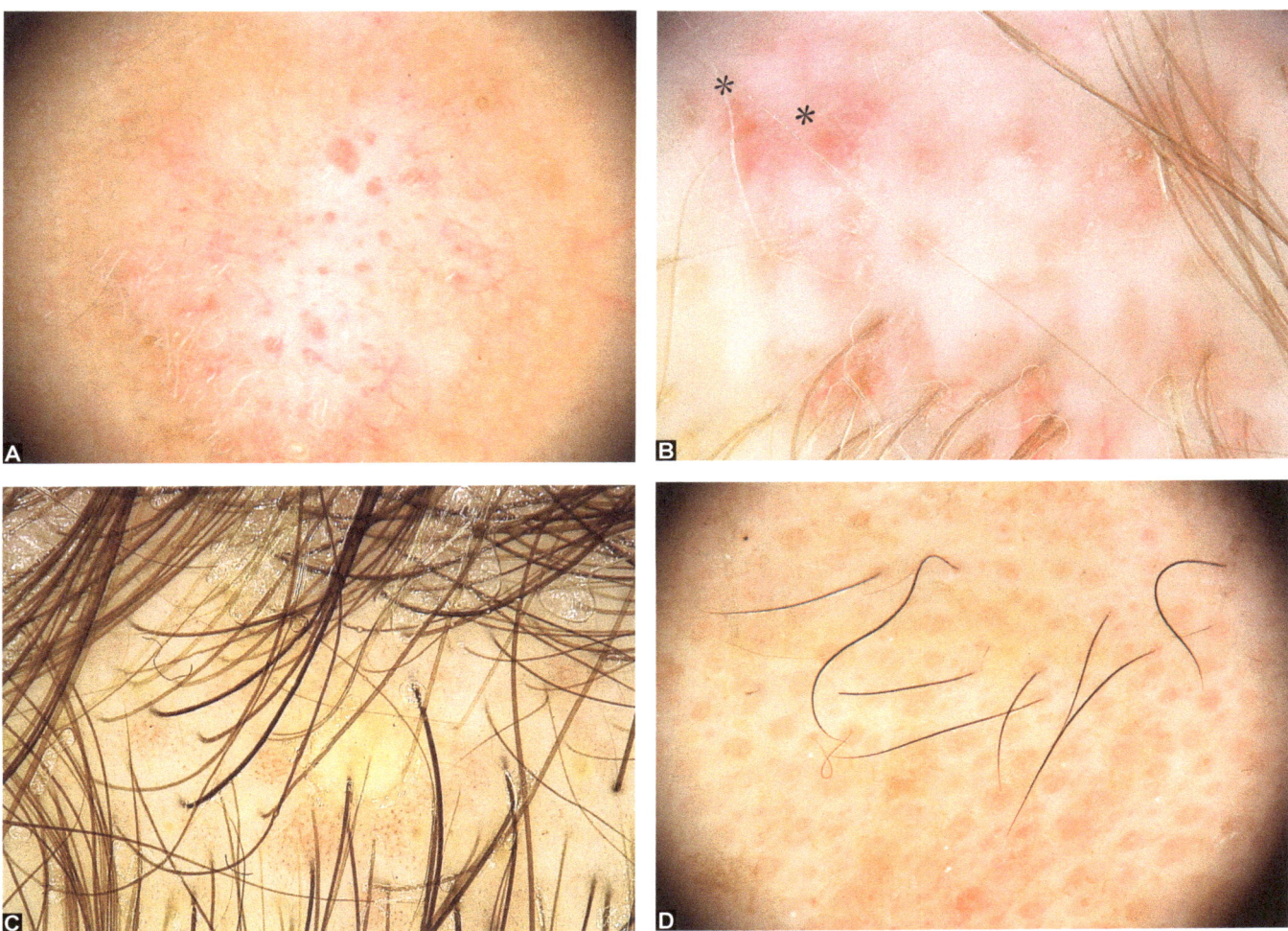

Figs. 3.5A to C: (A) Red dots in discoid lupus erythematosus. (B) Red dots surrounded by white scarring areas in a patient with discoid lupus erythematosus (*). (C) In low magnifications (20X), vessels arranged in multiple red dots can be seen in patients with scalp psoriasis. (D) Red and yellowish dots in the eyebrow of a patient with frontal fibrosing alopecia.
Source: (A, B, D) Division of Dermatology, Hospital das Clínicas, University of São Paulo Medical School.

Take-Home Message
- Red dots correspond to enlarged follicular openings surrounded by dilated vessels with blood extravasation.
- Red dots are characteristic of discoid lupus erythematosus.
- In discoid lupus, they are usually associated with good prognosis and the possibility of hair regrowth.
- Some patients with frontal fibrosing alopecia may present with red and yellowish dots on the glabella and eyebrows.
- In low magnifications, the presence of red dots associated with scales can be a sign of scalp psoriasis.

Gray-White Halos (Figs. 3.6A and B)

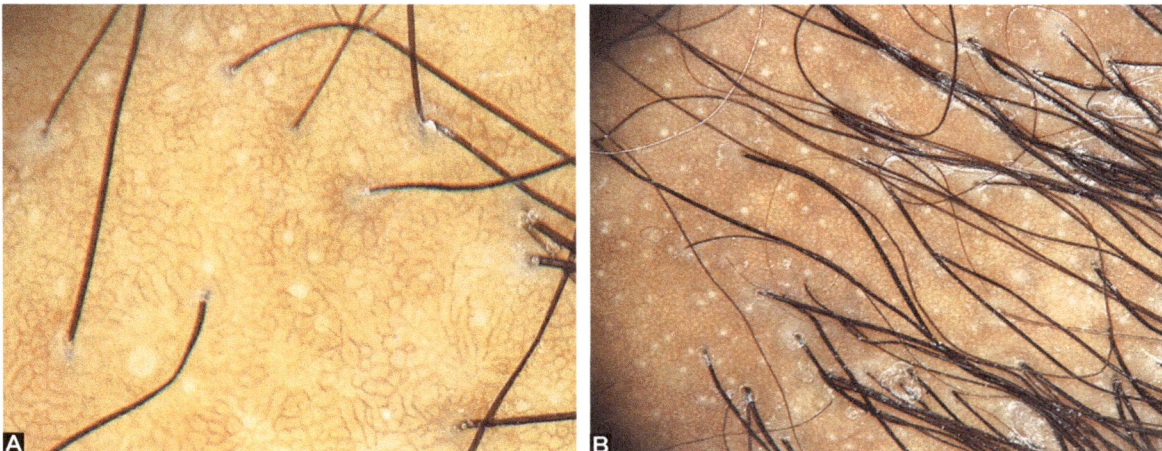

Figs. 3.6A and B: (A) Gray-white peripilar halos in central centrifugal cicatricial alopecia. (B) Gray-white halos in lichen planopilaris and Graham-Little syndrome.
Source: Division of Dermatology, Hospital das Clínicas, University of São Paulo Medical School.

> **Take-Home Message**
> - Gray-white halos correspond to the peripilar concentric and lamellar fibrosis.
> - They can be mostly seen in central centrifugal alopecia, although they are not specific.
> - Gray-white halos can also be present in traction alopecia and nonactive lichen planopilaris in black scalp.

Blue-gray Dots (Figs. 3.7A to D)

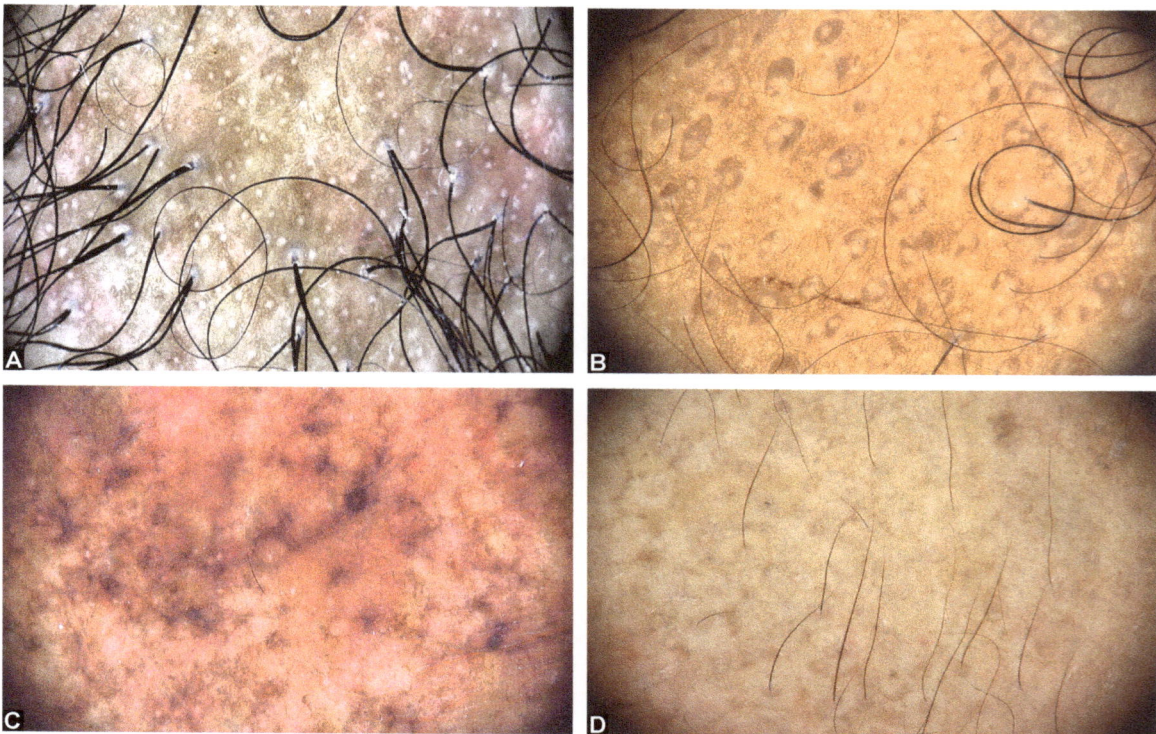

Figs. 3.7A to D: (A) Perifollicular blue-gray target dots in a patient with active central centrifugal cicatricial alopecia. (B) Variable hyperpigmentation (target pattern) in a dark-skinned patient with active traction alopecia. Note the presence of follicular openings and vellus hairs. (C) Blue-gray and violaceous dots (target pattern) on the face of a dark-skinned patient with lichen planus pigmentosum. (D) Blue-gray dots in target and specked patterns represent the interfollicular and follicular pigment incontinence that occurs in discoid lupus erythematosus.
Source: Division of Dermatology, Hospital das Clínicas, University of São Paulo Medical School.

Trichoscopy Patterns and Tips to Enhance Your Exam

Take-Home Message
- Blue-gray dots correspond to follicle inflammation and pigment incontinence in dark-skinned patients.
- They can be seen in active stages of scarring diseases especially lichen planopilaris and discoid lupus erythematosus.
- Some patterns of lichen planus pigmentosum may also present with blue-gray and violaceous dots (target pattern) on the face of dark-skinned patients.

Keratotic Plugs (Figs. 3.8A and B)

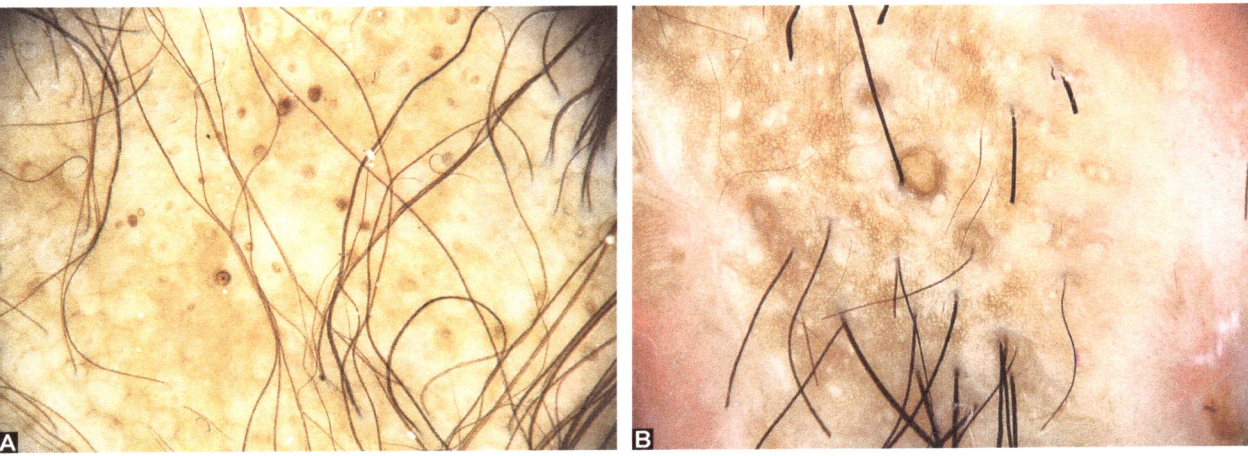

Figs. 3.8A and B: (A) Multiple small keratin plugs in discoid lupus erythematosus. (B) Larger isolated keratin plugs in dissecting cellulitis.
Source: Division of Dermatology, Hospital das Clínicas, University of São Paulo Medical School.

Take-Home Message
- Keratin plugs appear as yellow-brownish structures that correspond to the keratin masses filling follicular ostia caused by hyperkeratosis.
- Small and multiple keratin plugs highly suggest discoid lupus erythematosus.
- Larger and isolated keratin plugs highly suggest dissecting cellulitis.

Peripilar Sign (Brown Dots) (Figs. 3.9A and B)

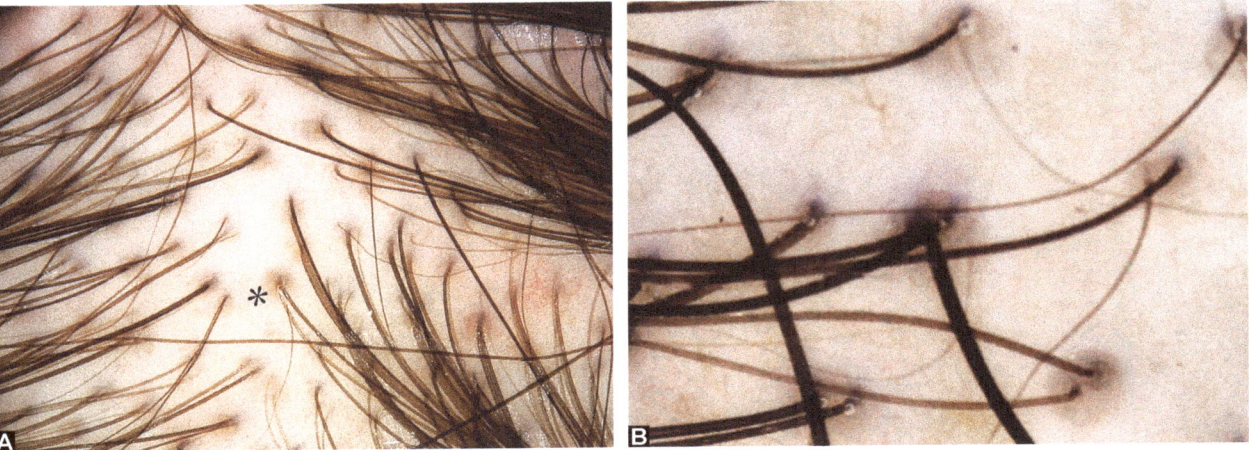

Figs. 3.9A and B: (A) Brownish halo (peripilar sign) (*) surrounding some intermediate and terminal hair shafts in androgenetic alopecia. Note the hair shaft diversity. (B) Note slightly depressed peripilar halo.

14 Fundamentals of Hair and Scalp Dermoscopy

> **Take-Home Message**
> - Peripilar sign is a brown halo that surrounds terminal or intermediate hair follicles.
> - Probably it corresponds to a mild perifollicular inflammation present in androgenetic alopecia.
> - Usually indicates early disease in patients with high or moderate hair density.

Peripilar Scale (Figs.3.10A to D)

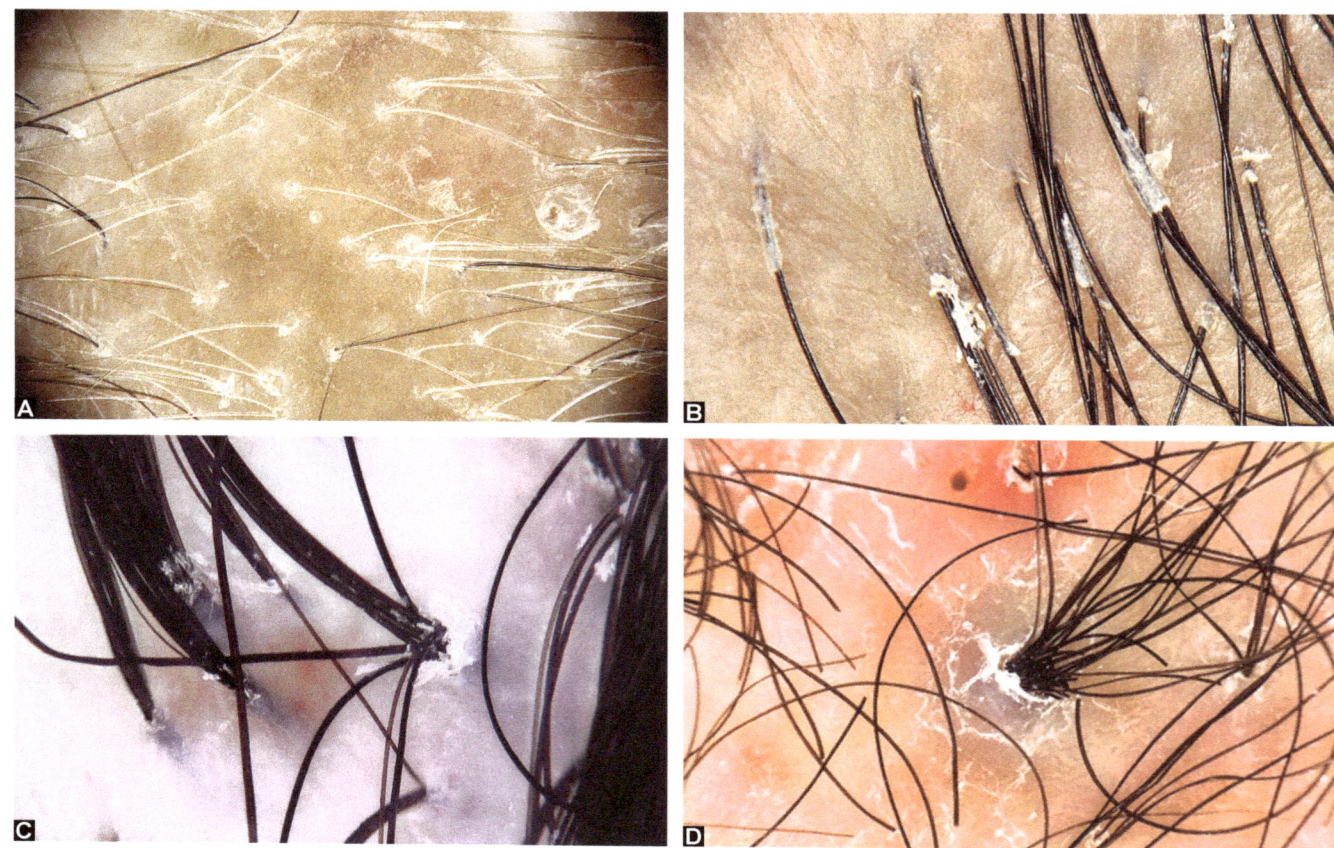

Figs. 3.10A to D: (A) Peripilar scales in lichen planopilaris. Scales can be better appreciated with dry dermoscopy. (B) Scales emerging from the base of the hair follicle and surrounding the hair shafts in lichen planopilaris. (C) Peripilar scale in folliculitis decalvans. Scales are thick and whitish. (D) Peripilar scale in folliculitis decalvans. On dry dermoscopy, note that scales may show a radiating pattern around the hair tufts (starburst-like pattern) due to intense fibrosis and epidermal hyperplasia.

Source: (A and B) Division of Dermatology, Hospital das Clínicas, University of São Paulo Medical School.

> **Take-Home Message**
> - Peripilar scales correspond to hyperkeratosis and are considered a sign of active inflammatory diseases.
> - They can be seen in all scarring diseases (active stage).
> - Usually perifollicular scales are associated with interfollicular scales in psoriasis, tinea capitis, seborrheic dermatitis, and folliculitis decalvans.

Exogen Substances (Figs. 3.11A and B)

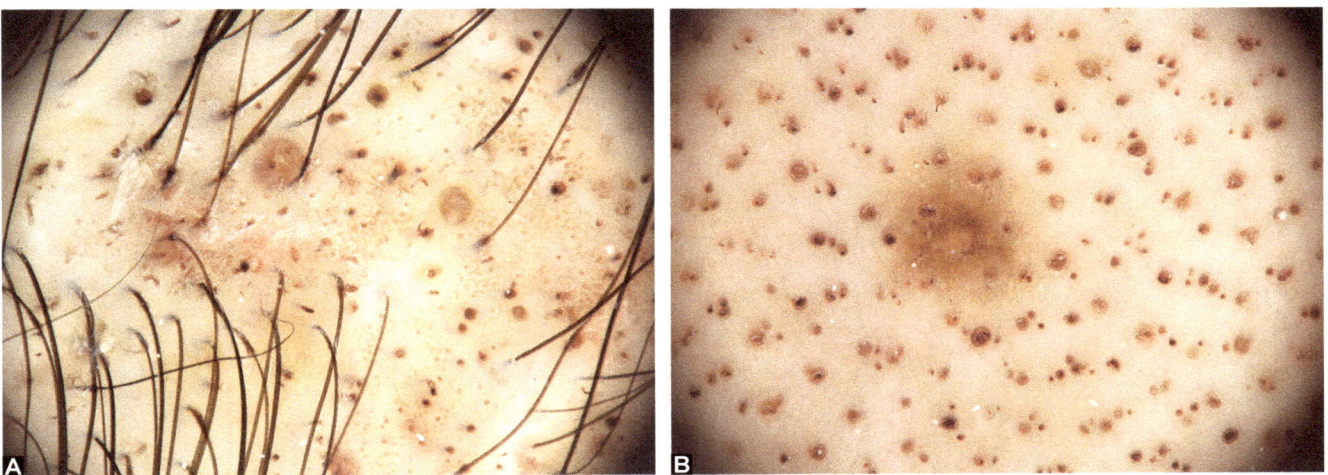

Figs. 3.11A and B: (A) Irregular residues of hair dye. (B) Note homogenous follicular pigmentation after anthralin treatment in alopecia areata.
Source: Division of Dermatology, Hospital das Clínicas, University of São Paulo Medical School.

Take-Home Message
• Exogen pigmentation can be caused by hair dyes and anthralin use. • In hair dye, the pigment is irregularly deposited in follicular and interfollicular areas of the scalp. • In anthralin use, the pigmentation is very uniform around almost all hair follicles.

Interfollicular Patterns

The interfollicular hair and scalp patterns are given in Box 3.2.

Box 3.2	Interfollicular hair and scalp patterns

• Interfollicular patterns
  – Scales
  – Vessels
  – Pigment
  – White (scarring) dots/patches
  – Exogen substances	

Scales (Figs. 3.12A to G)

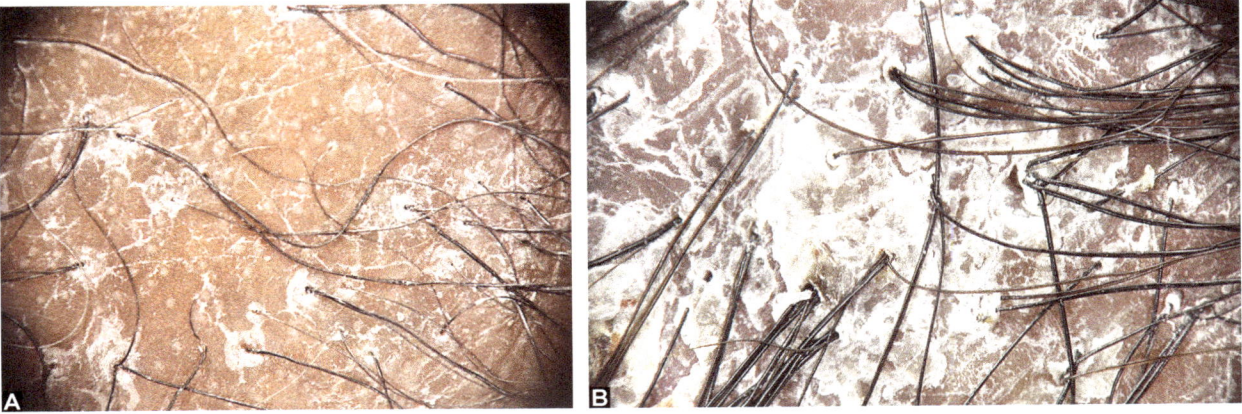

Figs. 3.12A and B.

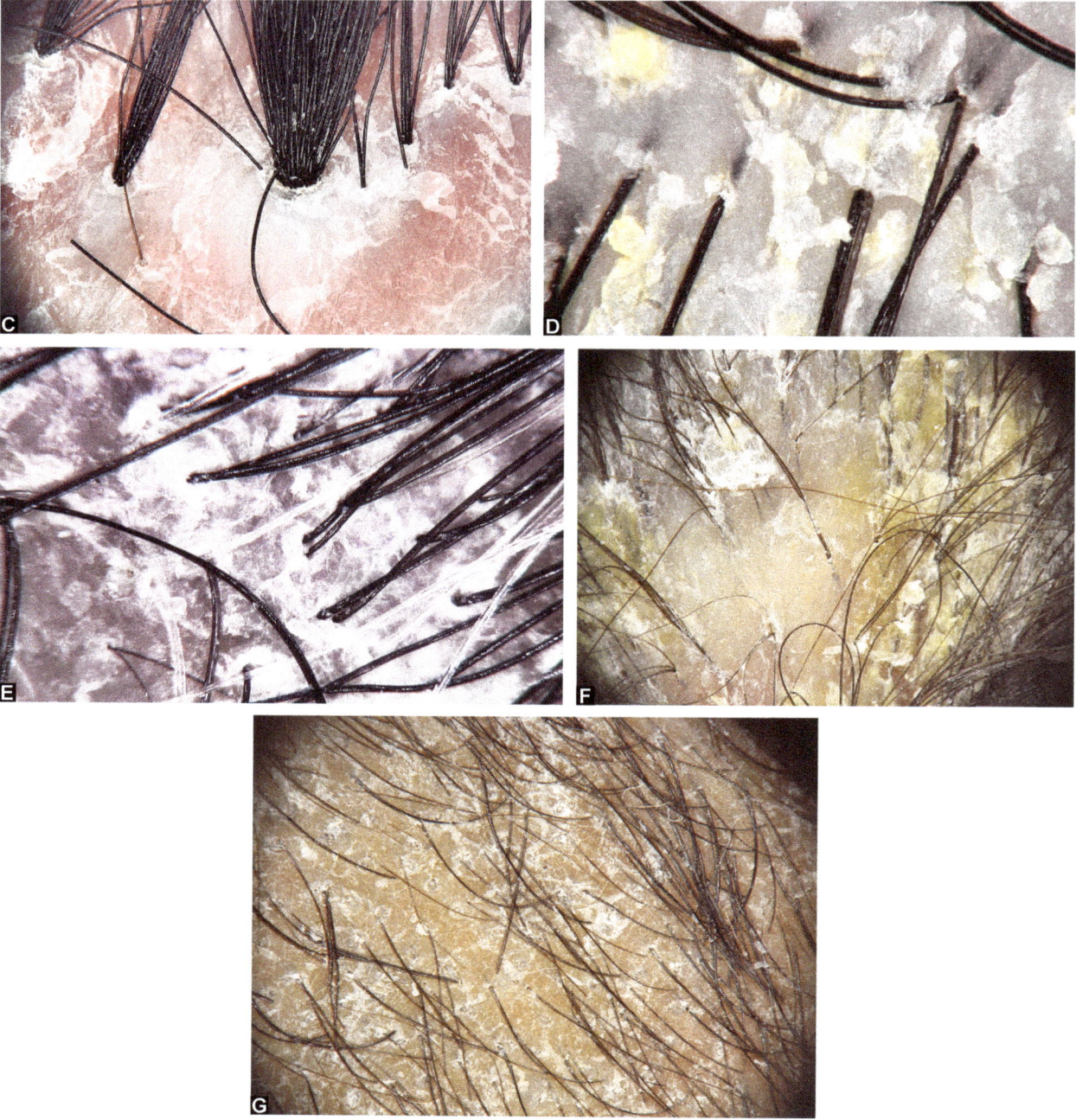

Figs. 3.12C to G.

Figs. 3.12A to G: (A) Although peripilar scales are more noticeable in lichen planopilaris, mild interfollicular scales also can be seen on dry dermoscopy. (B) Intense interfollicular scaling and crusts in lichen planopilaris with secondary infection. (C) Thicker scales in folliculitis decalvans. Note severe tuftings and scalp diffuse erythema. (D) Flaky yellowish interfollicular scales in seborrheic dermatitis. Note also perifollicular scales. (E) Gray-whitish scales in scalp psoriasis. (F) Intense perifollicular and interfollicular scales forming crusts in pityriasis amiantacea. The yellow color corresponds to the dessicated pustules and exudate. (G) Moderate interfollicular scales in tinea capitis. Specific findings of tinea capitis, such as comma and corkscrew hairs are hardly seen without fluid imersion.

Source: (A, B, F, G) Division of Dermatology, Hospital das Clínicas, University of São Paulo Medical School.

Trichoscopy Patterns and Tips to Enhance Your Exam

Take-Home Message

- Dry dermoscopy should be performed first to assess scales.
- Scales can be noted in interfollicular and perifollicular scalp and around the hair shafts (hair casts).
- Flaky, yellowish, and oily interfollicular scales may be a sign of seborrheic dermatitis, while gray-whitish thicker scales can indicate psoriasis.
- Scarring alopecias, such as discoid lupus erythematosus, folliculitis decalvans, and lichen planopilaris, may present interfollicular and follicular scales.
- Tinea capitis may also present hair casts and interfollicular scales.

Vessels (Figs. 3.13A to K)

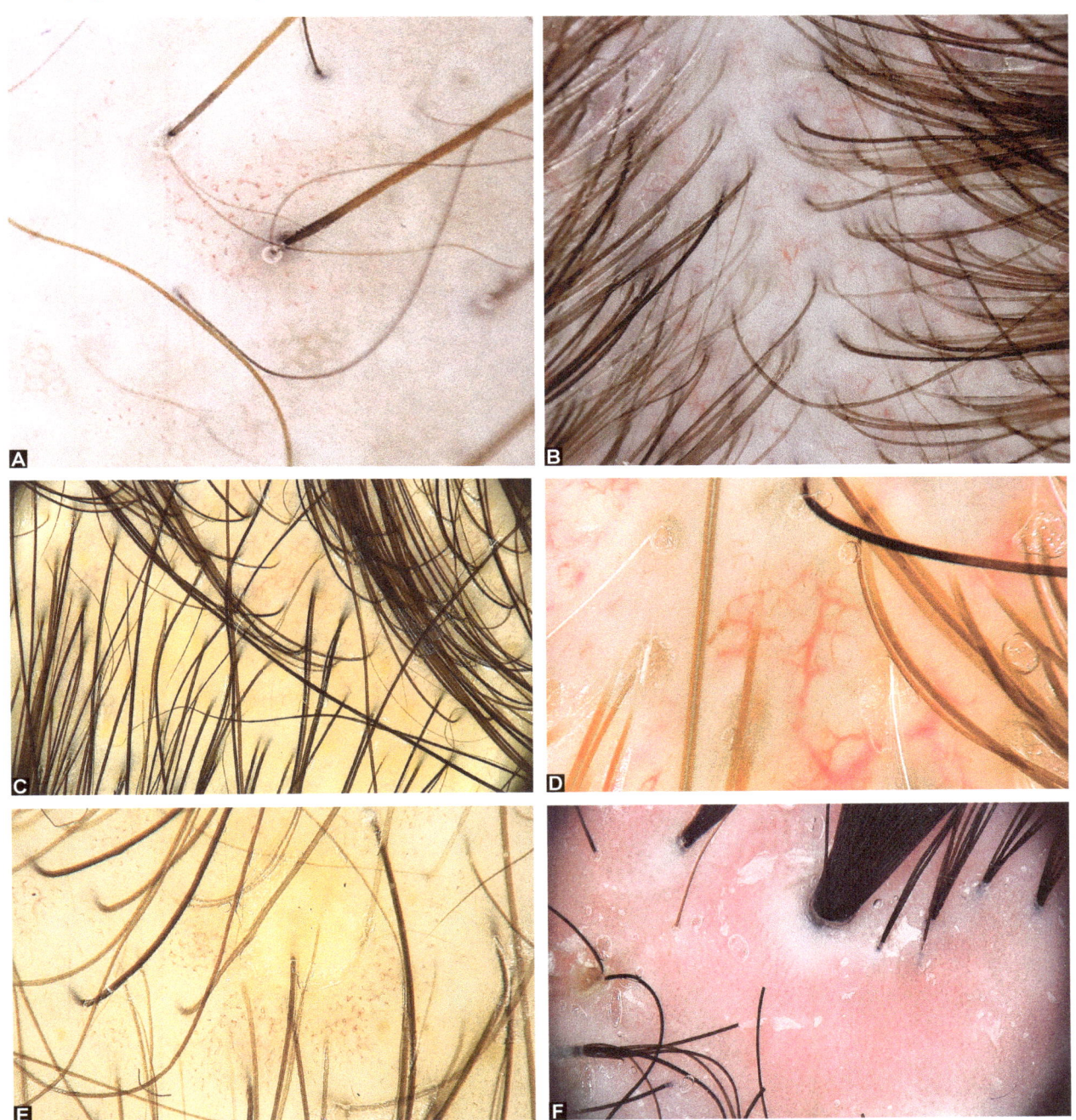

Figs. 3.13A to F.

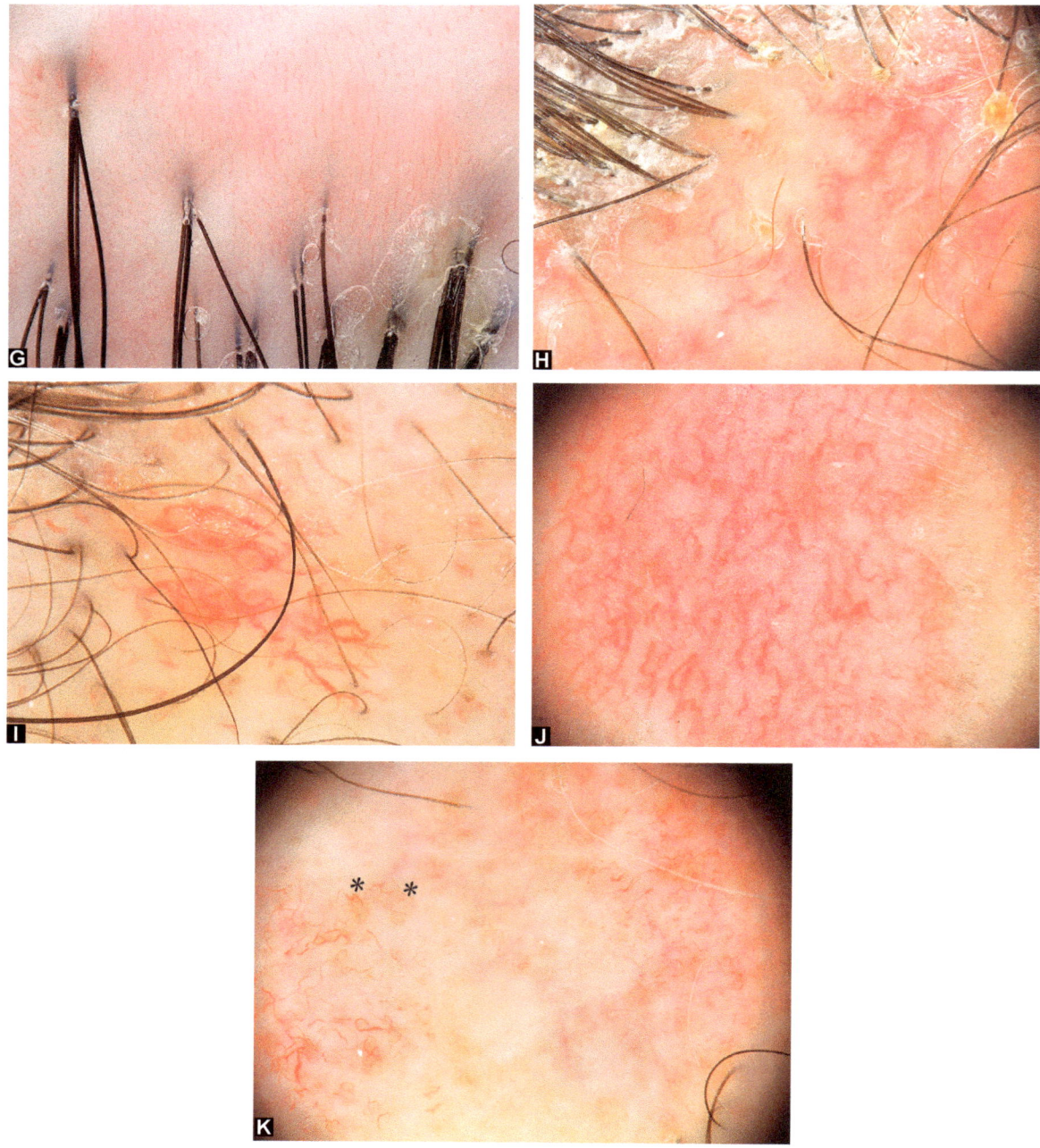

Figs. 3.13G to K.

Figs. 3.13A to K: (A) Small, dotted, linear (comma), and linear looped elongated (hairpin) vessels. These structures can be noted mostly in the frontal scalp from healthy subjects, seborrheic dermatitis, and psoriasis. (B) Simple red loops and thin arborizing vessel net are more evident in a normal occipital scalp in patients with low skin types. Note that vessels are not visible in the proximity of the follicles. (C) Prominent arborizing vessels in mild seborrheic dermatitis. Yellowish hues around some follicles correspond to increased sebum production. (D) Diffuse thin arborizing capillaries can be found in healthy individuals, atrophic scalp after chronic use of high-potency topical steroids, and in inflammatory scalp diseases, such as lichen planopilaris, and frontal fibrosing alopecia. (E) Twisted red loops in scalp psoriasis. (F, G) Twisted red loops and hairpin perifollicular vessels in folliculitis decalvans. Note scarring areas, intense perifollicular fibrosis surrounding big tuftings. (H) Thin capillaries can be noted within milky red areas in this patient with T-cell lymphoma. Note also some hairpin elongated perifollicular vessels. (I) Giant capillary vessels in systemic lupus erythematosus. In connective tissue disorders and basal cell carcinoma vessels can be enlarged and tortuous. (J) Thick root-like vessels in discoid lupus erythematosus. Note that differently from normal thick arborizing vessels, they do not have branchings. (K) Serpentine linear vessels in discoid lupus erythematosus. Note white scarring areas and absence of folicular openings. Some "red spiders" (thin arborizing vessels) surrounding yellow dots (*) can be seen and are suggestive of late stage of discoid lupus erythematosus.

Source: (G–K) Division of Dermatology, Hospital das Clínicas, University of São Paulo Medical School.

Take-Home Message

- Normal vessels in areas other than the occipital can only be examined in magnifications above 20X.
- Simple red loops, and thin arborizing vessels may be normal findings in the occipital and temporal scalp areas.
- Seborrheic dermatitis may increase the amount of thin arborizing vessels, mainly on the temporal regions of the scalp.
- Small dotted, linear curved (comma), and linear looped (hairpin) vessels can be found in healthy individuals, seborrheic dermatitis, sebopsoriaris, and mild eczema.
- In low magnifications (20X), multiple red dots can indicate psoriasis. In high magnifications (40X), twisted red loops and glomerular vessels can be noted.
- Multiple elongated hairpin vessels concentrated in the perifollicular area may be noted in folliculitis decalvans, and T-cell lymphoma.
- Enlarged vessels can be seen in atrophic scalp, discoid lupus, connective tissue disorders, and surrounding some tumors, as basal cell carcinoma.
- Giant and tortuous vessels usually suggest lupus erythematosus.

Pigment (Figs. 3.14A to D)

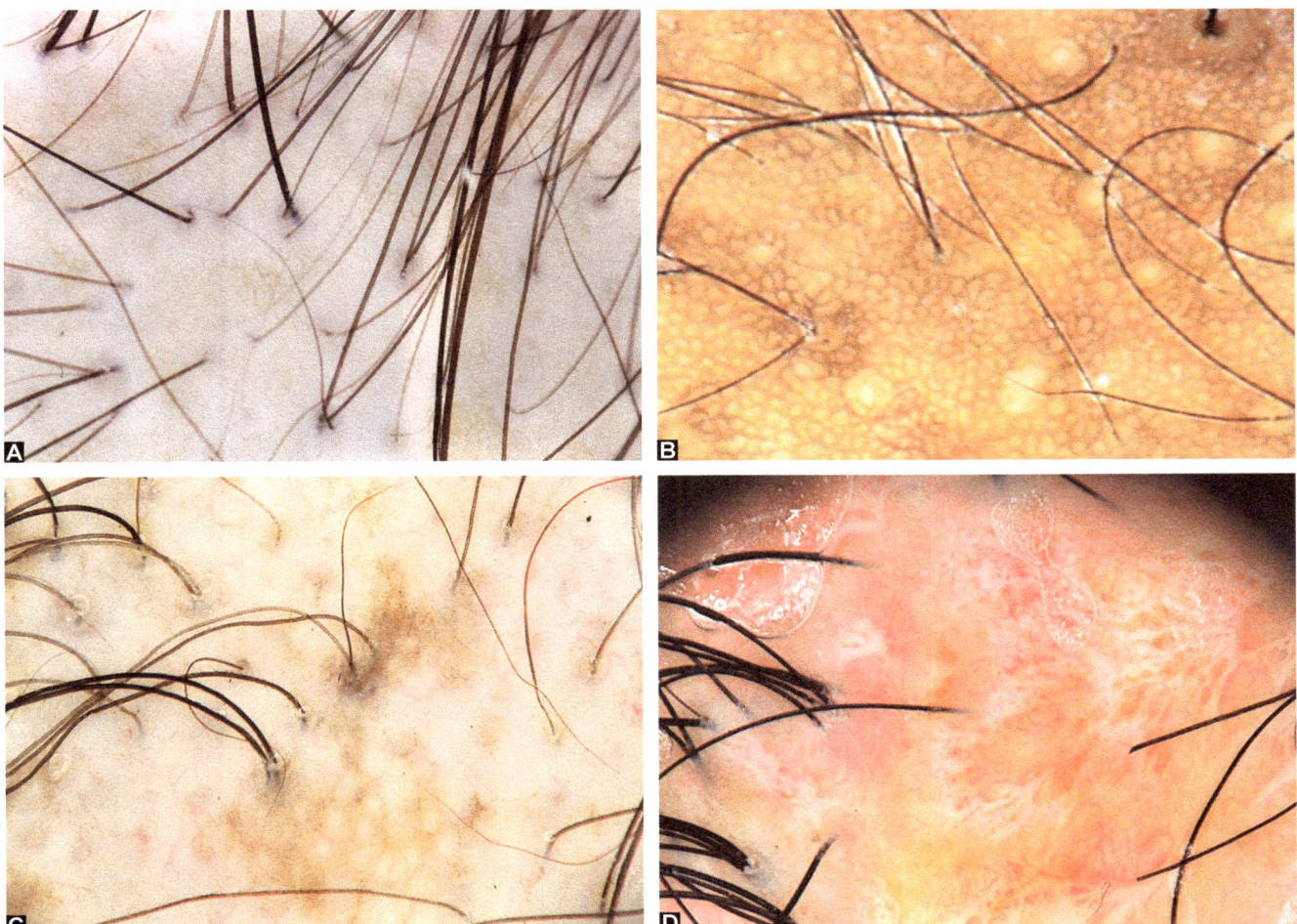

Figs. 3.14A to D: (A) Honeycomb pattern in sun-exposed scalp of a patient with androgenetic alopecia. (B) Honeycomb pattern in a black scalp. Honeycomb pattern can be easily seen in pigmented and high skin types. (C) Note disrupted honeycomb pattern and scattered brown skin pigmentation in discoid lupus erythematosus. (D) Note extensive golden-brown honeycomb pigment pattern with white scarring areas in advanced folliculitis decalvans.
Source: (C and D) Division of Dermatology, Hospital das Clínicas, University of São Paulo Medical School

Take-Home Message

- Honeycomb pattern is usually seen in sun-exposed areas or pigmented scalp.
- It corresponds to melanin-deposition on the rete ridges, involving central areas of hypopigmented epidermis on the tip of dermal papillae.
- In nonscarring alopecias, the honeycomb pattern is regularly distributed on the scalp.
- In scarring alopecias, as discoid lupus erythematosus, and folliculitis decalvans the honeycomb pattern is disrupted on the scalp.
- Scattered brown pigmentation is highly suggestive of discoid lupus erythematosus, and corresponds to pigment incontinence due to partial epidermal destruction.

White (Scarring) Dots/Patches (Figs. 3.15A and B)

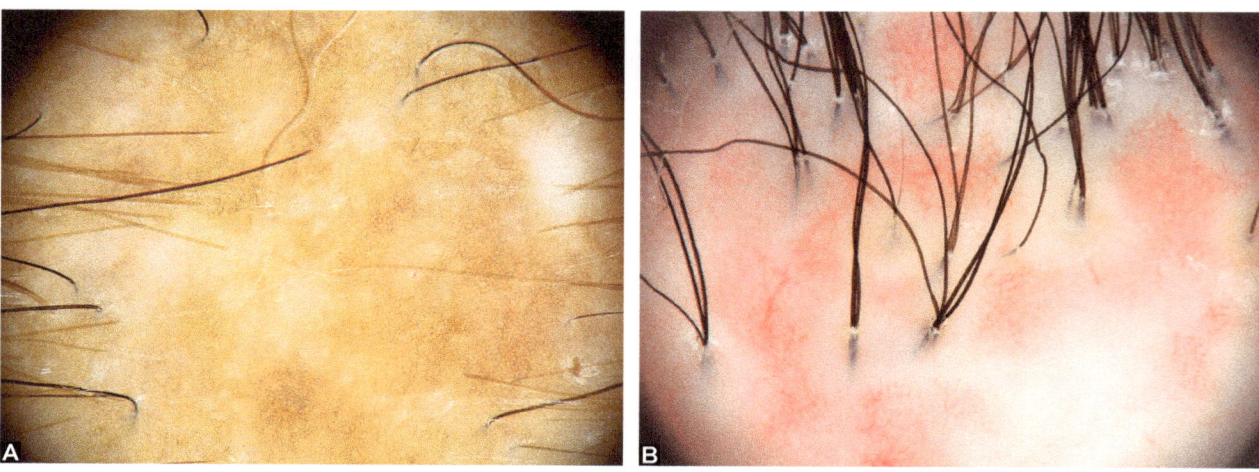

Figs. 3.15A and B: (A) White irregular patches in lichen planopilaris. (B) Large white scarring areas devoid of hairs, follicular openings, and vessels in folliculitis decalvans.
Source: Division of Dermatology, Hospital das Clínicas, University of São Paulo Medical School.

Take-Home Message

- White scarring patches are typical of chronic scarring alopecia.
- They are characterized by irregular areas with absence of follicular openings and vessels, and correspond to intense dermal fibrosis.
- They are more noticeable in high skin types.

Exogen Substances (Figs. 3.16A to C)

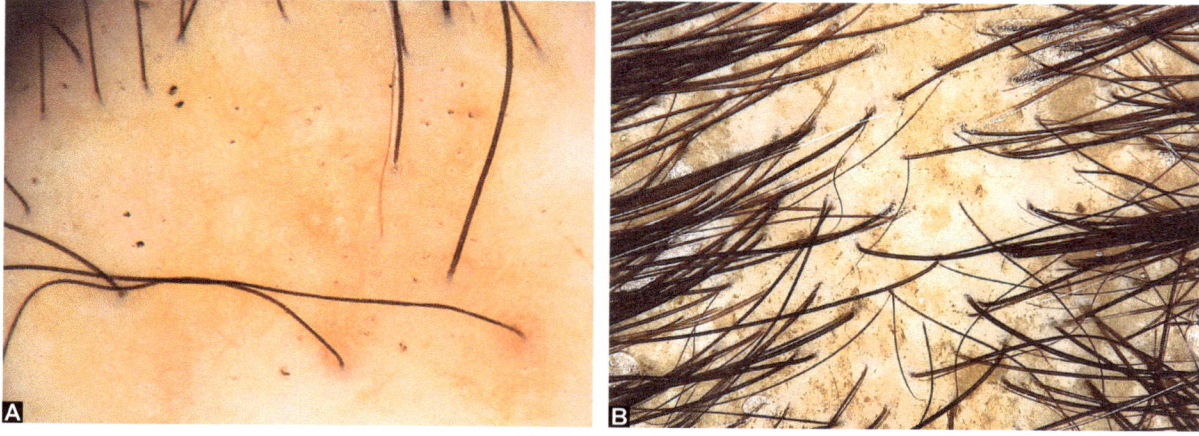

Figs. 3.16A and B.

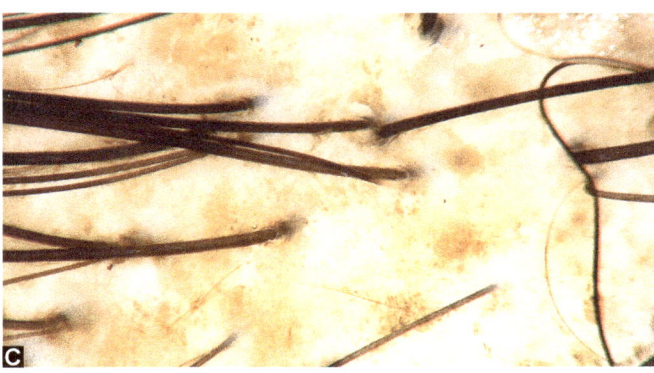

Fig. 3.16C.

Figs. 3.16A to C: (A) Dirty dots irregularly distributed on the scalp. (B) Note clogs of hair dye irregularly deposited on the scalp surface. (C) High magnification can help to detect hair dye penetration into the hair follicle and clogs on the scalp surface.

Source: (A) Division of Dermatology, Hospital das Clínicas, University of São Paulo Medical School.

Take-Home Message
- Exogen substances usually have an irregular format, size, and distribution on the scalp.
- Dirty dots are a normal finding in children and elderly people.
- Dirty dots correspond to small particles from the environment, and can be easily removed after shampooing.
- Hair dye is irregularly deposited in the interfollicular and perifollicular areas of the scalp.
- Hair dye is not easily removed from the scalp.

Hair Shafts

The patterns of hair shafts are given in Box 3.3.

Box 3.3 Patterns of hair shafts.
- Hair shafts
  - Hair density
  - Hair diameter/variability
  - Short hairs
  - Broken and dystrophic hairs
  - Curls and twists
  - Hair tuftings
  - Hair concretions

Hair Density (Figs.3.17A to E)

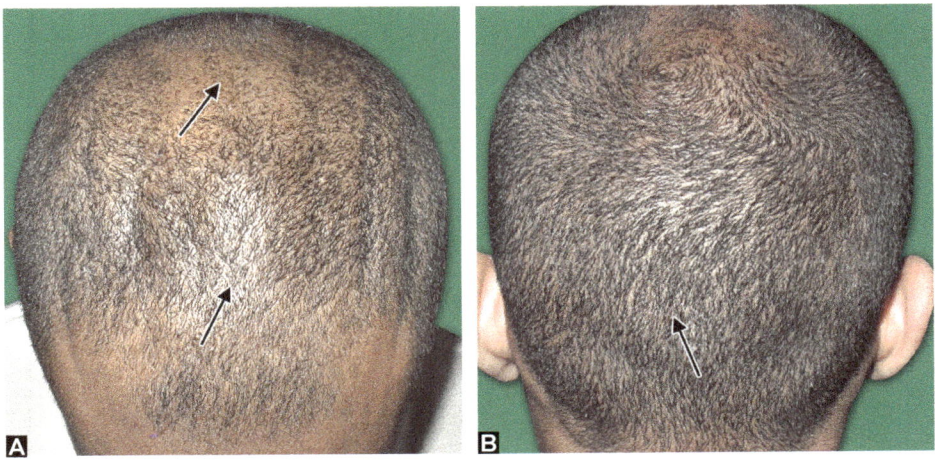

Figs. 3.17A and B.

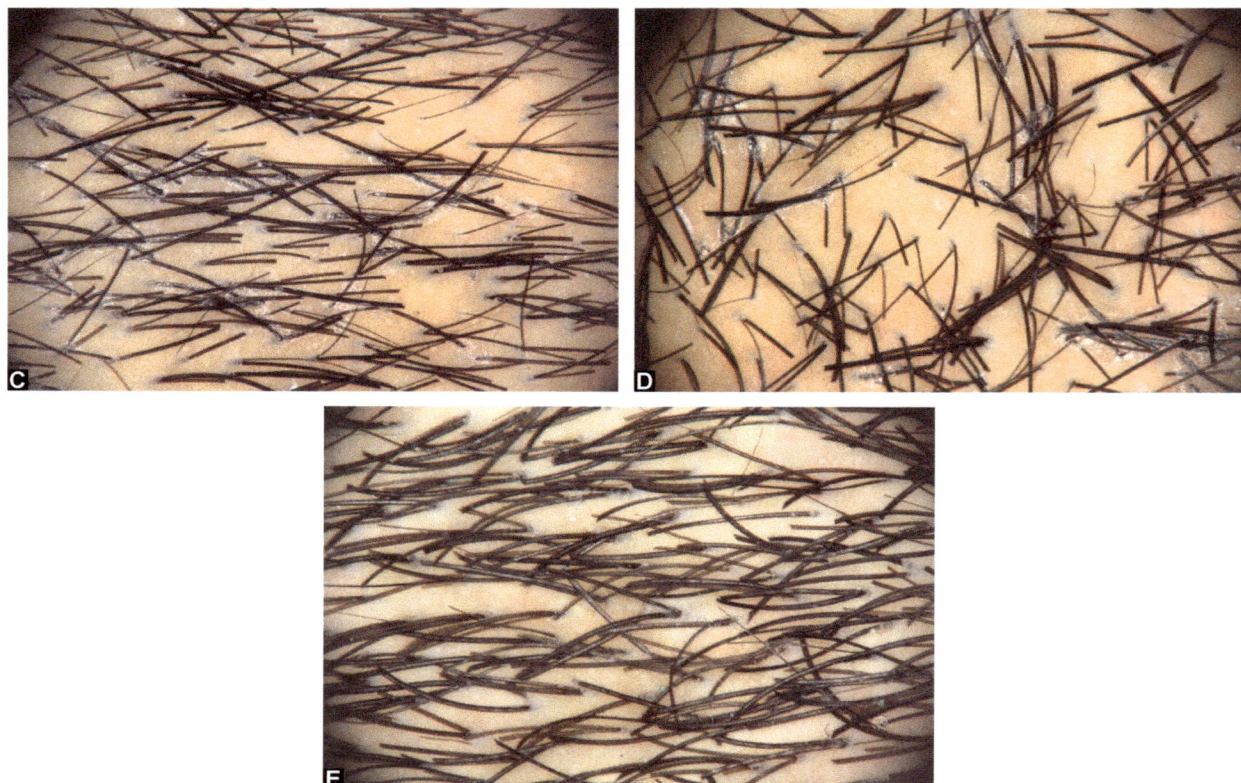

Figs. 3.17C to E.

Figs. 3.17A to E: Hair density in the anterior and occipital scalp areas. Decreased hair density mostly of the mid-area of the scalp can be noted in this patient with mild male pattern androgenetic alopecia. Occipital area presents with a normal hair density.

Source: Division of Dermatology, Hospital das Clínicas, University of São Paulo Medical School.

> **Take-Home Message**
> - Hair density in the anterior, mid and occipital scalp areas should be assessed.
> - Avoid comparing temporal areas where the hairs are normally shorter and thinner.

Hair Diameter/Variability (Figs. 3.18A and B)

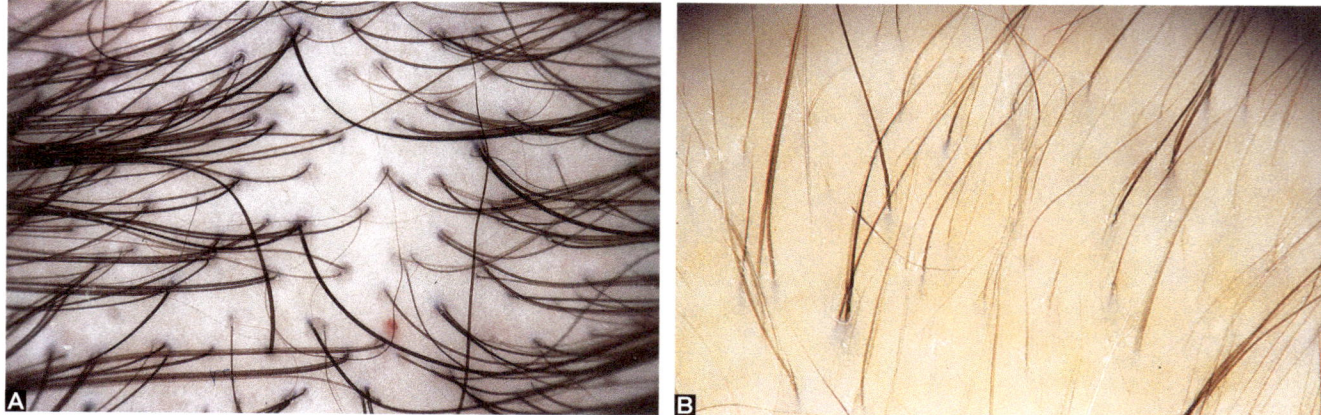

Figs. 3.18A and B: (A) Hair diameter variability in mild androgenetic alopecia. Note hair shafts with different thicknesses (anisotrichosis) and peripilar sign, suggestive of an early disease. (B) Note no hair variability in this patient with alopecia areata. Most hairs are thin and have almost the same thickness.

Source: (B) Division of Dermatology, Hospital das Clínicas, University of São Paulo Medical School.

Take-Home Message
- Hair diameter variability reflects hair miniaturization and is a sign of androgenetic alopecia (AGA).
- Hair diameter variability involving more than 20% of the hairs in the frontal-mid areas strongly suggests AGA.
- In alopecia areata, the hair variability is not increased, because all hairs are homogeneously miniaturized.

Short Hairs (Figs. 3.19A to C)

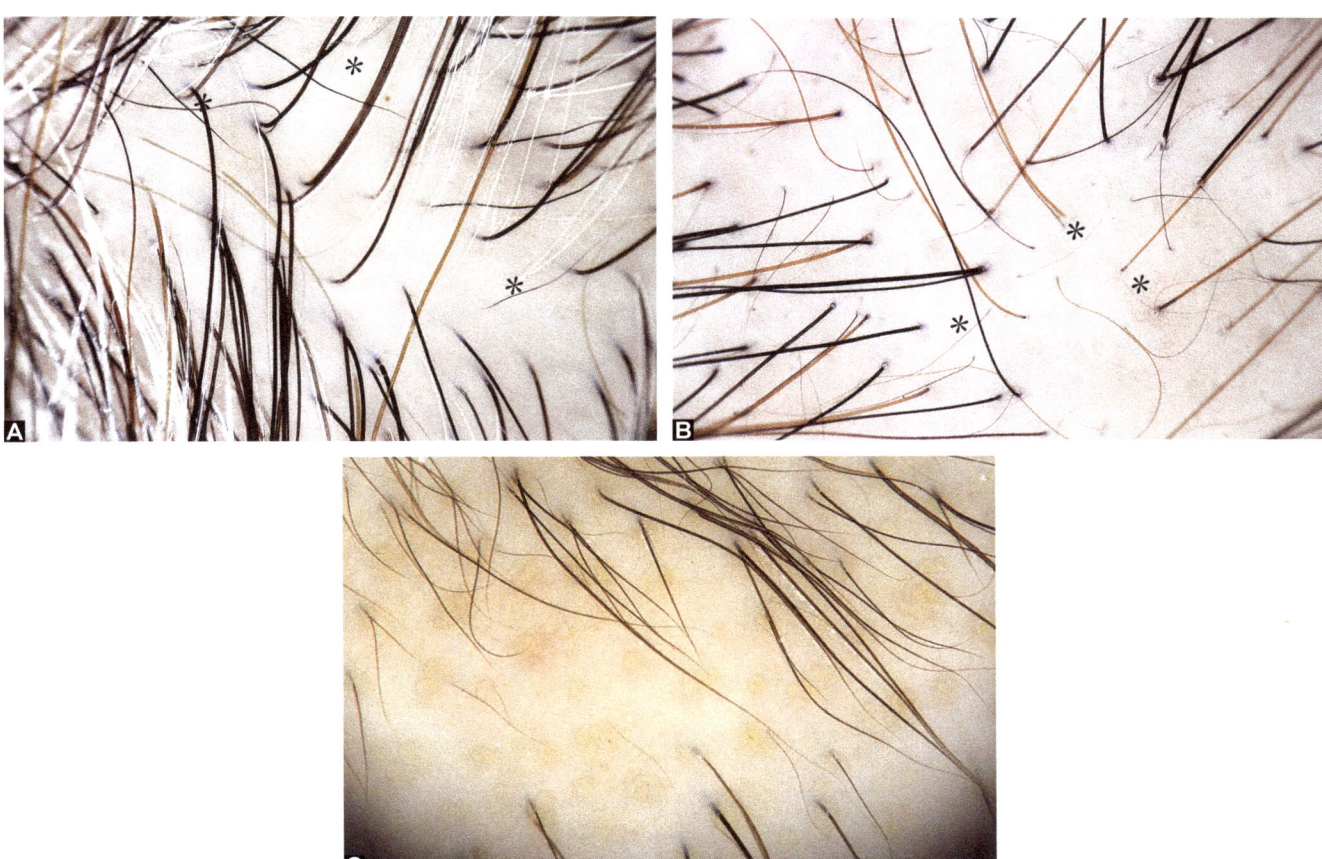

Figs. 3.19A to C: (A) Short regrowing hairs (*) with normal thickness (more than 0.03 mm) distributed within long terminal hairs in telogen effluvium. (B) Short vellus hairs (*) are hypopigmented, thin (less than 0.03 mm) and short (less than 3 cm) in androgenetic alopecia. (C) Note short regrowing hairs with normal thickness, vellus hairs and yellow dots in alopecia areata.
(*Source:* (C) Division of Dermatology, Hospital das Clínicas, University of São Paulo Medical School).

Take-Home Message
- Short regrowing hairs have normal thickness (> 0.03 mm) and are typical of telogen effluvium, and regrowing patches of alopecia areata.
- Short vellus hairs have reduced pigmentation, thickness (< 0.03 mm) and lenght (up to 3 cm), and are typical of androgenetic alopecia and active alopecia areata.

24 Fundamentals of Hair and Scalp Dermoscopy

Broken and Dystrophic Hairs (Figs. 3.20A to N)

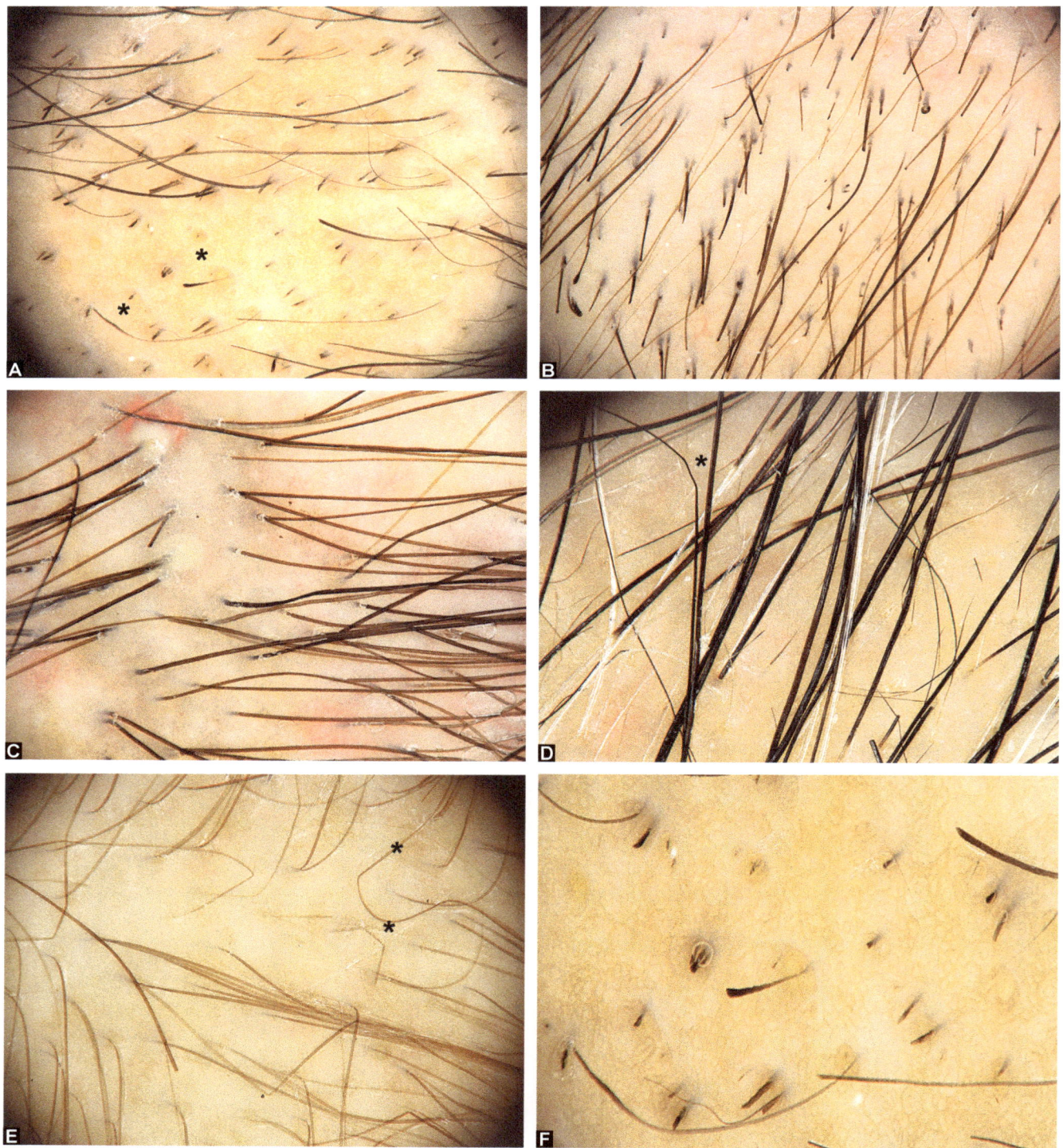

Figs. 3.20A to F.

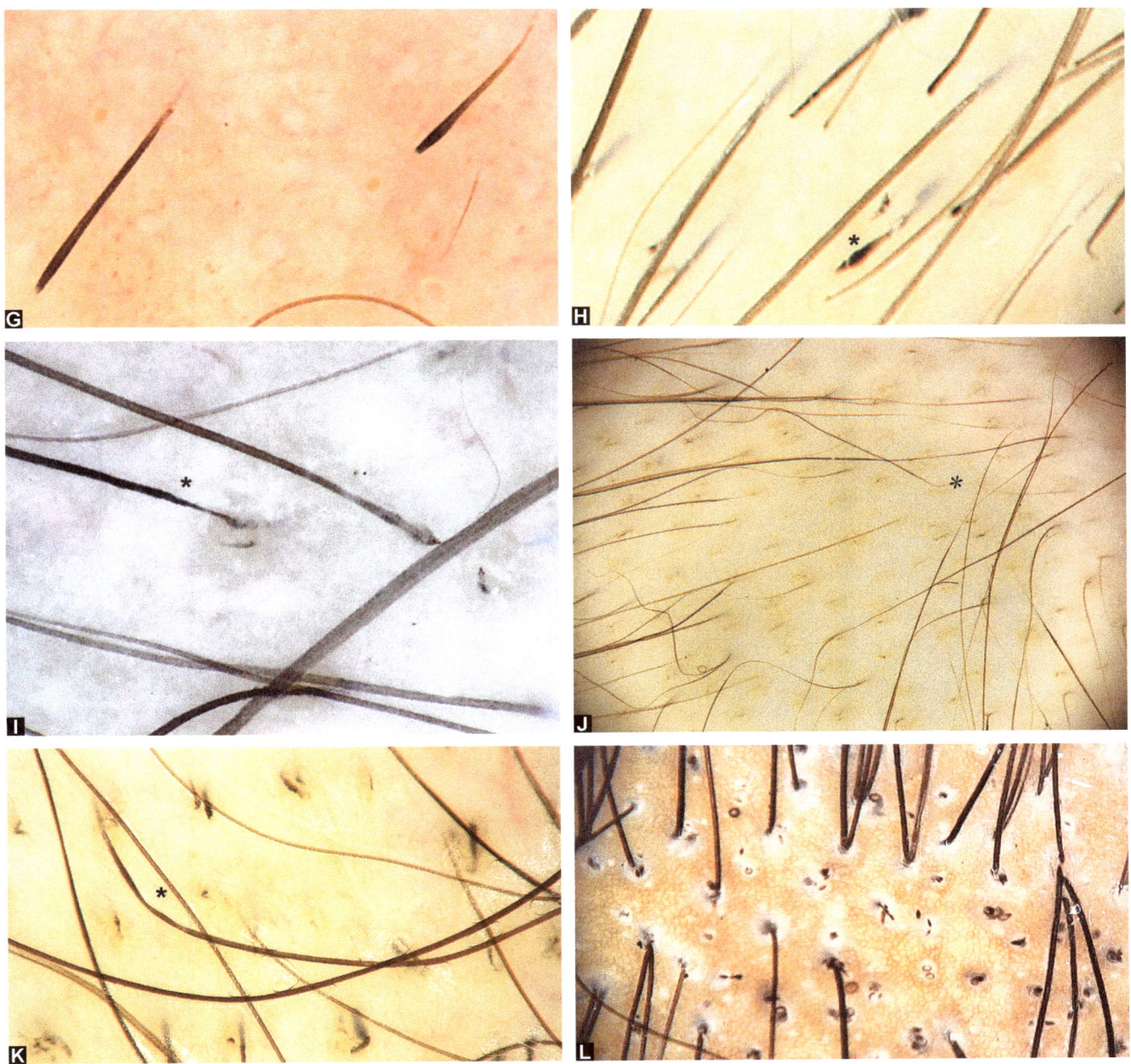

Figs. 3.20G to L.

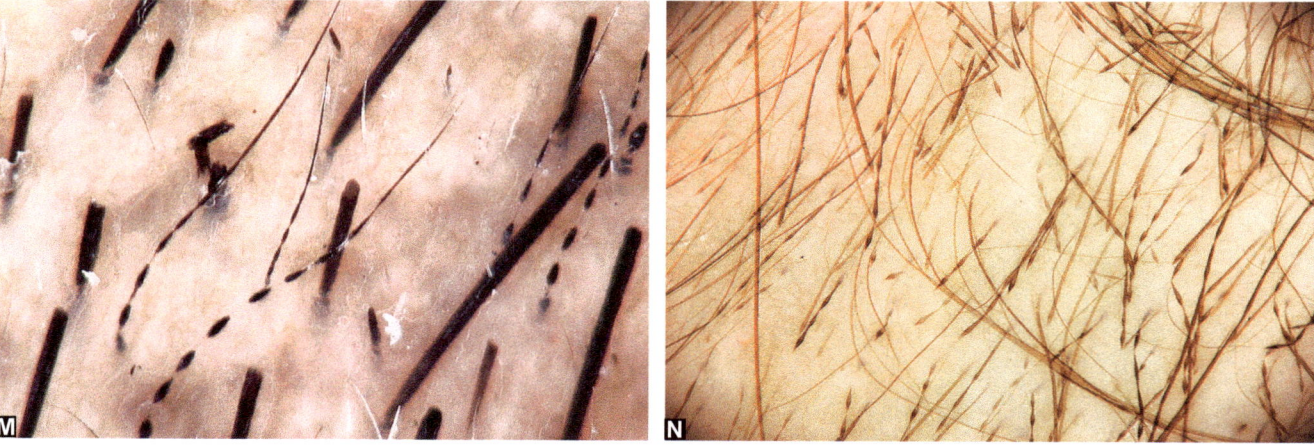

Figs. 3.20M and N.

Figs. 3.20A to N: (A) Multiple broken hairs, black dots and some dystrophic hairs (*) in a patient with alopecia areata. (B) Multiple tulip hairs fractured at different lengths in trichotillomania. Tulip hairs correspond to broken hairs with dark distal ends and are highly suggestive of trichotillomania. (C) Few broken hairs can be found in scarring alopecias, such as lichen planopilaris. Note peripilar casts surrounding one broken hair, few pili torti, and two pustules. (D) Zigzag hair in alopecia areata. It corresponds to hair with multiple areas of partial breakage (*). (E) Zigzag hairs in this rare case of asymptomatic syphilitic alopecia (*). (F) Exclamation mark hair surrounded by many broken hairs in active alopecia areata. This is a broken telogen hair with a darker, frayed, and thicker tip and a hypopigmented proximal portion. It is not specific of alopecia areata. It can also be present in all anagen effluvium, as chemotherapy-induced alopecia, radiation therapy, pressure alopecia, and pemphigus vulgaris. (G) Note the frayed and darker tips of exclamation mark hairs in alopecia areata. (H) Exclamation mark hair (*) in trichotillomania. (I) Caudability or tapered hair (*). Note a normal-looking hair tapered at the proximal end. This is highly indicative of alopecia areata and usually can be found in the edges of enlarging active patches. (J) Caudability hairs (*) in alopecia areata. They can break at the proximal portion due to hair fragility. (K) Pseudomonilethrix or monilethrix-like hairs (Pohl-Pinkus constrictions). Hair shafts with irregular narrowings can be seen in alopecia areata. These hairs can be fractured at the site of the narrowings. Moniletrix-like hairs can also be seen in lichen planopilaris, or in patients undergoing chemotherapy. (L and M) Monilethrix with intense hair breakage on the level of the scalp surface. Note short regular intervals of narrowing. (N) Monilethrix. Hair shafts with regular narrowings. Hair breakage can occur in any site of narrowing. Note one black dot (bottom right).
Source: (A-N, except K) Division of Dermatology, Hospital das Clínicas, University of São Paulo Medical School.

> **Take-Home Message**
> - Broken hairs can be fractured at different lengths from the follicular opening.
> - Black dots (cadaverized hairs) are broken hairs in the level of follicle emergence.
> - Multiple broken hairs can be seen in alopecia areata, trichotillomania, chemotherapy-induced alopecia, and tinea capitis.
> - Few isolated broken hairs can be seen in scarring alopecias.
> - Tulip hairs are specific broken hairs highly suggestive of trichotillomania.
> - Exclamation mark hairs are telogen dystrophic broken hairs that can be mostly seen in alopecia areata.
> - Caudability hairs are very long exclamation mark hairs with distal normal thickness and proximal tapered end. They may sometimes bend at the proximal tapered end. They are typical of active alopecia areata enlarging patches.
> - Zigzag and pseudomonilethrix hairs are partially fractured hairs in multiple levels without breakage.
> - Differently from pseudomonilethrix, in monilethrix the hair narrowings occur in regular intervals.

Curls and Twists (Figs. 3.21A to H)

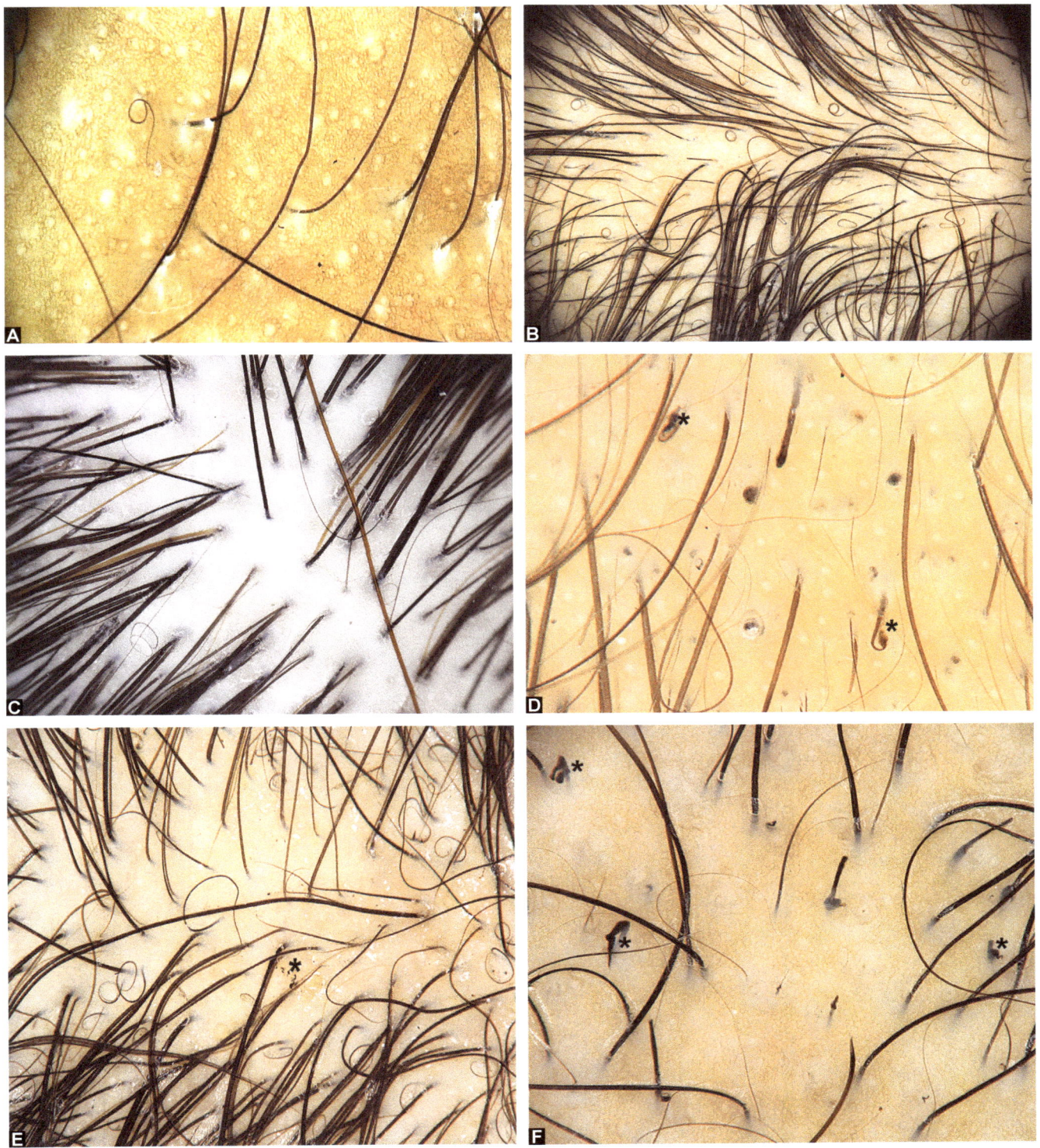

Figs. 3.21A to F.

28 Fundamentals of Hair and Scalp Dermoscopy

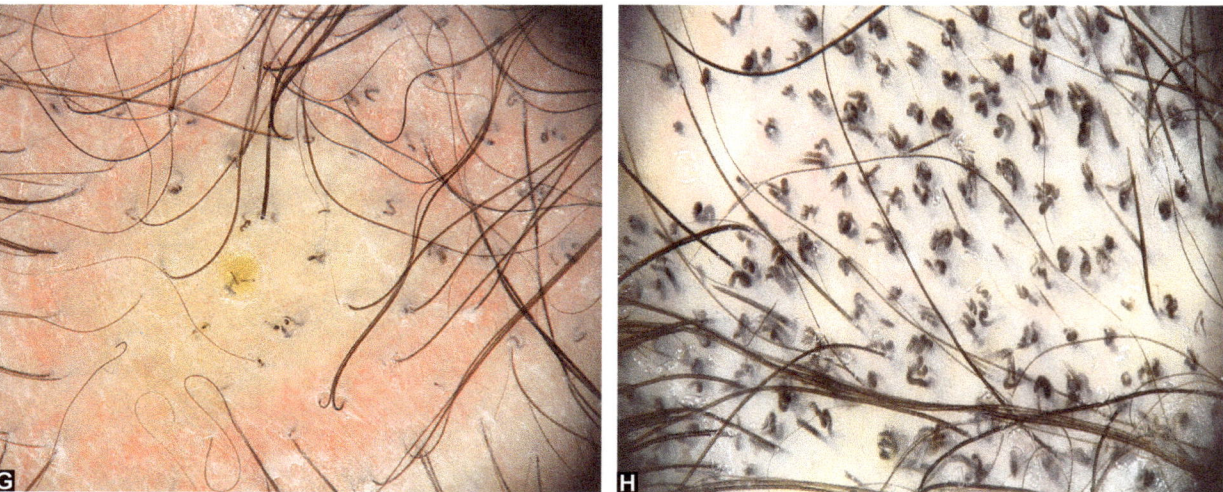

Figs. 3.21G to H.

Figs. 3.21A to H: (A) Isolated coiled hairs in traction alopecia. Coiled hairs can also be seen in normal black scalp due to hair pulling during hair styling. (B) Multiple circle hairs (pigtail hairs) in alopecia areata. Sometimes multiple circle hairs (usually more than 6 in 20X) can be the only finding of the disease. (C) Isolated circle hairs can be seen in androgenetic alopecia, especially in mild cases. (D) Question mark hairs (Hook hairs) in trichotillomania (*). Note the short coiled hairs with a thin tip. (E) Residues of a flame hair in alopecia areata. Flame hairs are formed by wavy, cone-shaped hair residue structures. Note multiple circle hairs. They can also be found in chemotherapy-induced alopecia and trichotillomania. (F) Flame hairs can have multiple forms in trichotillomania (*). (G) Comma hairs in the scalp of a child with tinea capitis. (H) Corkscrew hairs in tinea capitis. Although corkscrew hairs can be seen more often in African descents due to curly hair, they can also be found in association with comma hairs in all hair ethnicities.

Source: (A-G, except C) Division of Dermatology, Hospital das Clínicas, University of São Paulo Medical School.

> **Take-Home Message**
> - Isolated coiled hairs can be seen in normal black scalp.
> - Circle hairs are thin-coiled regrowing hairs that can occur in androgenetic alopecia and alopecia areata.
> - Few isolated circle hairs can be found in androgenetic alopecia.
> - Multiple circle hairs are highly suggestive of alopecia areata, and sometimes can be the sole finding of the disease.
> - Question mark hairs are short hairs with a coiled tip, very typical of trichotillomania due to hair pulling.
> - Flame hairs are diverse cone-shaped structures contaning hair residues, highly suggestive of trichotillomania due to hair pulling.
> - Comma and corkscrew hairs are elliptical hairs specific of tinea capitis.

Tuftings (Figs. 3.22A to D)

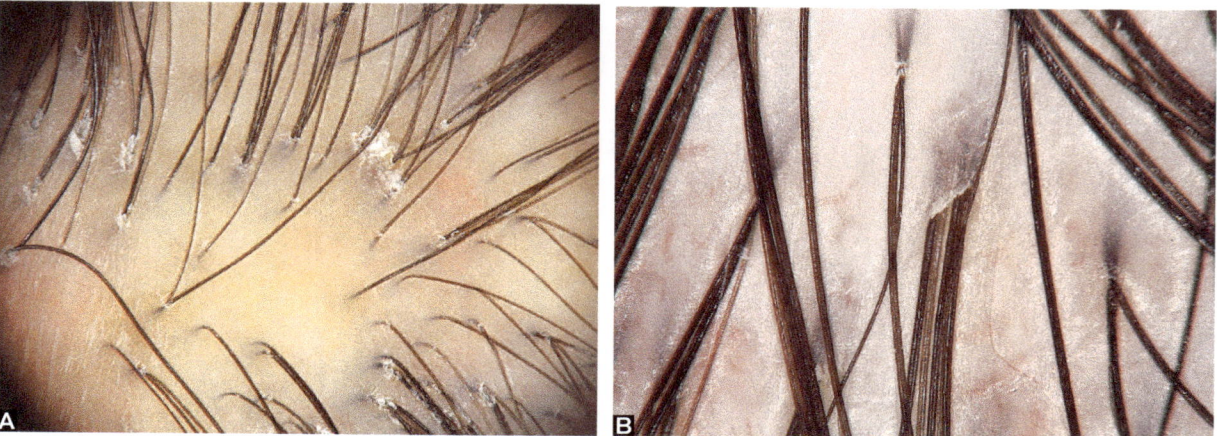

Figs. 3.22A and B.

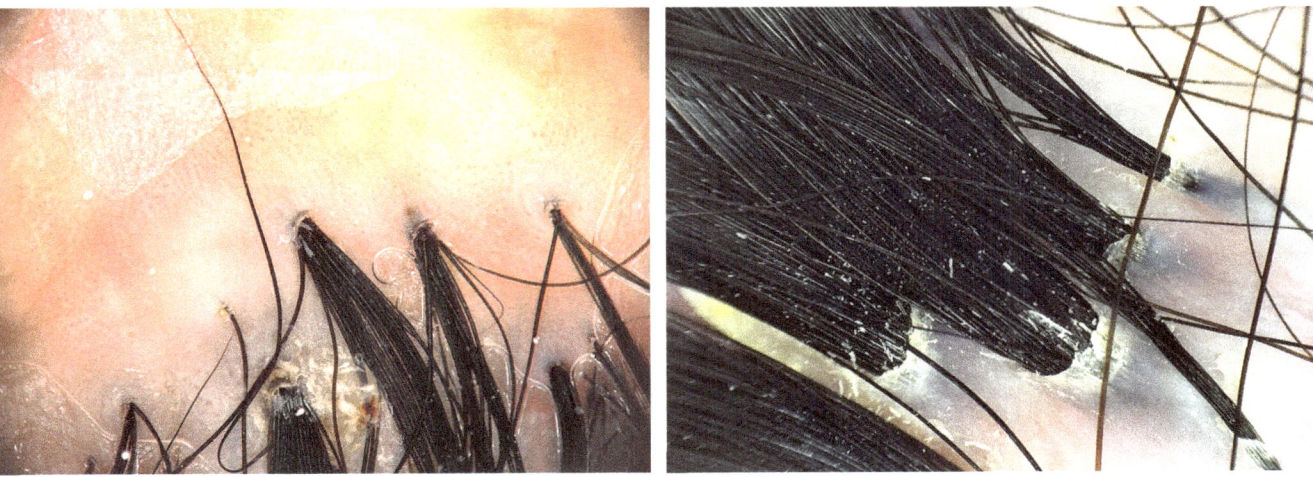

Figs. 3.22C and D.

Figs. 3.22A to D: (A) Hair tufts in lichen planopilaris. Note small tufts of hairs (less than 6) surrounded by peripilar scale. (B) Hair tufts in occipital scalp of a patient with lichen planopilaris. Small tufts and peripilar scale can occasionally be present in "normal appearing" areas of scarring alopecias. (C) Hairs tufts in folliculitis decalvans (more than 6). (D) Multiple and extense hair tufts in folliculitis decalvans. Note peripilar scale and intense skin atrophy.

Source (A and C): Division of Dermatology, Hospital das Clínicas, University of São Paulo Medical School.

> **Take-Home Message**
> - Hair tuftings are indicative of scarring alopecias.
> - Tuftings containing more than 6 hairs are indicative of folliculitis decalvans.
> - Small tuftings (less than 6 hairs) may be present in lichen planopilaris, mainly in lesions with secondary infection.
> - Small tuftings may be present in "normal-appearing" areas of scarring alopecia despite the absence of alopecia.
> - Some healthy subjects may present 4 hair shafts emerging from the same follicular openings.
> - Hair tuftings are usually associated with peripilar scales and hair casts.

Concretions (Figs. 3.23A to D)

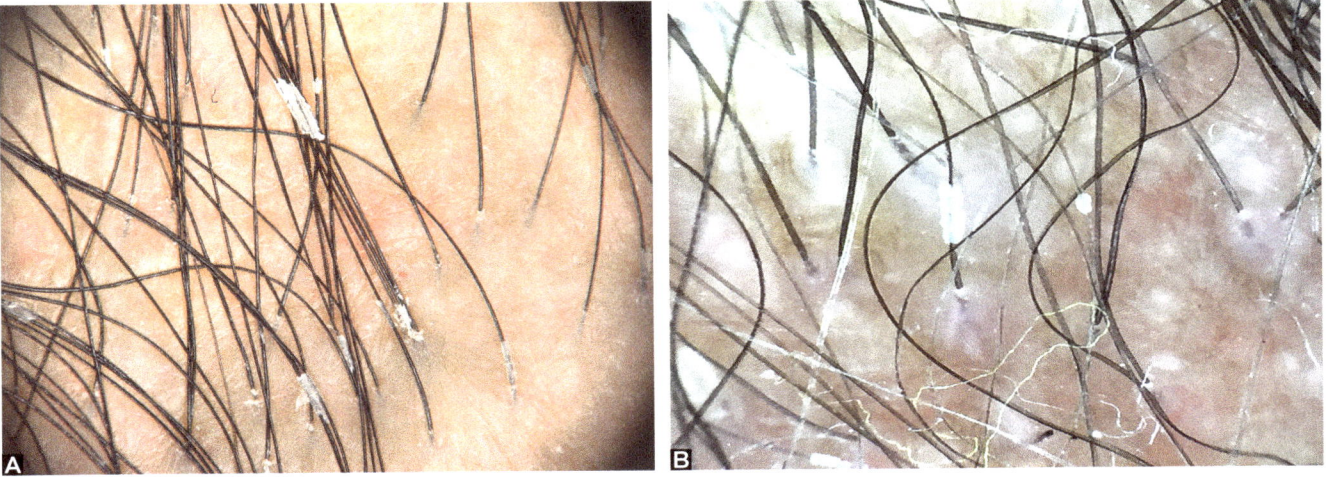

Figs. 3.23A and B.

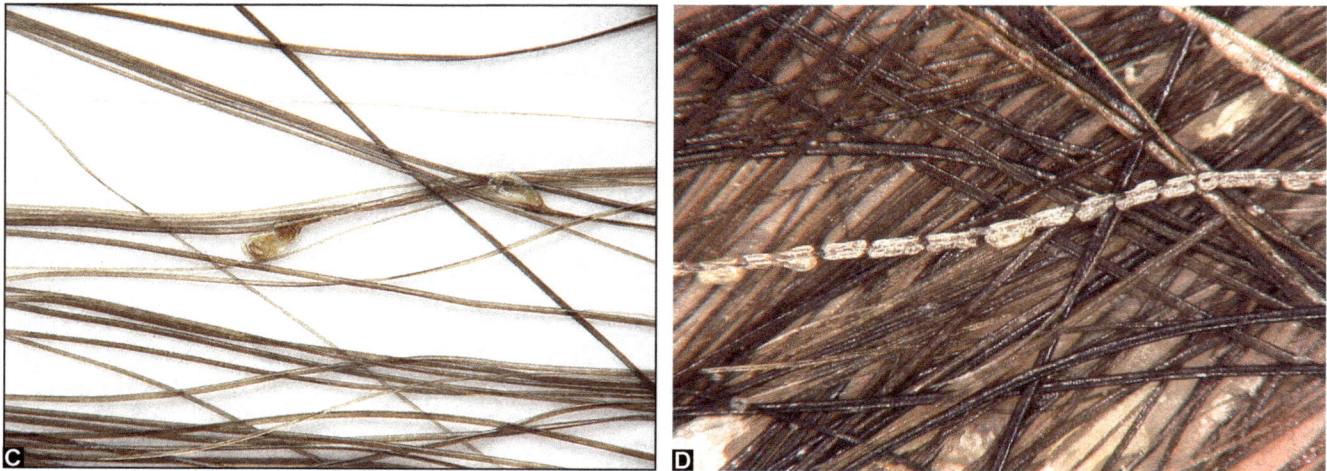

Figs. 3.23C and D.

Figs. 3.23A to D: (A) Hair casts in lichen planopilaris. Scales can detach from the follicular openings and surround the hairs shafts. (B) Hair casts in traction alopecia. Note translucent color of the hair casts encircling all the shafts. (C) Nits. Hair casts should not be confused with nits, a sign of lice infection. Note that nits attach to the hair shaft but do not encircle it. (D) Pseudocasts from hair sprays.
Source: (A and C) Division of Dermatology, Hospital das Clínicas, University of São Paulo Medical School; *(D):* Dr Antonella Tosti.

> **Take-Home Message**
> - Hair casts are concretions that encircle the hair shafts.
> - Casts are firm, tubular, and whitish structures that can move along the hair shaft.
> - They can be present in many inflammatory conditions, such as seborrheic dermatitis, psoriasis, tinea capitis, traction alopecia, and scarring alopecias.
> - Casts should not be misdiagnosed as nits, which attach to the hair shaft but do not encircle it.
> - Pseudocasts due to hair sprays, deodorants, and dry shampoos may form irregular structures similar to casts and nits.

Hair Roots

The patterns of hair roots are given in Box 3.4.

> **Box 3.4** Patterns of hair roots.
> - Hair roots
>   - Anagen
>   - Telogen
>   - Dystrophic

Hair roots from hairs that are shed and extracted from the scalp should be examined. Anagen and telogen plucked hairs may be difficult to distinguish based on their microscopic appearance. The root ends of plucked anagen hairs turn red when stained with 4-dimethylaminocinnamaldehyde, while those of plucked telogen hairs do not (Fig. 3.24). The red color results from a reaction with citrulline-containing proteins in the inner root sheath, responsible for anchoring the hair shaft within the follicle (Figs. 3.25A and B). This method provides an easy, quick, and effective manner to determine the anagen/telogen ratio in plucked hairs from the trichogram (Fig. 3.26).

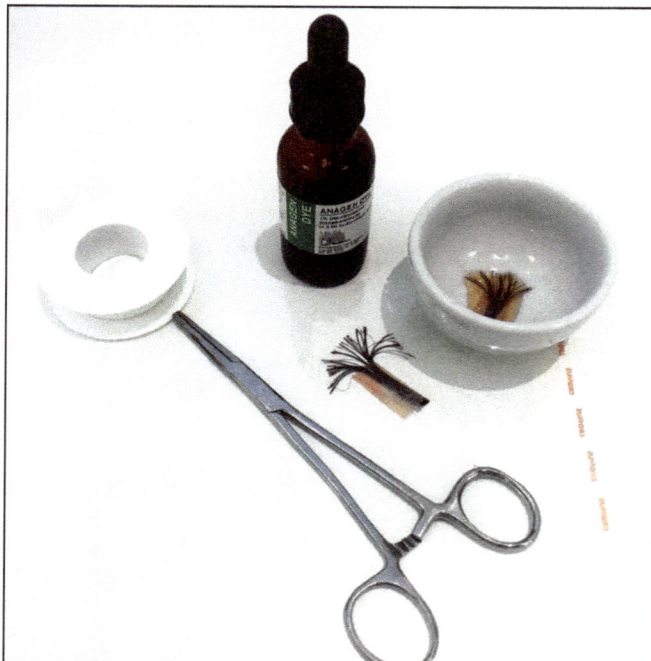

Fig. 3.24: Materials for the modified trichogram or "envelope trichogram," described by Dr Fernanda Torres. This method uses a dermoscope instead of a microscope to assess the type of roots in the trichogram. After 3–5 days without washing the hair, the patient is submitted to a hair plucking in two small scalp areas containg 30 to 50 hairs. Usually, we select one area from the anterior scalp and one from the posterior scalp for comparison. The plucked hairs are cut 5 cm from the roots and fixed with a tape. After 5 minutes of immersion in Anagen Hair Dye [1% Dimethylaminocinnamaldehyde (DACA), in 0.5N hydrochloric acid], from *Delasco Dermatologic Lab & Supply, USA*, the hairs are placed inside a plastic bag or envelope for dermoscopic analysis.

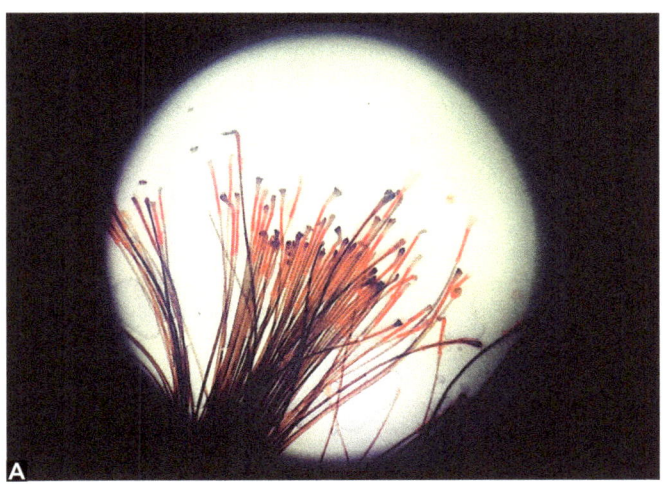 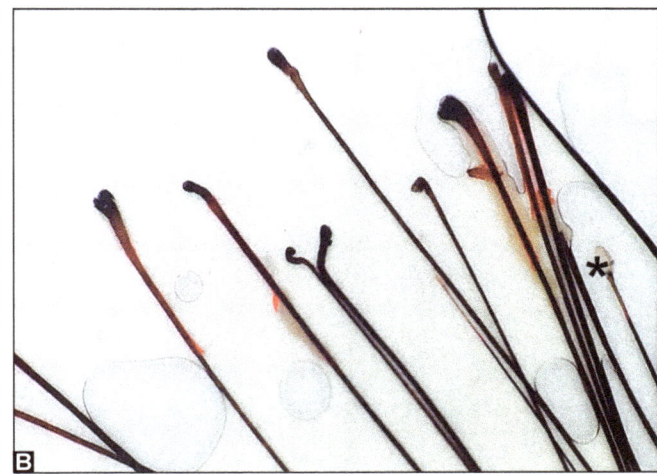

Figs. 3.25A and B: (A) Modified trichogram. Note anagen hair roots colored in red. (B) Note all anagen hairs deeply pigmented on the roots and one telogen hair (*).

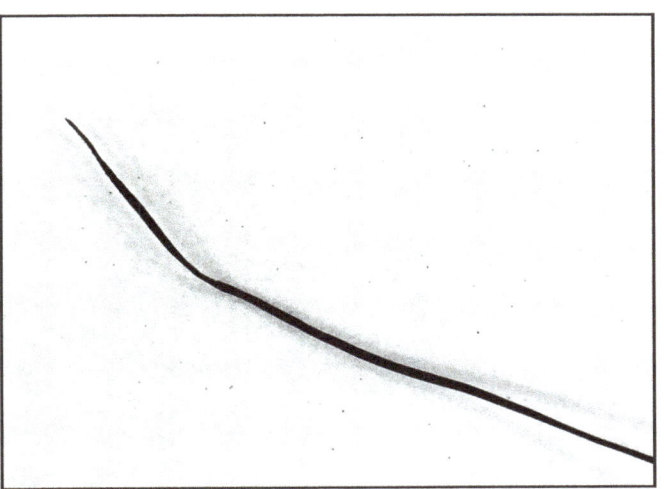 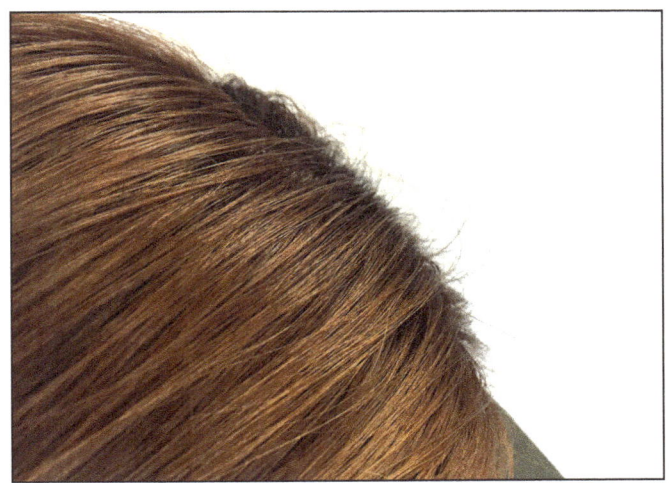

Fig. 3.26: Dystrophic anagen hair from a patient with alopecia areata. Note the tapered end and narrowings along the shaft.

Fig. 3.27: Multiple layers of high regrowth can be better appreciated using a white sheet as a background.

TEN TIPS TO ENHANCE YOUR EXAM

1. For scales, gray, blond, and vellus hairs, first perform dermoscopy without immersion fluid.
2. For immersion fluid, prefer the use of alcohol or water spray. The gel can get stuck on the lenses and produce artifacts and pseudonodes.
3. Ask patients about previous hair dye, hair powders, dry shampoos, hair sprays, or any camouflage products. These can be trichoscopy pitfalls and lead to misdiagnosis.
4. Avoid temporal areas to analyze hair diversity. Hairs from the temporal areas are normally shorter and thinner. Compare frontal to occipital scalp areas for hair diversity.
5. For diffuse and patterned hair loss, examine frontal, mid, and occipital scalp areas. For patchy hair loss, examine the center, borders, and perilesional areas. Use a white sheet to show the layers of hair regrowth to the patient (Fig. 3.27).
6. Examine hair roots from hairs that are shed and extracted from the scalp.
7. Avoid infected lesions with crusts and pustules. Use a plastic cap for contact dermoscopy in infected lesions. Perform dermoscopy after 2 weeks of keratolytic shampoos and/or antibiotic therapy to better assess the hair and scalp structures.

8. For vessels, do not pressure the scalp too much. Use noncontact dermoscopy or low-pressure contact dermoscopy.
9. Always examine nails, mucosa, eyebrows, and other skin lesions especially for alopecia areata, lichen planopilaris, frontal fibrosing alopecia, and genetic syndromes.
10. Examine the entire scalp, including "normal-appearing areas". In scarring alopecias, these areas may be affected as well and present typical perifollicular scale, erythema and small hair tufts despite the absence of clinically evident lesions.

SUGGESTED READINGS

1. Abedini R, Kamyab Hesari K, Daneshpazhooh M, et al. Validity of trichoscopy in the diagnosis of primary cicatricial alopecias. Int J Dermatol. 2016;55(10):1106-14.
2. Abraham LS, Pineiro-Maceira J, Duque-Estrada B, et al. Pinpoint White dots in the scalp: dermoscopic and histopathologic correlation. J Am Acad Dermatol. 2010;63(4):721-2.
3. Doche I, Vincenzi C, Tosti A. Casts and pseudocasts. J Am Acad Dermatol. 2016;75(4):e147-8.
4. Inui S. Trichoscopy for common hair loss diseases: algorithmic method for diagnosis. J Dermatol. 2011;38(1):71-5.
5. Kowalska-Oledzka E, Slowinska M, Rakowska A, et al. "Black dots" seen under trichoscopy are not specific for alopecia areata. Clin Exp Dermatol. 2012;37(6):615-9.
6. Lacarrubba F, Micali G, Tosti A. Scalp dermoscopy or tichoscopy. Curr Probl Dermatol. 2015;47:21-32.
7. Lencastre A, Tosti A. Role of trichoscopy in childrens` scalp and hair disorders. Pediatr Dermatol. 2013;30(6):674-82.
8. Mubki T, Rudnicka L, Olszewska M, et al. Evaluation and diagnosis of the hair loss patients: Part II. Trichoscopic and laboratory evaluations. J Am Acad Dermatol. 2014;71(3):431.e1-11.
9. Park J, Kim JI, Kim HU, et al. Trichoscopic findings of hair loss in Koreans. Ann Dermatol. 2015;27(5):539-50.
10. Rakowska A, Slowinska M, Kowalska-Oledzka E, et al. trichoscopy of cicatricial alopecia. J Drugs Dermatol. 2012;11(6):753-8.
11. Rudnicka L, Olszewska M, Rakowska A. Trichoscopic structures and patterns. In: Rudnicka L, Olszewska M, Rakowska A (Eds). Atlas of Trichoscopy. New York: Springer; 2011.
12. Rudnicka L, Olszewska M, Rakowska A, et al. Trichoscopy update 2011. J Dermatol Case Rep. 2011;5(4):82-8.
13. Rudnicka L, Rakowska A, Kerzeja M, et al. Hair shafts in trichoscopy: clues for diagnosis of hair and scalp diseases. Dermatol Clin. 2013;31(4):695-708.
14. Torres F, Tosti A. Trichoscopy: an update. G Ital Dermatol Venereol. 2014;149(1):83-91.
15. Tosti A. Trichoscopy patterns. In: Tosti A (Ed). Dermoscopy of Hair and Nails. Boca Raton: CRC Press; 2016.
16. Yin NC, Tosti A. A systematic approach to Afro-textured hair disorders: dermatoscopy and when to biopsy. Dermatol Clin. 2014;32(2):145-51.

CHAPTER 4

Nonscarring Alopecias

Patricia Damasco, Giselle Martins, Isabella Doche, Maria K Hordinsky, Emilie Jane Fowler, Antonella Tosti, Lidia Rudnicka

4.1 Androgenetic Alopecia or Male-Pattern Hair Loss

Patricia Damasco, Giselle Martins, Isabella Doche

MALE-PATTERN HAIR LOSS

Male-pattern hair loss (MPHL) is a common condition characterized by progressive thinning of scalp hairs. The disease occurs in all races, although the prevalence in Caucasians is little higher comparing to Asians and African descents.

Pathogenesis if MPHL is related to increased conversion of testosterone to dihydrotestosterone by the 5-α-reductase type II enzyme, leading to a progressive hair miniaturization in androgen-sensitive hair follicles. Also, there is a continuous reduction in the duration of the anagen phase over the course of successive hair cycles. The length of the telogen phase remains constant or is prolonged and, over time, the anagen phase becomes so short that the hairs fail to achieve sufficient length to reach the surface of the skin, resulting in empty follicular openings.

Most affected men present with bilateral frontotemporal recession and decreased hair density in the frontal and vertex scalp areas (Hamilton–Norwood Classification) (Figs. 4.1.1A to D).

Dermoscopy shows increased hair shaft diameter diversity (more than 20%), variable yellow dots, peripilar sign (perifollicular brown discoloration), increased proportion of single follicular units and vellus hairs (Figs. 4.1.2 to 4.1.6). In severe cases, scalp pigmentation with a honeycomb-pattern appearance and pinpoint white dots are usually seen (Fig. 4.1.7).

Topical minoxidil and oral finasteride (5-α-reductase type II inhibitor) are the only approved treatments. Hair transplantation can be an option for severe cases.

Fundamentals of Hair and Scalp Dermoscopy

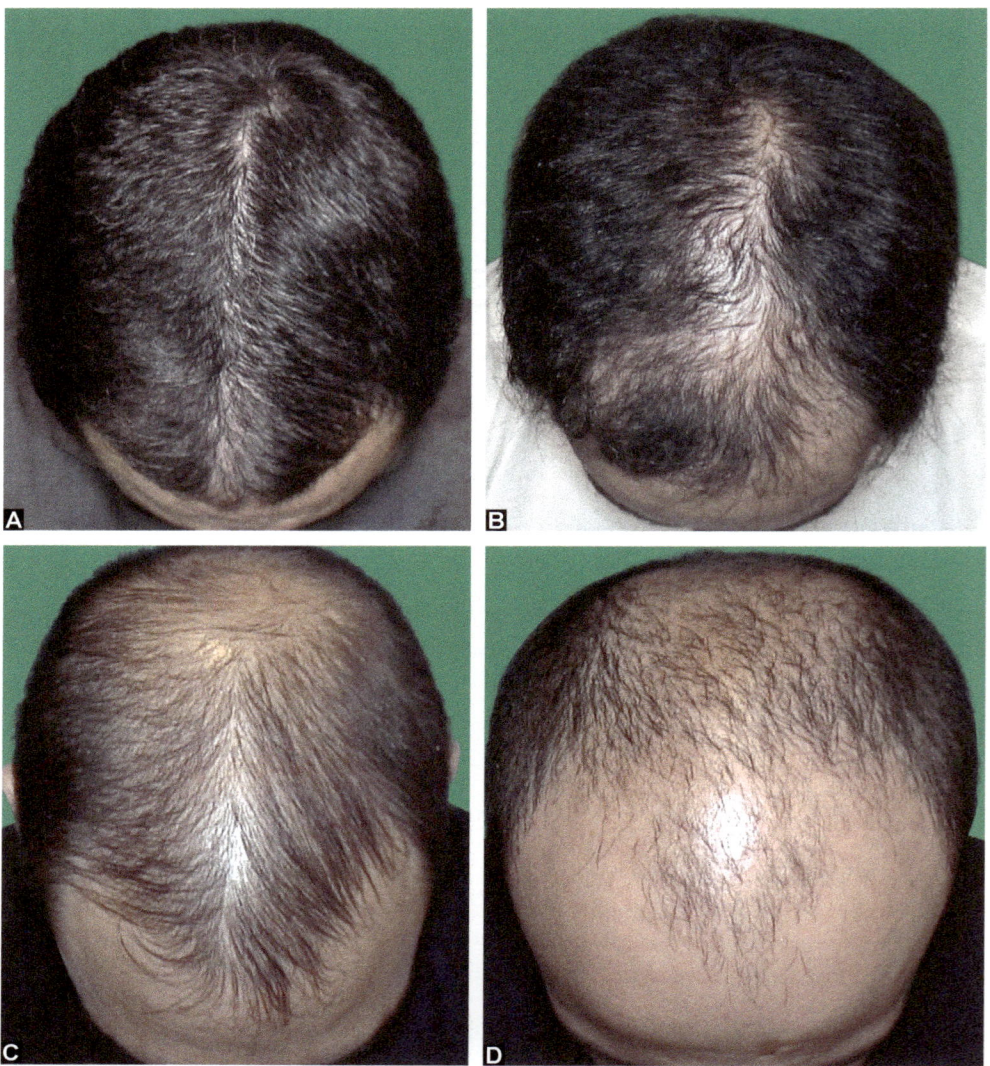

Figs. 4.1.1A to D: Male-pattern hair loss. (A) Frontotemporal recession with mild thinning in the frontal and mid-scalp areas (Norwood–Hamilton II). (B) Moderate frontotemporal recession (Norwood–Hamilton type III). (C) Diffuse hair thinning, mostly on the vertex scalp area (Norwood–Hamilton V). (D) Severe diffuse hair thinning (Norwood–Hamilton VI).

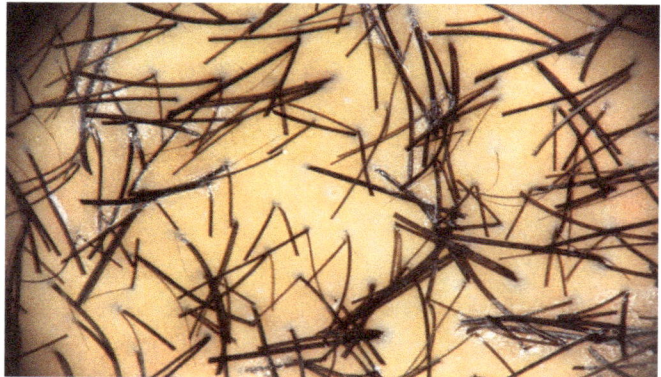

Fig. 4.1.2: Early male-pattern hair loss. Mild decreased hair density and increased hair diameter variability in the vertex scalp from an African-descent patient. Some areas present a more prominent honeycomb pattern.

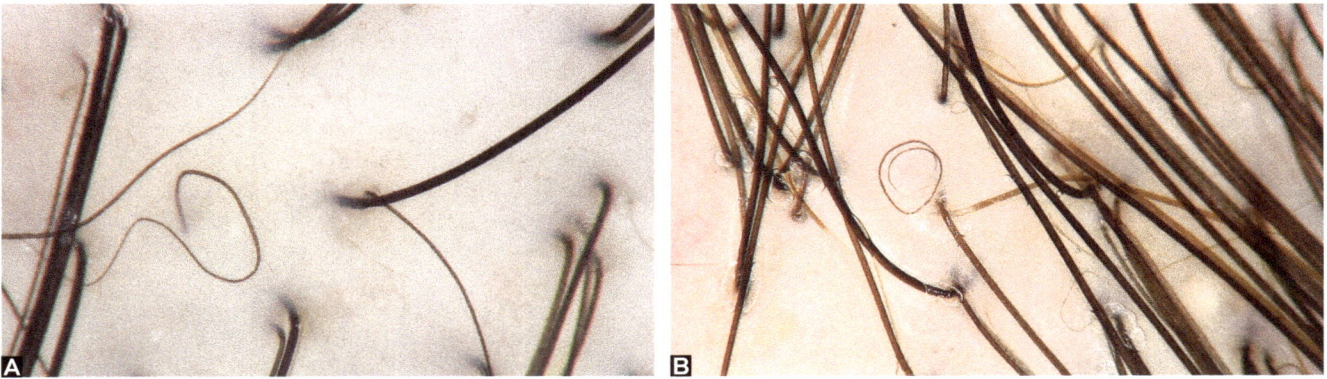

Figs. 4.1.3A and B: Early male-pattern hair loss. Circle or pigtail hairs and wavy hairs are regrowing hairs that appear as thin, isolated coiled hairs surrounded by terminal and intermediate hairs.

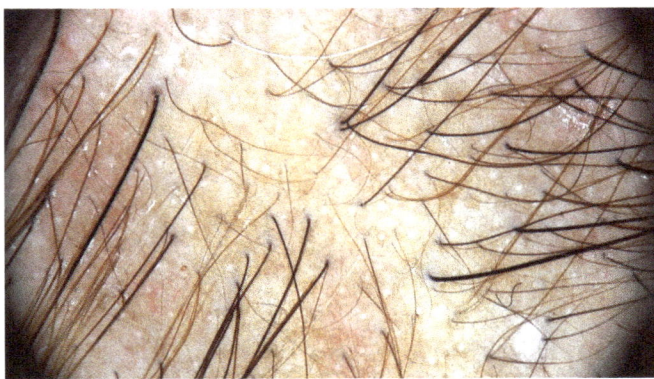

Fig. 4.1.4: Moderate male-pattern hair loss. Increased hair shaft thickness variability. Note thin, intermediate, and thick hairs simultaneously in the field.

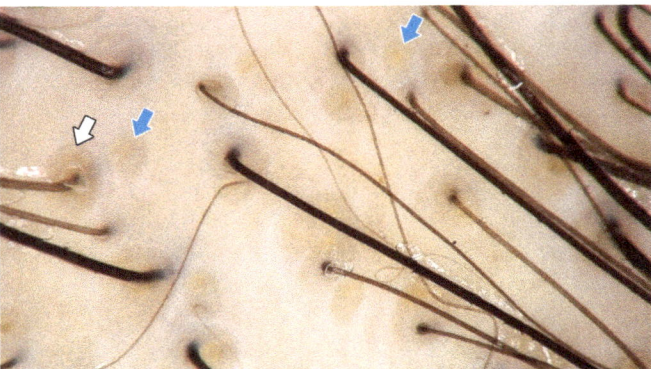

Fig. 4.1.5: Moderate male-pattern hair loss. Multiple small yellow dots (blue arrows) filled with keratotic material and devoid of hair shafts. Note large yellowish oily hues (white arrow) caused by the remains of sebaceous debris encircling terminal hairs.

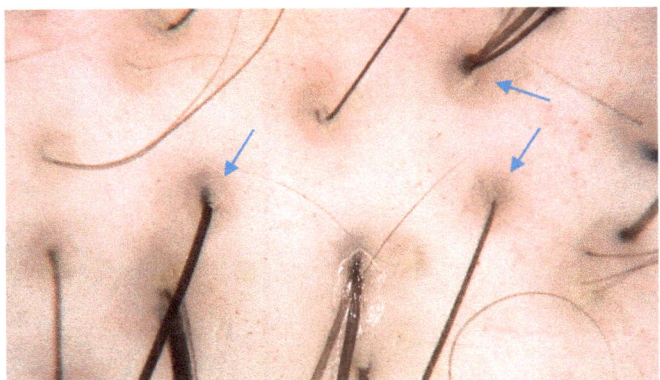

Fig. 4.1.6: Moderate male-pattern hair loss. Vellus hairs and peripilar sign (blue arrows), a slightly depressed brownish halo surrounding some terminal hairs.

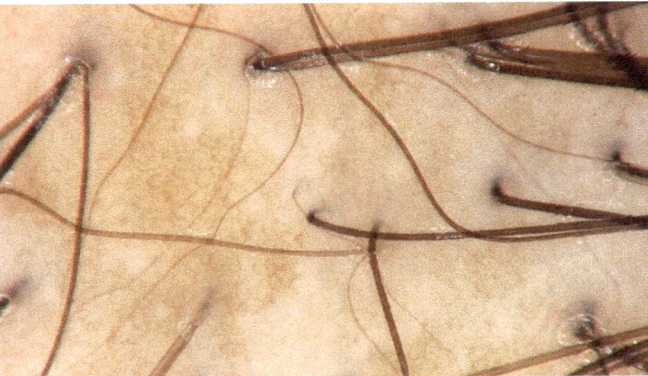

Fig. 4.1.7: Severe male-pattern hair loss. Honeycomb pattern due to chronic sun exposure and pinpoint white dots.

Take-Home Message
- Male androgenetic alopecia is a very frequent condition with progressive thinning of frontal and mid scalp hairs.
- Follicular miniaturization is the hallmark of the disease.
- Dermoscopy shows increased hair diameter variability, variable yellow dots, peripilar sign, increased vellus hairs, and single follicular units.
- Honeycomb network can be seen in more severe cases.

SUGGESTED READING

1. Adil A, Godwin M. The effectiveness of treatments for androgenetic alopecia: a systematic review and meta-analysis. J Am Acad Dermatol. 2017;77(1):136-41.e5.
2. Hu R, Xu F, Han Y, et al. Trichoscopic findings of androgenetic alopecia and their association with disease severity. J Dermatol. 2015;42(6):602-7.
3. Jain N, Doshi B, Khopkar U. Trichoscopy in alopecias: diagnosis simplified. Int J Trichology. 2013;5(4):170-8.
4. Lacarrubba F, Micali G, Tosti A. Scalp dermoscopy or trichoscopy. Curr Probl Dermatol. 2015;47:21-32.
5. Lee WS, Lee HJ. Characteristics of androgenetic alopecia in Asian. Ann Dermatol. 2012;24(3):243-52.
6. Lolli F, Pallotti F, Rossi A, et al. Androgenetic alopecia: a review. Endocrine. 2017;57(1):9-17.
7. Miteva M, Tosti A. Hair and scalp dermatoscopy. J Am Acad Dermatol. 2012;67(5):1040-8.
8. Mubki T, Rudnicka L, Olszewska M, et al. Evaluation and diagnosis of the hair loss patient: part II. Trichoscopic and laboratory evaluations. J Am Acad Dermatol. 2014;71(3):431.e1-431.e11.
9. Rathnayake D, Sinclair R. Male androgenetic alopecia. Expert Opin Pharmacother. 2010;11(8):1295-304.
10. Rudnicka L, Malgorzata O, Rakowska A, et al. Trichoscopy update 2011. J Dermatol Case Rep. 2011;5(4):82-8.
11. Rudnicka L, Rakowska A, Olszewska M. Trichoscopy. How it may help the clinician. Dermatol Clin. 2013;31(1):29-41.
12. Sinclair R, Torkamani N, Jones L. Androgenetic alopecia: new insights into the pathogenesis and mechanism of hair loss. 2015;4:585.
13. Varothai S, Bergfeld WF. Androgenetic alopecia: an evidence-based treatment update. Am J Clin Dermatol. 2014;15(3):217-30.

4.2 Female-Pattern Hair Loss

Giselle Martins, Patricia Damasco, Isabella Doche

FEMALE-PATTERN HAIR LOSS

Female-pattern hair loss (FPHL) is a diffuse nonscarring alopecia affecting women with scalp hair thinning and miniaturization. In fact, around 40% of women by the age of 50 years are affected by FPHL. The exact etiology of FPHL still remains uncertain, although a polygenic inheritance mode with genes inherited from both parents is acceptable. As it is not clear if androgens play a putative role in this kind of hair loss, the term FPHL is preferred instead of "female androgenetic alopecia."

Female-pattern hair loss presents quite differently from male-pattern hair loss (MPHL), which usually begins with a receding frontal hairline that progresses to a bald area over the vertex scalp (Figs. 4.2.1A to C). These signs are very uncommon in woman, unless hyperandrogenism is present. Usually, patients with FPHL present with diffuse hair thinning and decreased hair density (Ludwig Classification). Some patients complain of increased hair shedding, which should be differentiated from telogen effluvium and alopecia areata incognita.

Dermoscopy of the anterior scalp shows the same features as in MPHL. An increased proportion of vellus and fine hairs (hair diameter variability), yellow dots, perifollicular discoloration (peripilar sign), isolated circle and wavy hairs, and follicular units with only one hair shaft are commonly seen (Figs. 4.2.2 and 4.2.3). In long-standing cases, honeycomb pattern, pinpoint white dots, and focal atrichia can be seen (Fig. 4.2.4). It is very important to compare the anterior and posterior scalp hairs, as temporal hairs are normally thinner and shorter.

Recently some trichoscopic criteria were described by Rakowska et al. and have been used to help the early diagnosis of FPHL with 98% of specificity.

MAJOR CRITERIA

1. More than four yellow dots in four images at 70X in the frontal area.
2. Lower average hair thickness in the frontal area in comparison with the occiput (calculated from not less than 50 hairs from each area).
3. More the 10% of thin hairs (below 0.03 mm) in the frontal area.

MINOR CRITERIA

1. A ratio of single-hair unit percentage in the frontal area to the occiput greater than 2:1.
2. A ratio of number of vellus hairs in the frontal area to the occiput greater than 1.5:1.

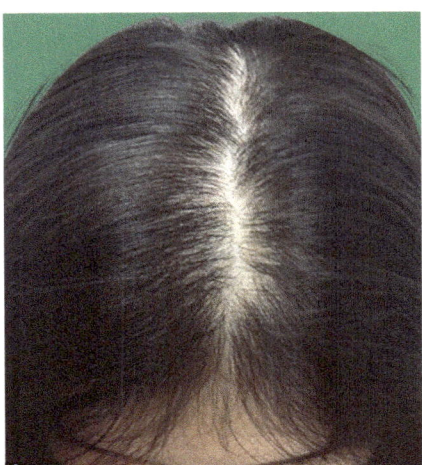 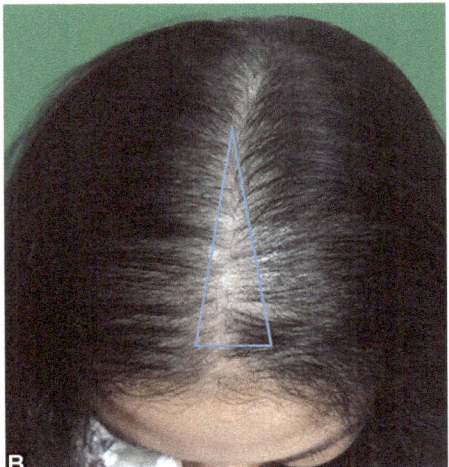 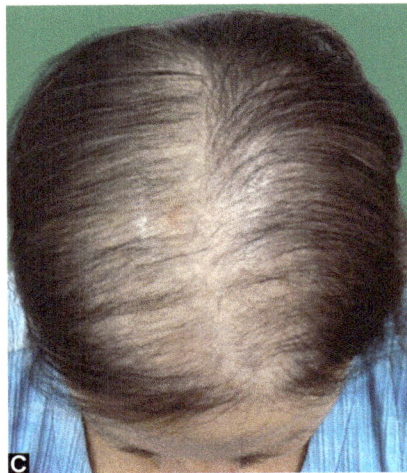

Figs. 4.2.1A to C: Female-pattern hair loss. (A) Mild frontal hair thinning (Ludwig I). (B) Moderate hair thinning, forming the "Christmas-tree pattern" (blue triangle) (Ludwig II). (C) Severe and diffuse hair thinning (Ludwig III). Note focal atrichia with small alopecic areas. After making a central parting, note the maintenance of the frontal hairline despite the severity of the disease.

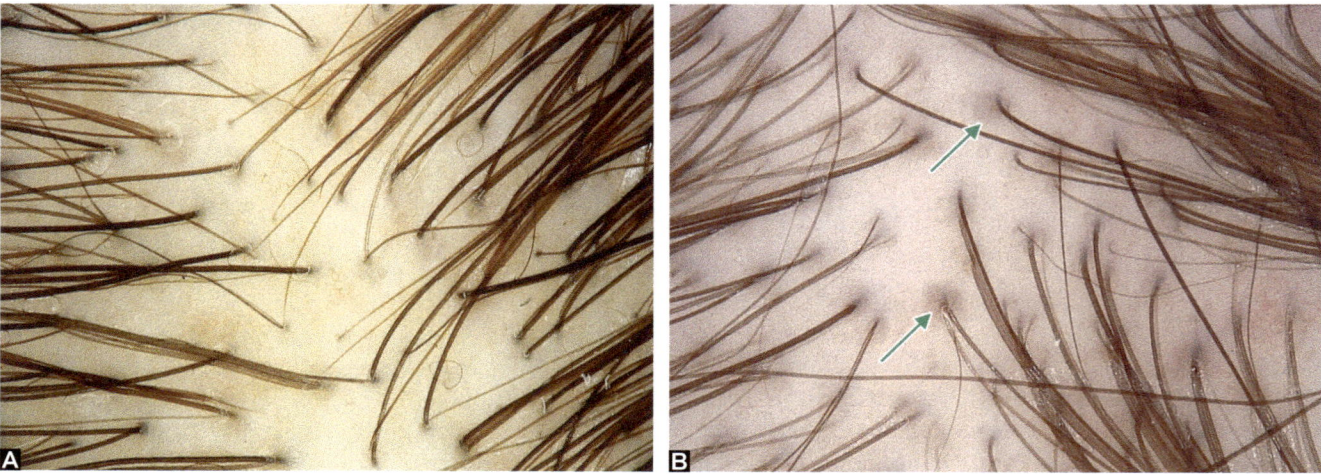

Figs. 4.2.2A and B: Mild female-pattern hair loss. (A). Hair shaft variability (>20%), isolated circle hairs, and single follicular units (hair follicles with one hair shaft) in the frontal scalp area. (B) Peripilar sign (green arrows), a slightly depressed brownish follicular halo can sometimes be seen surrounding some terminal and intermediate hair follicles in early cases. It corresponds to the mild infundibular inflammation and tends to disappear after treatment.

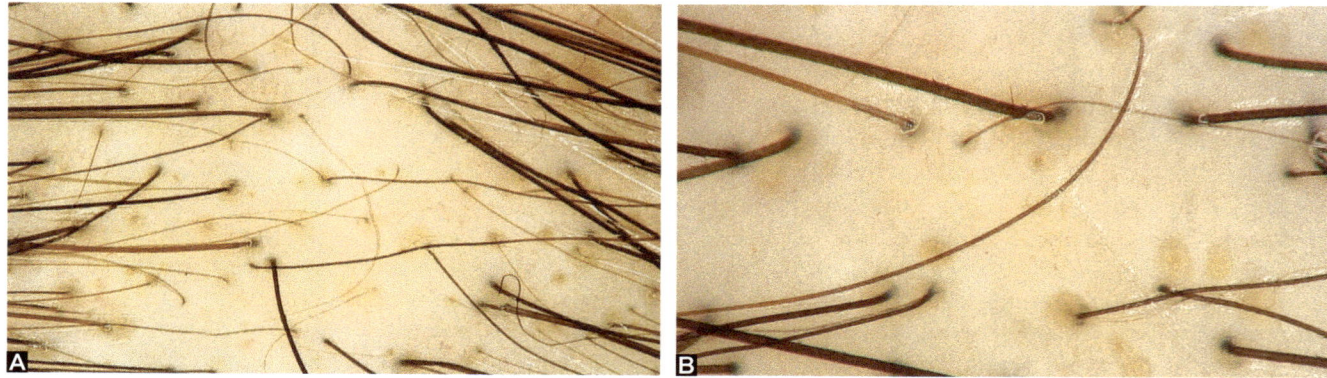

Figs. 4.2.3A and B: Moderate female-pattern hair loss. (A) Decreased hair density, increased hair diameter variability with multiple vellus and fine hairs. (B) Yellow dots irregularly distributed in the scalp and increased hair diameter variability.

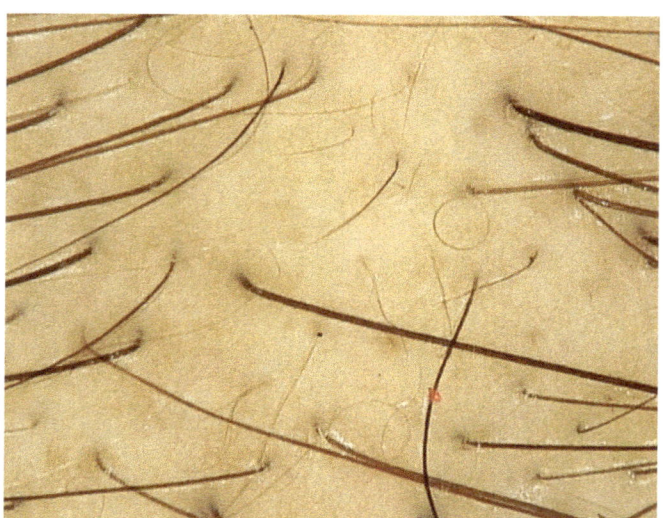

Fig. 4.2.4: Severe female-pattern hair loss. Focal atrichia that corresponds to small alopecic areas with preserved follicular openings, vellus, and short hairs.

3. A ratio of hair follicles with perifollicular discoloration in the frontal area to occiput greater than 3:1.

Fulfillment of two major criteria or one major and two minor criteria is required to diagnose FPHL based on trichoscopy.

Female-pattern hair loss (FPHL) should be differentiated from senescent or senile alopecia, which normally occurs in patients over 60 years of age. Irregular areas of central hair loss, perifollicular scale, and perifollicular erythema may suggest fibrosing alopecia in a pattern distribution, a scarring process.

As MPHL, FPHL has no cure and it is very important to manage expectations when starting treatment, as the main aim is to stop or slow hair thinning, and not promoting hair regrowth. Anti-androgens drugs (e.g. spironolactone, cyproterone, finasteride) associated with topical minoxidil (2% solution or 5% foam) can be used with variable results.

Take-Home Message

- Dermoscopy of frontal and vertex scalp areas shows increased hair shaft diameter variability (>20%), yellow dots, vellus hairs, short regrowing hairs, isolated and few circle or wavy hairs.
- Peripilar sign, single follicular units, and vellus hairs in the frontal scalp indicate early androgenetic alopecia.
- Long-standing disease shows honeycomb pattern, pinpoint white dots, and areas with focal atrichia.
- Main differential diagnosis includes senescent or senile alopecia, alopecia areata incognita, telogen effluvium, and fibrosing alopecia in a pattern distribution.

SUGGESTED READING

1. Asz-Sigall D, González-de-Cossio-Hernández AC, Rodríguez-Lobato E, et al. Differential diagnosis of female pattern hair loss. Skin Appendage Disord. 2016;2(1-2):18-21.
2. Blume-Peytavi U, Hillmann K, Dietz E, et al. A randomized, single-blind trial of 5% minoxidil foam once daily versus 2% minoxidil solution twice daily in the treatment of androgenetic alopecia in women. J Am Acad Dermatol. 2011;65(6):1126-34.
3. De Lacharrière O, Deloche C, Misciali C, et al. Hair diameter diversity: a clinical sign reflecting the follicle miniaturization. Arch Dermatol. 2001;137(5):641-6.
4. Gupta AK, Charrette A. Topical minoxidil: systematic review and meta-analysis of its efficacy in androgenetic alopecia. Skin Med. 2015;13(3):185-9.
5. Herskovitz I, de Sousa IC, Tosti A. Vellus hair in the frontal scalp in early female pattern alopecia. Int J Trichol. 2013;5(3):118-20.
6. Lee WS, Lee HJ. Characteristics of androgenetic alopecia in Asian. Ann Dermatol. 2012;24(3):243-52.
7. Martínez-Velasco MA, Vázquez-Herrera NE, Maddy AJ, et al. The hair shedding visual scale: a quick tool to assess hair loss in women. Dermatol Ther (Heidelb). 2017;7(1):155-65.
8. McCoy J, Goren A, Kovacevic M, et al. Minoxidil dose response study in female pattern hair loss patients determined to be non-responders to 5% topical minoxidil. J Biol Regul Homeost Agents. 2016;30(4):1153-5.
9. Mubki T, Rudnicka L, Olszewska M, et al. Evaluation and diagnosis of the hair loss patient: part II. Trichoscopic and laboratory evaluations. J Am Acad Dermatol. 2014;71(3):431.e1-431.e11.
10. Rakowska A, Slowinska M, Kowalska-Oledzka E, et al. Dermoscopy in female androgenetic alopecia: method standardization and diagnostic criteria. Int J Trichol. 2009;1(2):123-30.
11. Redler S, Messenger AG, Betz RC. Genetics and other factors in aetiology of female pattern hair loss. Exp Dermatol. 2017;26(6):510-7.
12. van Zuuren EJ, Fedorowicz Z. Interventions for female pattern hair loss. JAMA Dermatol. 2017;153(3):329-30.

4.3 Senescent or Senile Alopecia

Isabella Doche

SENILE ALOPECIA

Senescent or senile alopecia (SA) is the diffuse and permanent scalp hair thinning in patients over 60 years with no family history of androgenetic alopecia (AGA). Patients present with diffuse scalp thinning and decreased hair volume (Fig. 4.3.1). Dermoscopy shows diffuse decreased hair thinning and density, and multiple hair shafts with one follicle, mostly on the top of the scalp. Hair diameter variability and yellow dots are usually absent (Fig. 4.3.2).

Although SA and AGA may coexist in the same patient, the concept of whether SA and AGA are distinct disorders remains controversial.

Microarray comparison of age-matched subjects with AGA, SA, and normal controls without hair loss has shown differences in gene expression profiles, suggesting that AGA and SA may represent two independent hair disorders and that nonandrogen pathways may also contribute to hair loss. AGA genes related to follicle homeostasis and hair cycling were underexpressed compared to SA genes. Also, the androgen receptor is upregulated in AGA, but not in SA. In contrast, SA revealed changes in genes important to apoptosis processes.

These genetic differences can have significant implications in terms of treatment of hair loss at different ages. Topical treatments, such as minoxidil and laser devices can benefit patients with senescent or age-related thinning, although beneficial results with finasteride remain ascertained.

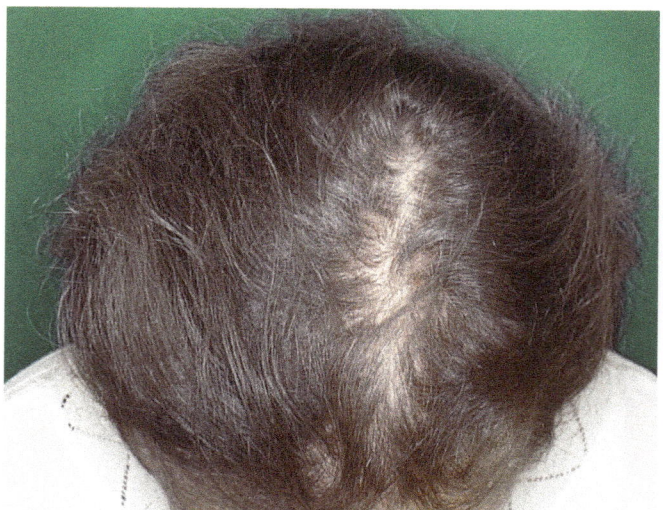

Fig. 4.3.1: Senescent alopecia. Diffuse hair thinning in a 68-year-old female patient.

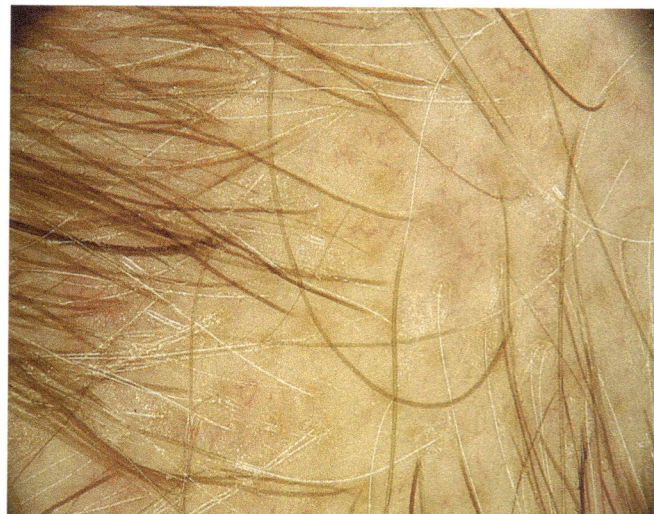

Fig. 4.3.2: Senescent alopecia. Decreased hair density and multiple single hair units (follicular units with only one hair shaft) on the vertex area of the scalp. Note the lack of hair diameter variability, no thin or vellus hairs, and no yellow dots.

> **Take-Home Message**
> - Senile alopecia is the diffuse hair thinning in people older than 60 years and no family history of androgenetic alopecia.
> - AGA and SA can coexist in the same patient.
> - Although SA and AGA show different gene profile expression, there is no consensus on whether SA is in the spectrum of AGA.
> - Dermoscopy shows diffuse decreased hair thinning and density that can be more pronounced on the vertex area.
> - Absent or mild hair miniaturization and variability with a few vellus hairs can be often present.

SUGGESTED READING

1. Chen W, Yang CC, Todorova A, et al. Hair loss in elderly women. Eur J Dermatol. 2010;20(2):145-51.
2. Karnik P, Shah S, Dvorkin-Wininger Y, et al. Microarray analysis of androgenetic and senescent alopecia: comparison of gene expression shows two distinct profiles. J Dermatol Sci. 2013;72(2):183-6.
3. Mirmirani P. Age-related hair changes in men: mechanisms and management of alopecia and graying. Maturitas. 2015;80(1):58-62.
4. Torres F. Androgenetic, diffuse and senescent alopecia in men: practical evaluation and management. Curr Probl Dermatol. 2015;47:33-44.
5. Trueb RM. Aging of hair. J Cosmet Dermatol. 2005;4(2):60-72.
6. Van Neste D, Tobin DJ. Hair cycle and hair pigmentation: dynamic interactions and changes associated with aging. Micron. 2004;35(3):193-200.
7. Whiting DA. How real is senescent alopecia? A histopathologic approach. Clin Dermatol. 2011;29(1):49-53.

4.4 Telogen Effluvium

Patricia Damasco, Giselle Martins, Isabella Doche

TELOGEN EFFLUVIUM

Telogen effluvium (TE) is a nonscarring and diffuse hair loss. Acute TE occurs usually 3 months after a triggering event and is self-limiting, lasting about 6 months. Many potential triggers have been implicated in the pathogenesis of TE, including starting and stopping sex hormone therapy, parturition, major illness, surgery, rapid weight loss or poor nutrition, thyroid dysfunction, high fever, hemorrhage, and acute psychosocial stressors. In acute cases, there is severe hair shedding with variable decrease in hair density. Hair pull test is usually positive with more than 6 telogen hairs.

Chronic telogen effluvium (CTE) is an idiopathic condition, presenting with diffuse scalp hair loss and a fluctuating course that persists for more than 6 months, without any widening of the central part of the scalp or follicular miniaturization (Figs. 4.4.1 and 4.4.4). Although some cases of CTE may follow TE with a known trigger, in most cases, a specific trigger cannot be identified. It typically affects middle-aged women presenting with insidious onset and alternating periods of spontaneous remissions and relapses that can last for several years. Chronic hair loss may produce diffuse thinning of scalp hairs, decreased hair volume, and bitemporal recession (Fig. 4.4.1B). Some patients may refer a painful or burning sensation in the scalp (trichodynia). Shorter and regrowing frontal hairs may be seen in patients with resolving effluvium (Fig. 4.4.1C). Hair pull test is usually negative.

Dermoscopy is usually inespecific. However, some short and upright regrowing hairs may be found (Fig. 4.4.2). Hair shaft variability can be seen in patients with associated androgenetic alopecia (Fig. 4.4.3). Club hairs, a hair in the final stage of a telogen phase, can be rarely found (Fig. 4.4.5). Trigger causes should be identified and treated specifically. However, in many cases a causal factor cannot be identified.

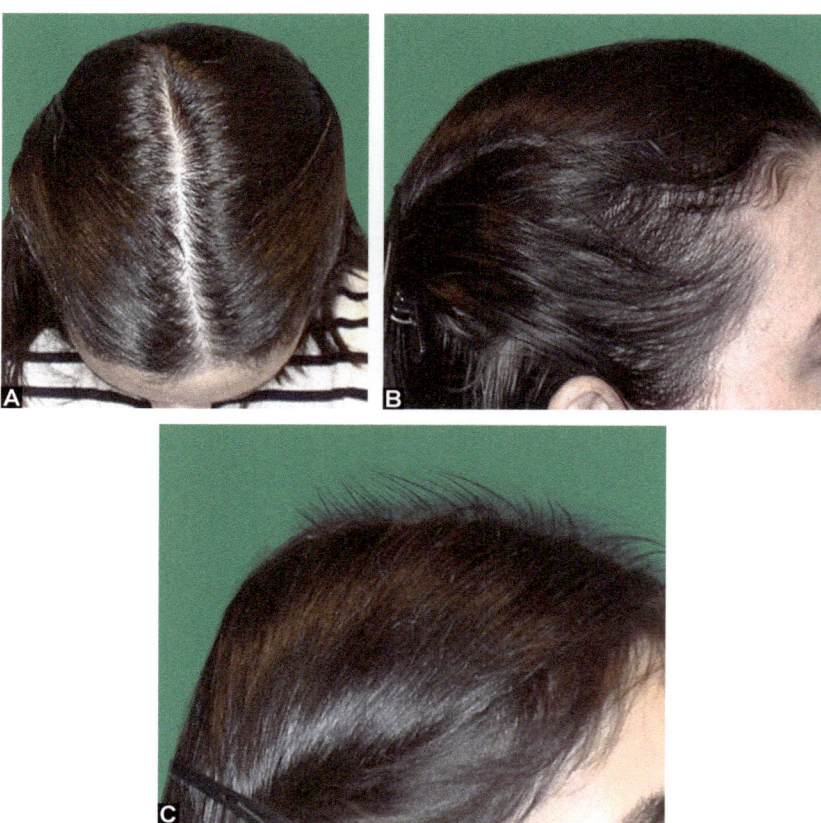

Figs. 4.4.1A to C: Chronic telogen effluvium. (A) No evident hair thinning. (B) Note the temporal recession. (C) Hair regrowth after treatment.

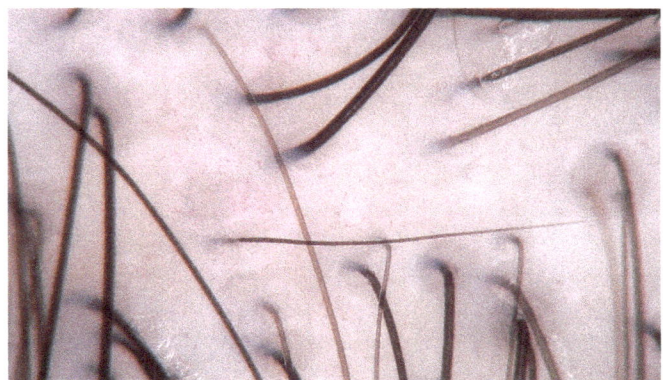

Fig. 4.4.2: Acute telogen effluvium. Note a short or upright regrowing hair of normal thickness.

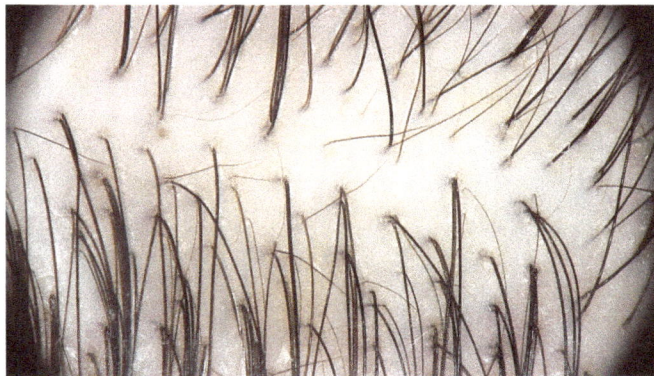

Fig. 4.4.3: Acute telogen effluvium. Multiple short and upright regrowing hairs of normal thickness, vellus hairs, yellow dots, and hair shaft variability in a patient with associated mild androgenetic alopecia.

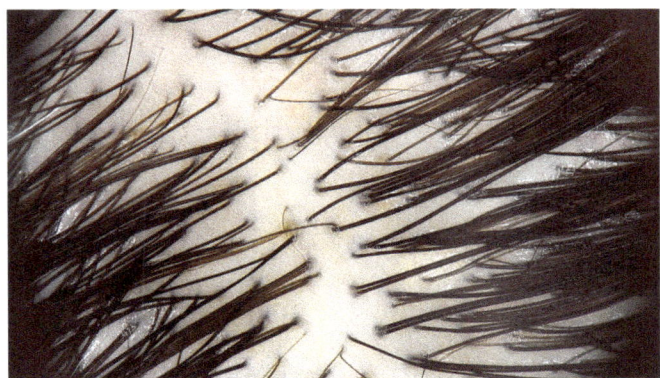

Fig. 4.4.4: Chronic telogen effluvium. Note the absence of hair shaft variability.

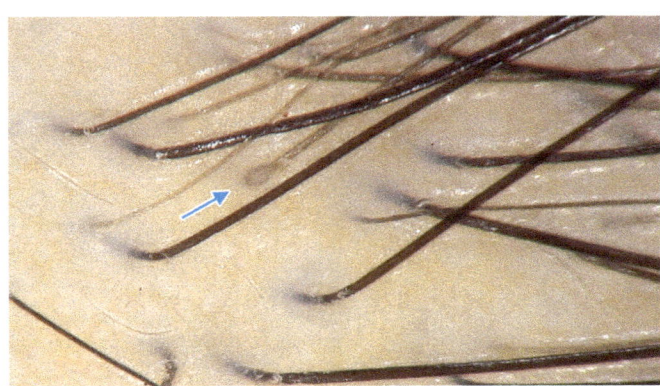

Fig. 4.4.5: Telogen effluvium. Club hairs (blue arrow) can be rarely found in telogen effluvium. They are the final product of a hair in the telogen stage.

Take-Home Message

- Telogen effluvium is a diffuse and nonscarring hair loss.
- Acute telogen effluvium usually occurs 3 months after a triggering event, lasting up to 6 months. Severe shedding and variable decrease in hair density are present.
- In chronic telogen effluvium, diffuse shedding has a fluctuating course and lasts more than 6 months. Bitemporal recession, decreased hair volume and variable hair shedding can be noted.
- Trichoscopy is not specific. Short regrowing hairs may be seen in acute and chronic cases.

SUGGESTED READING

1. Grover C, Khurana A. Telogen effluvium. Indian J Dermatol Venereol Leprol. 2013;79(5):591-603.
2. Malkud S. Telogen effluvium: a review. J Clin Diagn Res. 2015;9(9):WE01-3.
3. McDonald KA, Shelley AJ, Colantonio S, et al. Hair pull test: evidence-based update and revision of guidelines. J Am Acad Dermatol. 2017;76(3):472-7.
4. Miteva M, Tosti A. Hair and scalp dermatoscopy. J Am Acad Dermatol. 2012;67(5):1040-8.
5. Ross EK, Shapiro J. Management of hair loss. Dermatol Clin. 2005;23(2):227-43.
6. Rudnicka L, Olszewska M, Rakowska A, et al. Trichoscopy update 2011. J Dermatol Case Rep. 2011;5(4):82-8.
7. Sinclair R. Chronic telogen effluvium: a study of 5 patients over 7 years. J Am Acad Dermatol. 2005;52(2 Suppl 1):12-6.
8. Torres F, Tosti A. Female pattern alopecia and telogen effluvium: figuring out diffuse alopecia. Semin Cutan Med Surg. 2015;34(2):67-71.
9. Trüeb R. Difuse hair loss. In: Blume-Peytavi U, Tosti A, Whiting D, Trueb R, (Eds). Hair growth and disorders. Leipzig: Springer; 2008. pp. 259-72.
10. Trüeb RM. Telogen effluvium: Is there a need for a new classification? Skin Appendage Disord. 2016;2(1-2):39-44.

4.5 Alopecia Areata

Isabella Doche, Maria K Hordinsky

ALOPECIA AREATA

Alopecia areata (AA) is a chronic, immune-mediated nonscarring alopecia that attacks anagen hair follicles. The disease affects around 2% of the population, both male and female patients at all ages. Clinically, it may appear as round or oval unique or multiple patches, diffuse scalp hair loss (alopecia totalis), diffuse scalp and body hair loss (alopecia universalis), or ophiasis pattern (alopecia in the lower occipital scalp and the region above the ears) (Figs. 4.5.1A to D). Patchy lesions may mimic tinea capitis, traction alopecia, loose anagen syndrome, aplasia cutis congenita, and pseudopelade (Fig. 4.5.1E). Other causes of acute alopecia may be ruled out in diffuse and extensive cases. Hair-regrowing lesions may show hypopigmented hair shafts (Fig. 4.5.1F).

When the AA is active, pull test is usually positive with dystrophic hairs. Partial or total eyebrow alopecia and nail abnormalities may occur, and nail pittings are the most reported feature.

Dermoscopy of active lesions shows exclamation mark hairs, broken hairs, vellus hairs, yellow dots, and black dots (Figs. 4.5.2 to 4.5.4) Caudability hairs, which is a long exclamation mark hair, are usually seen in the border of enlarging patches (Fig. 4.5.4B). Pseudomonilethrix/monilethrix-like hairs with irregular Pohl–Pinkus

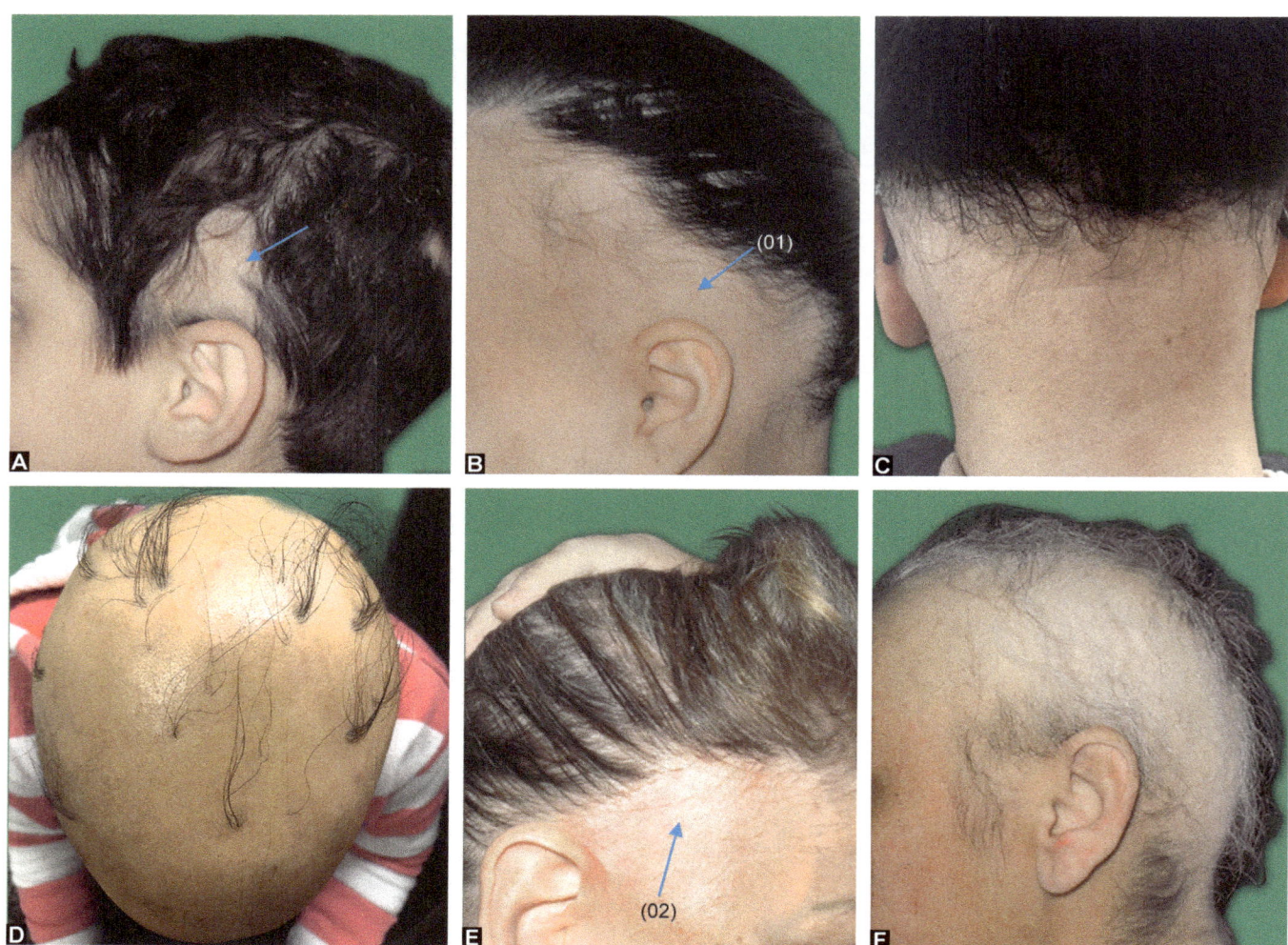

Figs. 4.5.1A to F: Alopecia areata. (A) Unique alopecic patch. (B and C) Ophiasis pattern. (D) Alopecia totalis with areas of hair regrowth. (E) Long-standing patch mimicking a scarring process. (F) Diffuse alopecia presenting hair regrowth and hypopigmented hair shafts.
Source: (A, B, E, F) Division of Dermatology, Hospital das Clínicas, University of São Paulo Medical School. (D) Dr Giselle Martins.

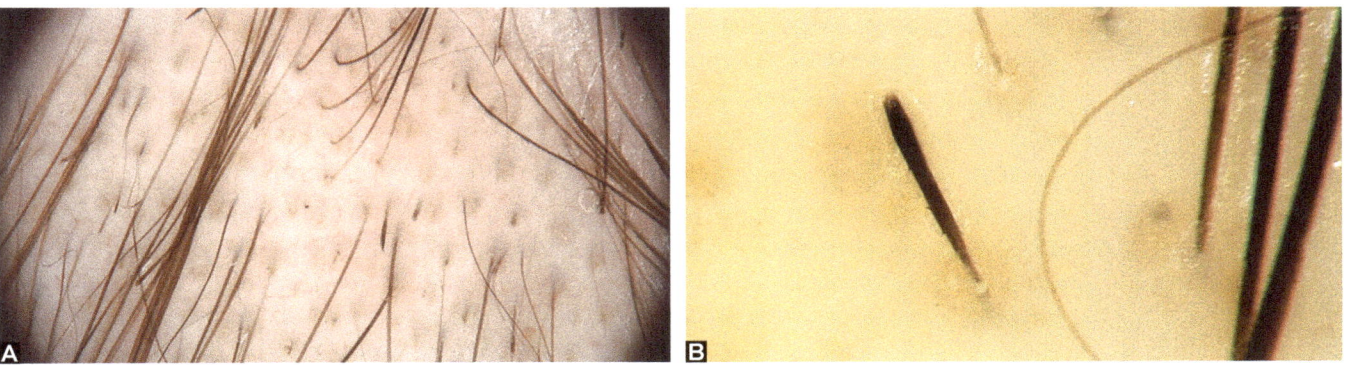

Figs. 4.5.2A and B: Alopecia areata. (A) Note multiple yellow dots, some empty and some containing broken hairs, black dots, and dystrophic hairs. (B) Exclamation mark hair contains a dark, frayed, and pigmented tip.

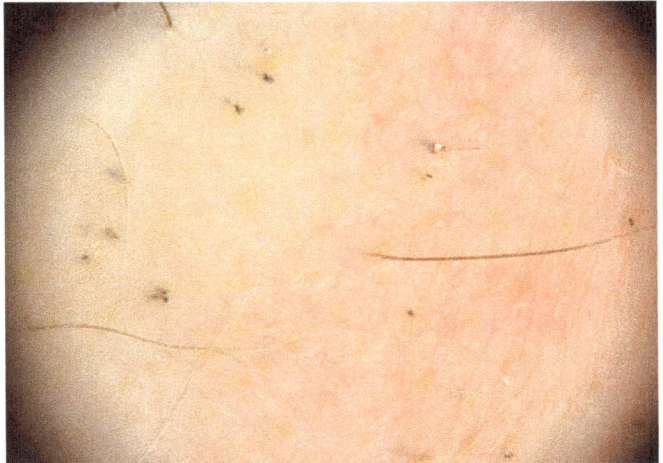

Fig. 4.5.3: Alopecia areata. Note multiple black dots and yellow dots. Although a few black dots can occur in active scarring alopecias, the presence of yellow dots and follicular openings helped the diagnosis of alopecia areata.
Source: Division of Dermatology, Hospital das Clínicas, University of São Paulo Medical School.

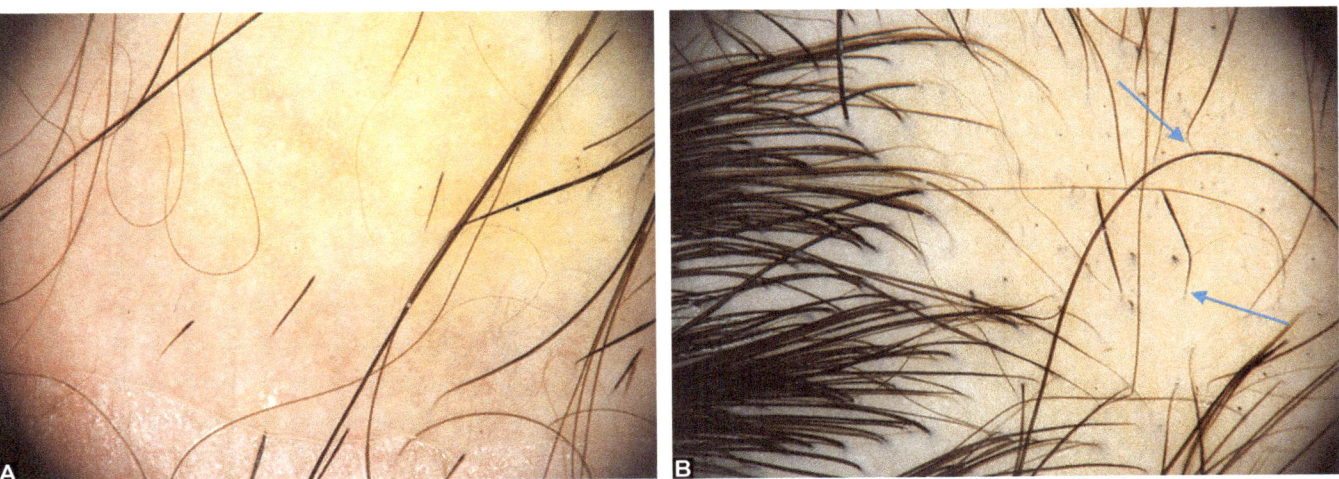

Figs. 4.5.4A and B: Alopecia areata. (A) Exclamation mark hairs, and vellus hairs. (B) Broken hairs, black dots and caudability hairs (blue arrows) in the border of an active patch. In children, yellow dots are hardly seen as follicular openings have the same color as the scalp.
Source: Division of Dermatology, Hospital das Clínicas, University of São Paulo Medical School.

constrictions along the hair shafts can be seen in a few hair shafts (Fig. 4.5.5). Short regrowing coiled hairs and flame hairs can be present in acute and chronic lesions (Figs. 4.5.6A and B). "Broom hair-like structures" may occur in multiple disorders and is not specific to alopecia areata (Fig. 4.5.7). In dark-skinned patients, pinpoint white dots can be empty or contain broken hairs, black dots, or dystrophic hairs. Chronic lesions show multiple yellow dots, vellus hairs, and the absence of dystrophic hairs (Fig. 4.5.8). Anthralin use should not be mistaken as black dots, which is a sign of active disease (Fig. 4.5.9). The presence of hypopigmented shafts indicates hair regrowth (Fig. 4.5.10).

There is no FDA-approved drug for the treatment of AA. Therapy strategy should be based on the disease extent, disease duration, previous treatment, history of atopy, and age of the patient. The most common treatment options include intralesional, topical, or oral steroids, topical minoxidil, and anthralin. Topical sensitizers, light therapy, biologicals, and methotrexate can be also tried alone or in combination therapies with variable results.

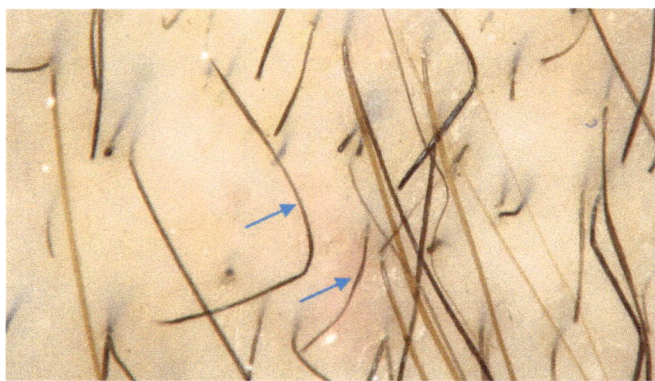

Fig. 4.5.5: Alopecia areata. Pseudomonilethrix/monilethrix-like hairs with irregular Pohl–Pinkus constrictions along the hair shaft (blue arrows). Note multiple broken hairs.
Source: Division of Dermatology, Hospital das Clínicas, University of São Paulo Medical School.

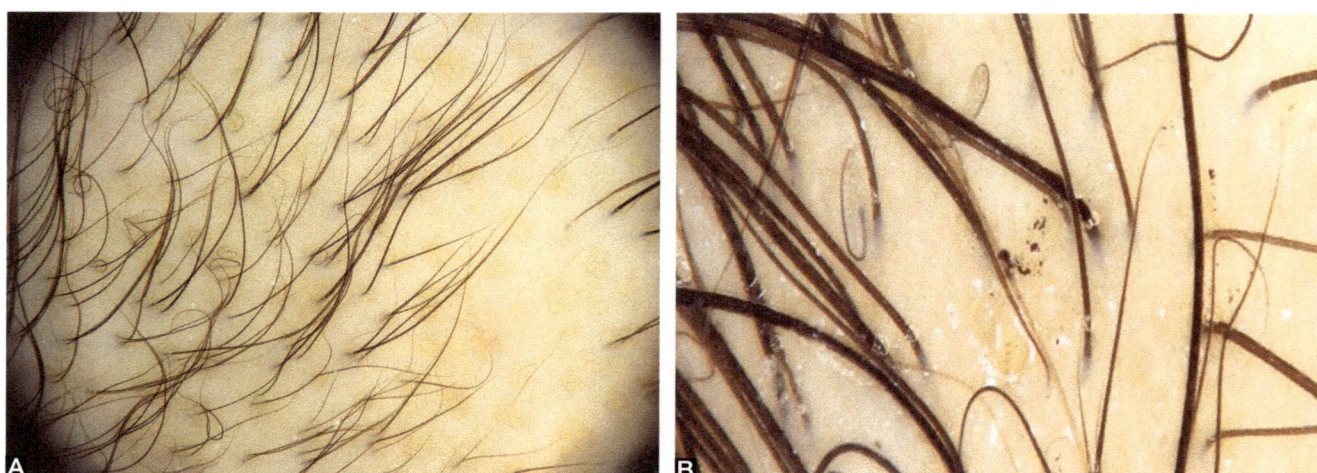

Fig. 4.5.6A and B: Alopecia areata. (A) Multiple circle or coiled hairs (pigtail hairs), vellus hairs, thinned hairs, and yellow dots. Short miniaturized hairs and coiled hairs can be seen in acute and chronic cases of alopecia areata. Although circular hairs are also seen in androgenetic alopecia, the presence of multiple circle hairs is highly indicative of alopecia areata. Sometimes they can be the unique finding of the disease. (B) Note a flame hair with wavy-hair residues.
Source: Division of Dermatology, Hospital das Clínicas, University of São Paulo Medical School.

Nonscarring Alopecias

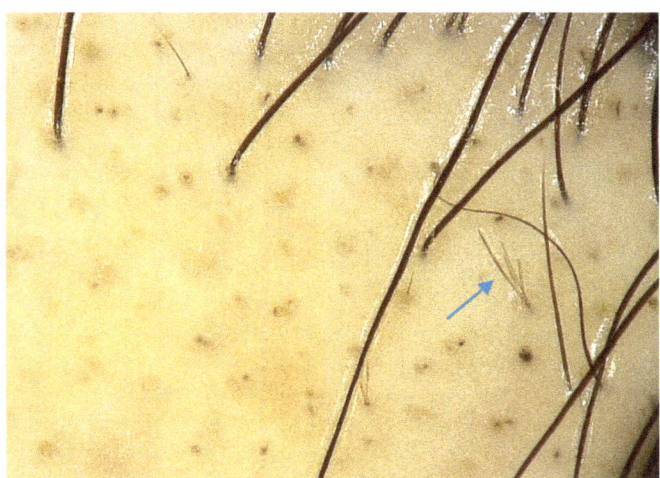

Fig. 4.5.7: Alopecia areata. "Broom hairs" (blue arrow) can sometimes be present in different entities, such as alopecia areata and trichotillomania.

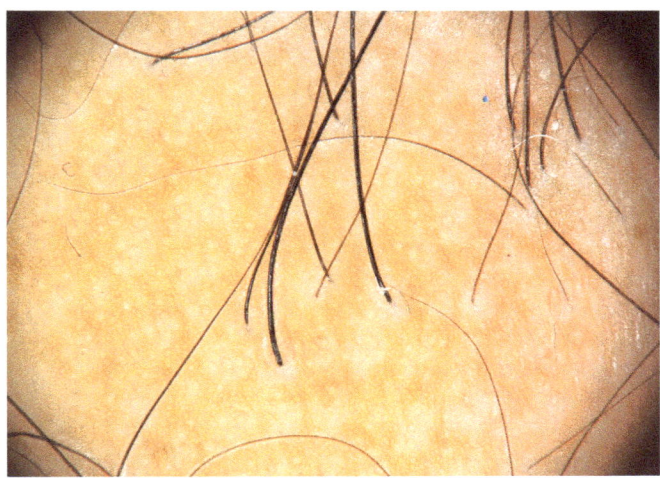

Fig. 4.5.8: Alopecia areata. Empty pinpoint white dots can be seen in dark-skinned patient with long-standing disease. Note the absence of broken hairs, dystrophic hair, and black dots.
Source: Division of Dermatology, Hospital das Clínicas, University of São Paulo Medical School.

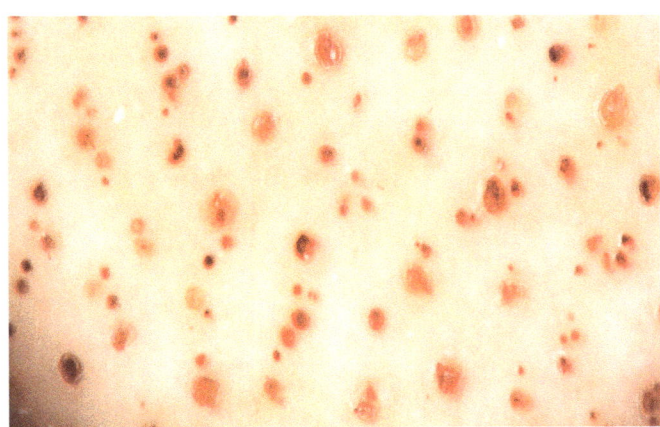

Fig. 4.5.9: Anthralin use in a patient with alopecia areata. In low magnifications, it may mimic black dots. In high magnifications, perifollicular hyperpigmented halos present as bigger structures that are diffusely and regularly distributed all over the scalp.
Source: Division of Dermatology, Hospital das Clínicas, University of São Paulo Medical School.

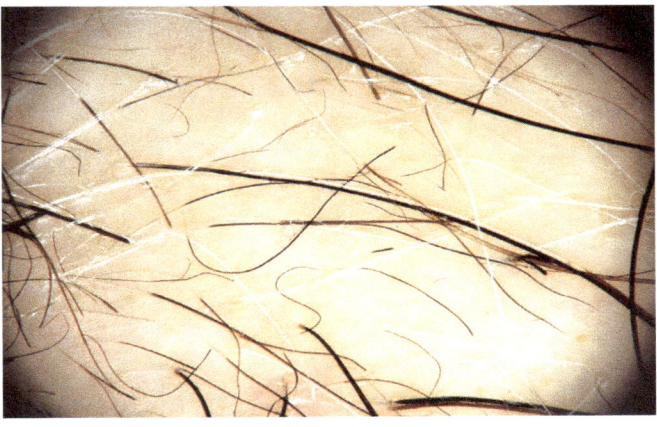

Fig. 4.5.10: Alopecia areata. Hypopigmented shafts are a sign of hair regrowth. A few broken hairs and dystrophic hairs can still be seen in this recovering stage of the disease.
Source: Division of Dermatology, Hospital das Clínicas, University of São Paulo Medical School.

Take-Home Message

- Alopecia areata is a nonscarring hair loss.
- Variable presentations with unique or multiple patches, diffuse scalp alopecia (alopecia totalis), total scalp and body alopecia (alopecia universalis) or ophiasis pattern.
- Eyebrow alopecia and nail abnormalities may occur.
- Dermoscopy of active lesions shows exclamation mark hairs, dystrophic hairs, black dots, broken hairs, yellow dots, caudability hairs, and vellus hairs.
- Coiled hairs, flame hairs, pseudomonilethrix, and broom hairs may be present.
- Dermoscopy is an important tool to assess disease activity and treatment efficacy.

SUGGESTED READING

1. Amer M, Helmy A, Amer A. Trichoscopy as a useful method to differentiate tinea capitis from alopecia areata in children at Zagazig University Hospitals. Int J Dermatol. 2017;56(1):116-20.
2. Bapu NG, Chandrashekar L, Munisamy M, et al. Dermoscopic findings of alopecia areata in dark skinned individuals: an analysis of 116 cases. Int J Trichology. 2014;6(4):156-9.
3. de Moura LH, Duque-Estrada B, Abraham LS, et al. Dermoscopy findings of alopecia areata in an African-American patient. J Dermatol Case Rep. 2008;2(4):52-4.
4. Inui S, Nakajima T, Itami S. Significance of dermoscopy in acute diffuse and total alopecia of the female scalp: review of twenty cases. Dermatology. 2008;217(4):333-6.

5. Inui S, Nakajima T, Itami S. Coudability hairs: a revisited sign of alopecia areata assessed by trichoscopy. Clin Exp Dermatol. 2010;35(4):361-5.
6. Inui S, Nakajima T, Nakagawa K, et al. Clinical significance of dermoscopy in alopecia areata: analysis of 300 cases. Int J Dermatol. 2008;47(7):688-93.
7. Johnson CM, Miteva M. Alopecia areata on vertex as a potential pitfall for misdiagnosis of central centrifugal cicatricial alopecia in african-american women. Int J Trichology. 2017;9(2):73-5.
8. Khunkhet S, Vachiramon V, Suchonwanit P. Trichoscopic clues for diagnosis of alopecia areata and trichotillomania in Asians. Int J Dermatol. 2017;56(2):161-5.
9. Lencastre A, Tosti A. Role of trichoscopy in children's scalp and hair disorders. Pediatr Dermatol. 2013:30(6): 674-82.
10. Park J, Kim JI, Kim HU, et al. Trichoscopy findings of hair loss in koreans. Ann Dermatol. 2015;27(5):539-50.
11. Pratt CH, King LE Jr, Messenger AG, et al. Alopecia areata. Nat Ver Dis Primers. 2017;3:17011.
12. Rudnicka L, Rakowska A, Kerzeja M, et al. Hair shafts in trichoscopy: clues for diagnosis of hair and scalp diseases. Dermatol Clin. 2013;31(4):695-708.

4.6 Alopecia Areata Incognito

Emilie Jane Fowler, Antonella Tosti

ALOPECIA AREATA INCOGNITO

Alopecia areata incognito (AAI) is a disorder characterized by diffuse hair loss of the scalp with an acute onset, occurring just over the course of a few weeks to months. It is most commonly seen in females, and is more common in the age range of 20–40 years. Differential diagnoses include telogen effluvium and androgenetic alopecia, which can be differentiated based on clinical history, dermatoscopic findings, and histological findings.

On clinical examination, patients with AAI present with diffuse hair thinning (Fig. 4.6.1). The typical patches of hair loss seen in classic alopecia areata are not present, and the patient's history is negative for known factors causing telogen effluvium. Examination of the skin and nails is normal, with no complaints of pain or burning sensation in the scalp. Pull test is positive in all patients, and microscopic examination of these hairs shows telogen roots in various stages of maturation, with a high predominance in early stages.

Dermoscopic examination shows polycyclic yellow dots that vary in size, located diffusely throughout the scalp (Figs. 4.6.2 to 4.6.3). Pathological data indicate that these yellow dots correspond to the dilated ostia of the nanogen and miniaturized hair follicles that contain keratin debris and sebum. Dermoscopy also reveals large numbers of regrowing, tapered terminal hairs diffusely spread throughout the scalp. Exclamation mark hairs, cadaverized hairs, and dystrophic hairs are usually not present. Although suggestive, dermoscopy is not diagnostic and it is always necessary to perform a scalp biopsy to confirm the diagnosis. AAI is usually treated with topical or systemic steroids, showing a good response in most cases.

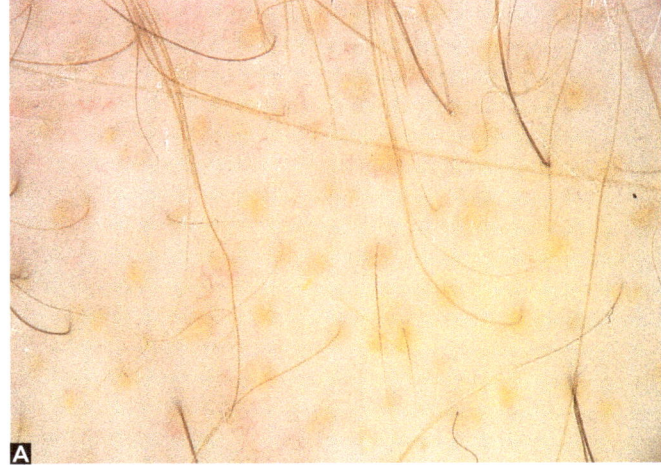
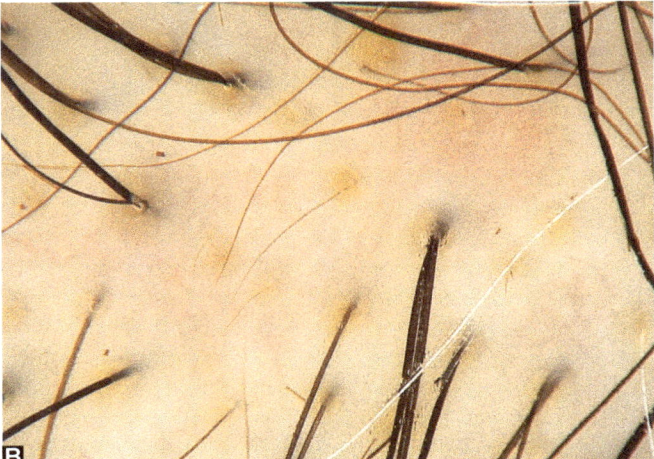

Fig. 4.6.2A and B: Alopecia areata incognito. Yellow dots and short regrowing hairs.

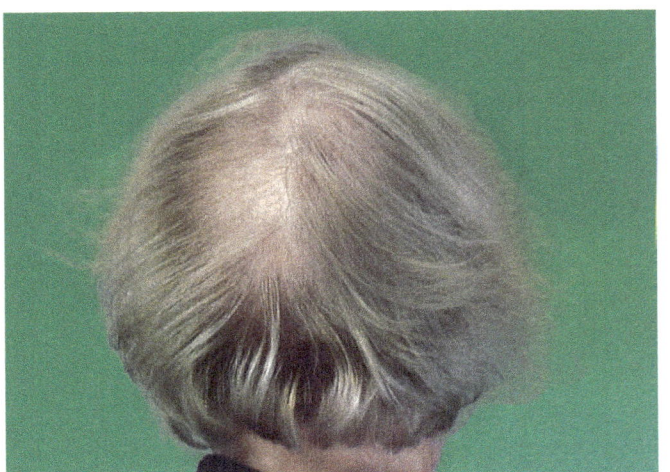

Fig. 4.6.1: Alopecia areata incognito. Diffuse hair thinning.

> **Take-Home Message**
> - Alopecia areata incognito is characterized by diffuse hair thinning.
> - On clinical examination, pull test is positive, and skin and nails appear normal.
> - Polycyclic yellow dots and tapered, short, regrowing terminal hairs are a consistent finding on dermoscopic examination.

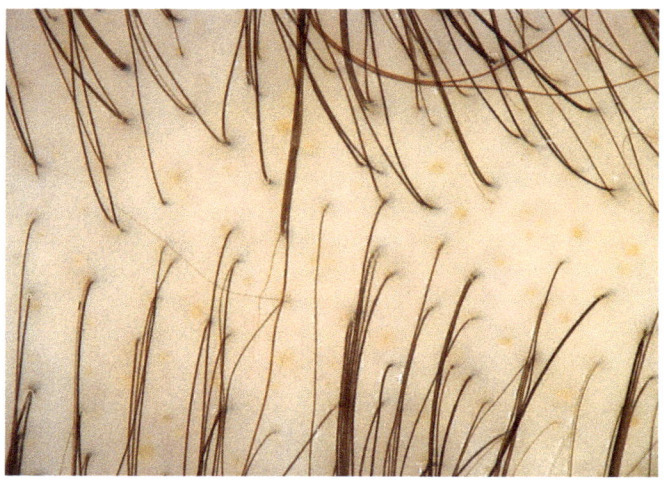

Fig. 4.6.3: Alopecia areata incognito. Note multiple yellow dots.

SUGGESTED READING

1. Asz-Sigall D, González-de-Cossio-Hernández AC, Rodríguez-Lobato E, et al. Differential diagnosis of female-pattern hair loss. Skin Appendage Disord. 2016;2(1-2):18-21.
2. Miteva M, Misciali C, Fanti PA, et al. Histopathologic features of alopecia areata incognito: a review of 46 cases. J Cutan Pathol. 2012;39(6):596-602.
3. Moftah NH, El-Barbary RA, Rashed L, et al. ULBP3: a marker for alopecia areata incognita. Arch Dermatol Res. 2016; 308(6):415-21.
4. Piraccini BM, Alessandrini A. Diffuse hair loss in a young female. Hair Ther Transplant. 2014;4(2):122.
5. Rebora A. Alopecia areata incognita. J Am Acad Dermatol. 2011;65(6):1228.
6. Tosti A, Whiting D, Iorizzo M, et al. The role of scalp dermoscopy in the diagnosis of alopecia areata incognita. J Am Acad Dermatol. 2008;59(1):64-7.

4.7 Trichotillomania

Lidia Rudnicka

TRICHOTILLOMANIA

Trichotillomania (hair pulling disorder) is a disease in which the patients are compulsively pulling hair. Usually scalp hairs, eyelashes or eyebrows are affected. Hair pulling may result in hairless patches or (less commonly) diffuse hair loss. Some data indicate that up to 4% of the population may experience trichotillomania in their lifetime. It usually begins in late childhood/early puberty. In childhood, it occurs about equally in boys and girls. By adulthood, 80–90% of reported cases are women.

From a psychiatric point of view trichotillomania is a complex syndrome, which includes: (1) recurrent pulling out of one's own hair, resulting in noticeable hair loss; (2) an increasing sense of tension immediately before pulling out the hair or when attempting to resist the behavior, (3) pleasure, gratification, or relief when pulling out the hair, (4) hair pulling that cannot be better accounted for by another mental disorder, and (5) significant distress or impairment in social, occupational, or other important areas of functioning.

This definition describes a mental disorder and is not consistent with the experience of dermatologists. From a dermatologist's point of view, trichotillomania is (episodic) self-induced hair loss due to the repetitive pulling of one's own hair. Most patients fulfill no other Diagnostic and Statistical Manual of Mental Disorders-Fourth Edition (DSM-IV) criteria. A similar clinical and trichoscopic manifestation will be associated with hair rubbing (trichoteiromania) or scratching (e.g. in scalp dysesthesia).

Clinically, patients present with patches of irregular-length hair or hairless areas. Commonly, the vertex is affected. Hair loss in this area creates the characteristic "tonsure trichotillomania," called also the "Friar Tuck sign" (Fig. 4.7.1). Another common location is the temporoparietal area from the side of the dominating hand. Patients may pull hair at multiple sites, including the eyebrows, eyelashes, face, arms, legs, and pubic area.

Pull test is negative. Histopathology may be helpful in doubtful cases.

Trichoscopy of trichotillomania is characterized by a chaotic pattern of diverse features related to hair fracturing. The most common feature is the presence of hairs broken at different lengths (Fig. 4.7.2). Short hairs with trichoptilosis ("split ends") and black dots are common. Irregular coiled hairs and flame hairs are most specific but least prevalent (Fig. 4.7.3).

A relatively specific feature of trichotillomania is the V-sign. It develops when two hairs in one follicular unit are being pulled at the same time in the same direction and break at a similar height. "Hair powder" (amorphous hair residues) is a residue of dark hair particles which remain after a hair has been destroyed. These particles are usually

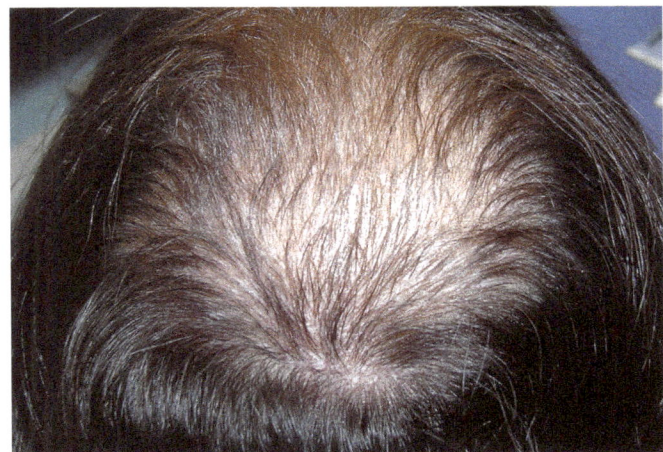

Fig. 4.7.1: Trichotillomania. Typical clinical appearance.

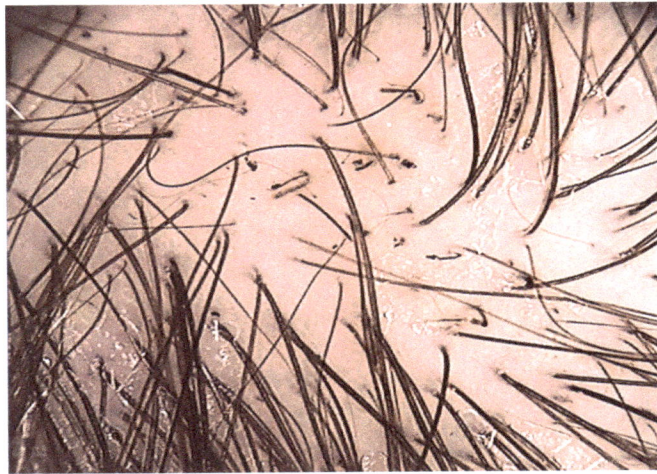

Fig. 4.7.2: Trichotillomania. Trichoscopy shows multiple hairs broken at different lengths.

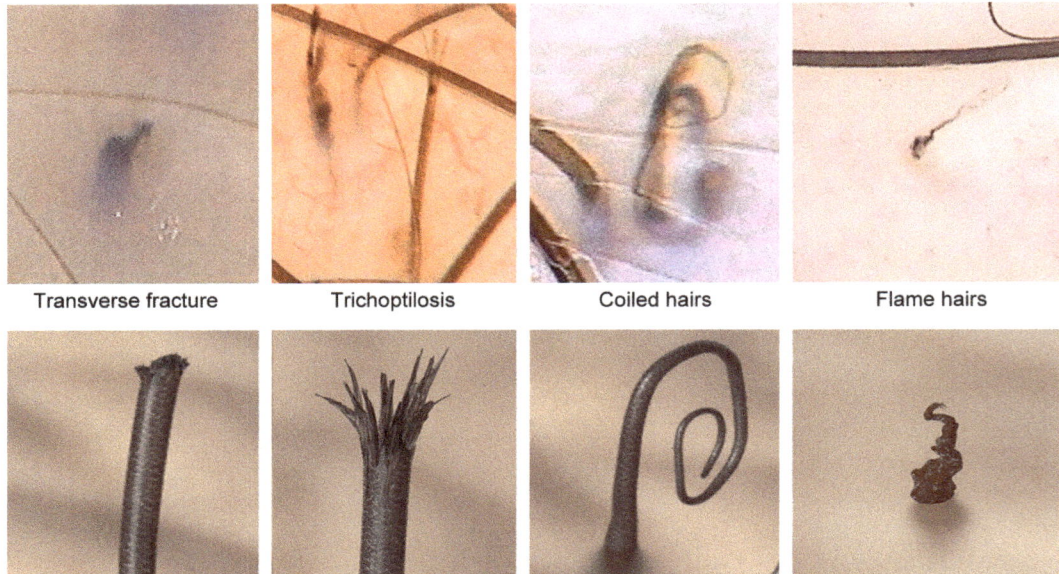

Fig. 4.7.3: The most characteristic trichoscopy features of trichotillomania.

not visible if the patients washed their hair directly before trichoscopy, and rather observed as a result of hair rubbing or scratching than pulling. The so-called tulip hairs develop when a hair shaft is broken diagonally.

Exclamation mark hairs are rare in trichotillomania, but they may be a diagnostic pitfall and lead to misdiagnosis of alopecia areata. Unlike active alopecia areata, which is characterized by an abundance of exclamation mark hairs, usually only few exclamation hairs are present. Scarce tapered hairs may be present. In doubtful cases, signs of scalp-skin injury (extravasations) may be indicative of trichotillomania. Yellow dots generally are not observed in trichotillomania, but yellow dots with black dot residues in the central part may be present. A recent study of self-induced alopecia in cats has documented similar findings as in humans and has shown that trichoscopy may be also a useful diagnostic tool in veterinary dermatology.

Traction alopecia, which is most commonly caused by hairstyling procedures or other mechanical trauma to hair may show similar features, but they are usually less prominent. Occasionally, hair casts may be present.

Treatment of trichotillomania is limited. However, behavioral therapies and drug intervention, such as antidepressants and antipsychotic agents and more recently, *N*-acetylcysteine, an amino acid that influences neurotransmitters related to mood, can be used with some results.

Take-Home Message

- Compulsive disorder characterized by recurrent hair pulling.
- Irregular areas of patchy alopecia mostly affecting the vertex of children.
- Eyebrows and eyelashes may be also affected.
- Alopecic areas show broken hairs at different lengths.
- Dermoscopy shows broken hairs, black dots, flame hairs, V-sign, trichoptilosis, coiled hairs, exclamation mark hairs.
- Alopecia areata is the main differential diagnosis.

SUGGESTED READING

1. Khunkhet S, Vachiramon V, Suchonwanit P. Trichoscopic clues for diagnosis of alopecia areata and trichotillomania in Asians. Int J Dermatol. 2017;56(2):161-5.
2. Mathew J. Trichoscopy as an aid in the diagnosis of trichotillomania. Int J Trichology. 2012;4(2):101-2.
3. Peralta L, Morais P. Photoletter to the editor: the Friar Tuck sign in trichotillomania. J Dermatol Case Rep. 2012;6(2):63-4.
4. Rakowska A, Slowinska M, Olszewska M, et al. New trichoscopy findings in trichotillomania: flame hairs, V-sign, hook hairs, hair powder, tulip hairs. Acta Derm Venereol. 2014;94(3):303-6.
5. Sah DE, Koo J, Price VH. Trichotillomania. Dermatol Ther. 2008;21(1):13-21.
6. Thakur BK, Verma S, Raphael V, et al. Extensive tonsure pattern trichotillomania-trichoscopy and histopathology aid to the diagnosis. Int J Trichology. 2013;5(4):196-8.

4.8 Dissecting Cellulitis (Initial Stage)

Isabella Doche

DISSECTING CELLULITIS

Dissecting cellulitis is a chronic and progressive inflammatory scalp disorder, most commonly affecting dark skinned-type men. This disease usually starts with sterile pustules on the vertex or occipital scalp and progresses to hair loss and nodules with pustular discharge (Figs. 4.8.1 and 4.8.2). Dissecting cellulitis may coexist with acne conglobata, pilonidal cysts, hidradenitis suppurativa, as part of the *follicular occlusion tetrad* or *triad*.

Dermoscopy of the initial alopecic patches shows nonscarring features as yellow dots, black dots, regrowing hairs, pustules, and scalp erythema (Figs. 4.8.3 to 4.8.7). Treatment options are oral isotretinoin, oral antibiotics, biological medications, steroids, and surgical excisions for scarring lesions. Early treatment is fundamental to avoid disease progression and cicatricial lesions.

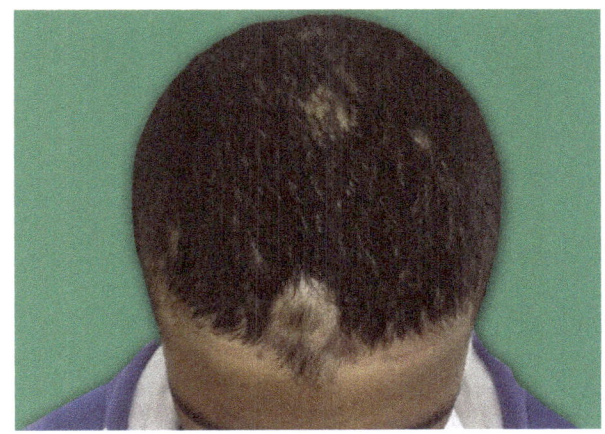

Fig. 4.8.1: Dissecting cellulitis (initial stage). Note an alopecic patch with a boggy nodule on the scalp.

Source: Division of Dermatology, Hospital das Clínicas, University of São Paulo Medical School.

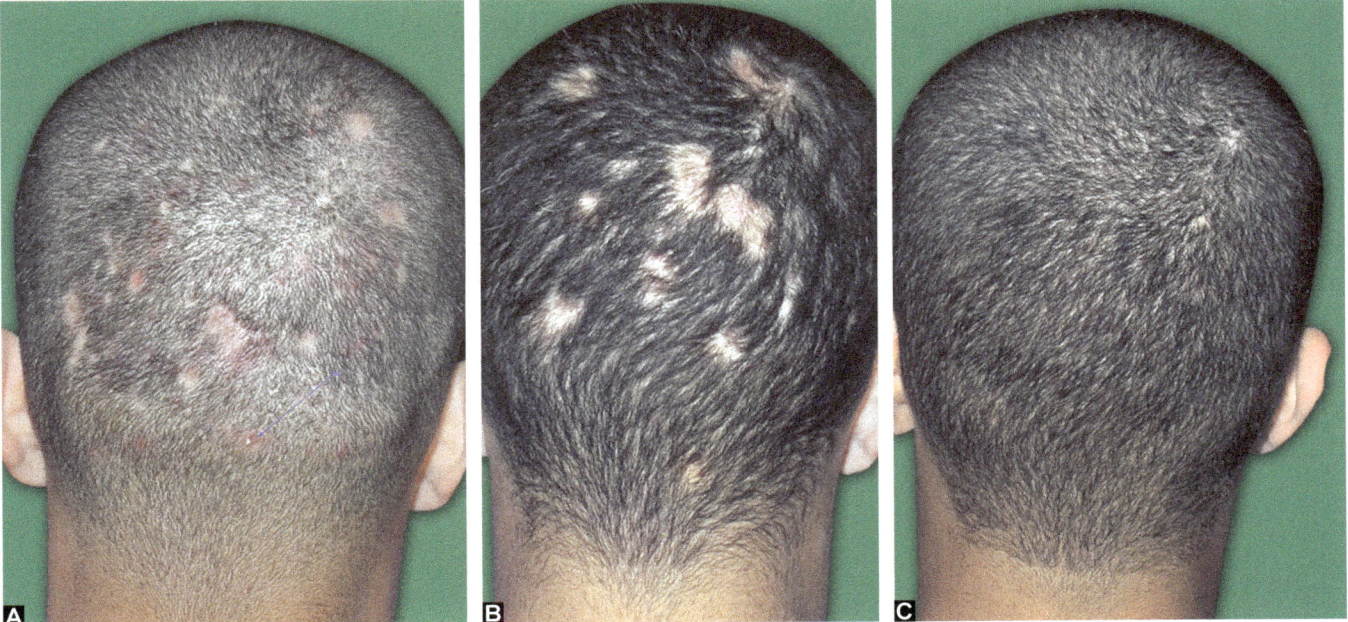

Figs. 4.8.2A to C: Dissecting cellulitis (initial stage). (A and B) In the early stages, the alopecia is nonscarring. Note some pustules on the scalp (blue arrow). (C) Note complete hair regrowth after treatment.

Source: Division of Dermatology, Hospital das Clínicas, University of São Paulo Medical School.

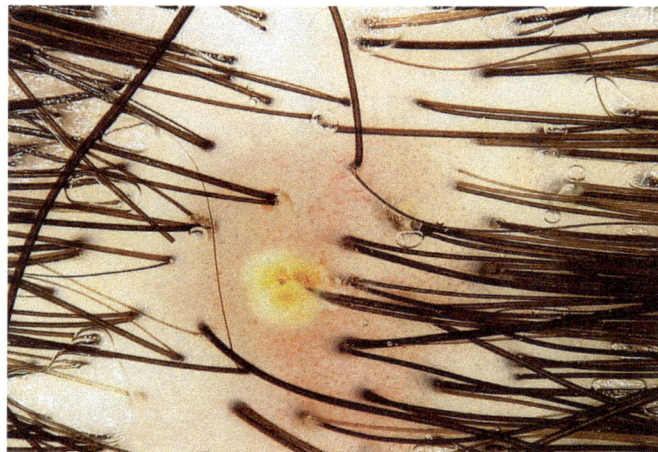

Fig. 4.8.3: Dissecting cellulitis (initial stage). Large perifollicular pustules are the earliest finding of the disease. Pustules may be misdiagnosed as a superficial folliculitis. Note some dotted vessels in this case of associated scalp psoriasis.

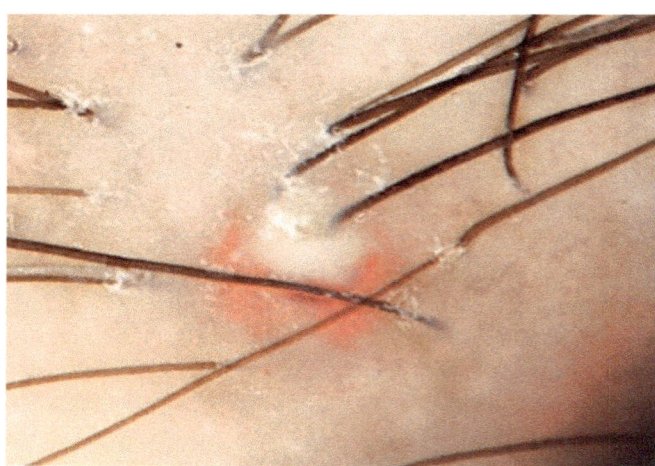

Fig. 4.8.4: Yellow pustules in bacterial folliculitis. Note a pronounced inflammatory reaction surrounding the hair follicle.
Source: Division of Dermatology, Hospital das Clínicas, University of São Paulo Medical School.

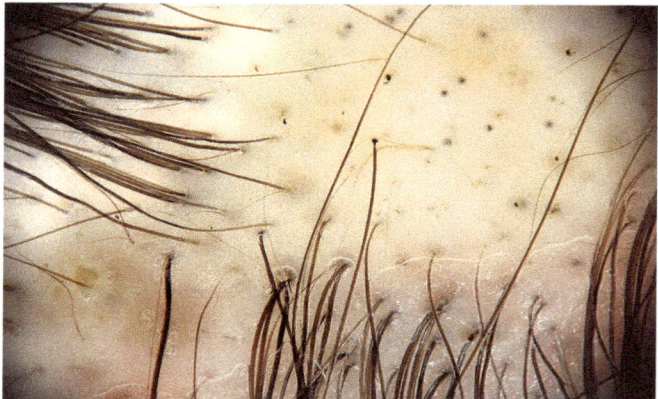

Fig. 4.8.5: Dissecting cellulitis (initial stage). Yellow dots, black dots, and vellus hairs.
Source: Division of Dermatology, Hospital das Clínicas, University of São Paulo Medical School.

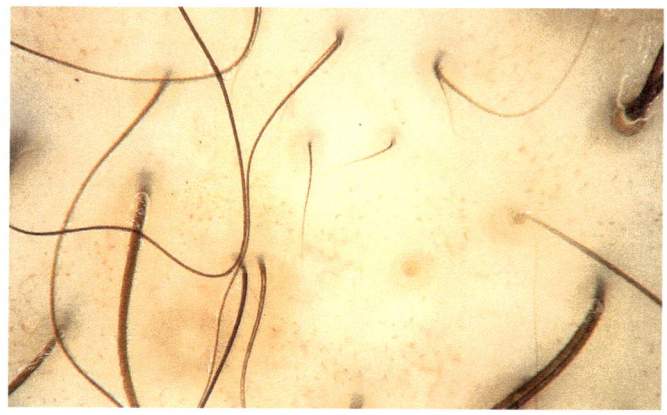

Fig. 4.8.6: Dissecting cellulitis (initial stage). Yellow 3D dots and regrowing hairs.
Source: Division of Dermatology, Hospital das Clínicas, University of São Paulo Medical School.

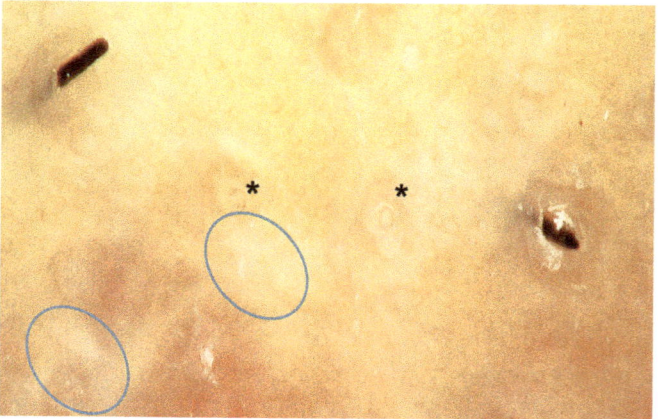

Fig. 4.8.7: Dissecting cellulitis. Yellow 3D dots (soap bubble dots) (*), broken hairs, yellow areas devoid of structures (blue rings), suggestive of a scarring evolutive phase.

> **Take-Home Message**
> - Initial stages of dissecting cellulitis are nonscarring and potentially reversible.
> - Multiple nonscarring patches with painful and boggy nodules on the scalp, mostly common in patients with dark skin types.
> - Large perifollicular pustules are usually the first sign of the disease.
> - Dermoscopy of initial stage shows vellus hairs, black dots, and yellow 3D dots. Erythema may be also present.
> - Main differentials of initial cases include alopecic and aseptic nodules of the scalp, superficial folliculitis and nonscarring alopecias, such as alopecia areata and tinea capitis.

SUGGESTED READING

1. Abdennader S, Janier M, Morel P. Alopecic and aseptic nodules of the scalp (pseudocyst of the scalp): a prospective

clinicopathological study of 15 cases. Dermatology. 2011;222(1):31-5.
2. Badaoui A, Reygagne P, Cavelier-Balloy B, et al. Dissecting cellulitis of the scalp: a retrospective study of 51 patients and review of literature. Br J Dermatol. 2016;174(2):421-3.
3. Bolduc C, Sperling LC, Shapiro J. Primary cicatricial alopecia: other lymphocytic primary cicatricial alopecias and neutrophilic and mixed primary cicatricial alopecias. J Am Acad Dermatol. 2016;75(6):1101-17.
4. Gaopande VL, Kulkarni MM, Joshi AR, et al. Perifolliculitis capitis abscedens et suffodiens in a 7 years old male: a case report with review of literature. Int J Trichology. 2015;7(4):173-5.
5. Garelli V, Didona D, Paolino G, et al. Dissecting cellulitis: response to topical steroid and oral clindamycin. G Ital Dermatol Venereol. 2017;152(3):324-5.
6. Lacarrubba F, Micali G. Regarding trichoscopy of dissecting cellulitis of the scalp. J Am Acad Dermatol. 2017; 76(6):e213.
7. Marquis K, Christensen LC, Rajpara A. Dissecting cellulitis of the scalp with excellent response to isotretinoin. Pediatr Dermatol. 2017;34(4):e210-1.
8. Martin-García RF, Rullán JM. Refractory dissecting cellulitis of the scalp successfully controlled with adalimumab. P R Health Sci J. 2015;34(2):102-4.
9. Mubki T, Rudnicka L, Olszewska M, et al. Evaluation and diagnosis of the hair loss patient: part II. Trichoscopic and laboratory evaluations. J Am Acad Dermatol. 2014;71(3):431.e1-431.e11.
10. Powers MC, Mehta D, Ozog D. Cutting Out the Tracts: Staged Excisions for Dissecting Cellulitis of the Scalp. Dermatol Surg. 2017;43(5):738-40.
11. Scheinfeld N. Dissecting cellulitis (Perifolliculitis Capitis Abscedens et Suffodiens): a comprehensive review focusing on new treatments and findings of the last decade with commentary comparing the therapies and causes of dissecting cellulitis to hidradenitis suppurativa. Dermatol Online. 2014;20(5):22692.
12. Tosti A, Torres F, Miteva M. Dermoscopy of early dissecting cellulitis of the scalp simulates alopecia areata. Actas Dermosifiliogr. 2013;104(1):92-3.
13. Verzì AE, Lacarrubba F, Micali G. Heterogeneity of trichoscopy findings in dissecting cellulitis of the scalp: correlation to disease activity and duration. Br J Dermatol. 2017;177(6):e331-e332.

4.9 Chemotherapy-induced Alopecia

Giselle Martins, Patricia Damasco, Isabella Doche

Chemotherapy-induced alopecia can occur as a result of many antineoplasis drugs. Usually, patients develop an acute and severe anagen effluvium 1–3 weeks after drug administration due to abrupt suppression of mitotic activity in the follicle. Anagen effluvium is usually reversible with complete hair regrowth within a few weeks after the drug is stopped. However, in rare cases, some patients may develop dose-dependent permanent alopecia. The most common drugs related to permanent alopecia are taxanes (docetaxel) for breast cancer, busulfan for acute myelogenous leukemia, and cisplatin and etoposide for lung cancer.

Acute and diffuse hair shedding may involve all body hairs, including eyebrows and eyelashes (Fig. 4.9.1A). Patients with permanent alopecia complain of hair thinning mostly over the androgenic-dependent scalp areas that lasts more than 6 months after the end of chemotherapy regimen (Fig. 4.9.1B). Regrowing hairs may show a different color and texture for many years after treatment.

Dermoscopy of anagen effluvium shows similar features to alopecia areata, such as yellow dots, black dots, broken hairs, dystrophic hairs, circle or pigtail hairs and monilethrix-like hairs (Pohl–Pinkus constrictions) (Figs. 4.9.2 and 4.9.3). Grain-like structures can be found surrounding defective regrowing hair shafts (Fig. 4.9.4). Permanent alopecia shows a nonscarring process, diffuse decrease in hair density, empty follicles, vellus, and thin hairs, mostly on the androgenic areas of the scalp, very similar to androgenetic alopecia (Figs. 4.9.5A and B).

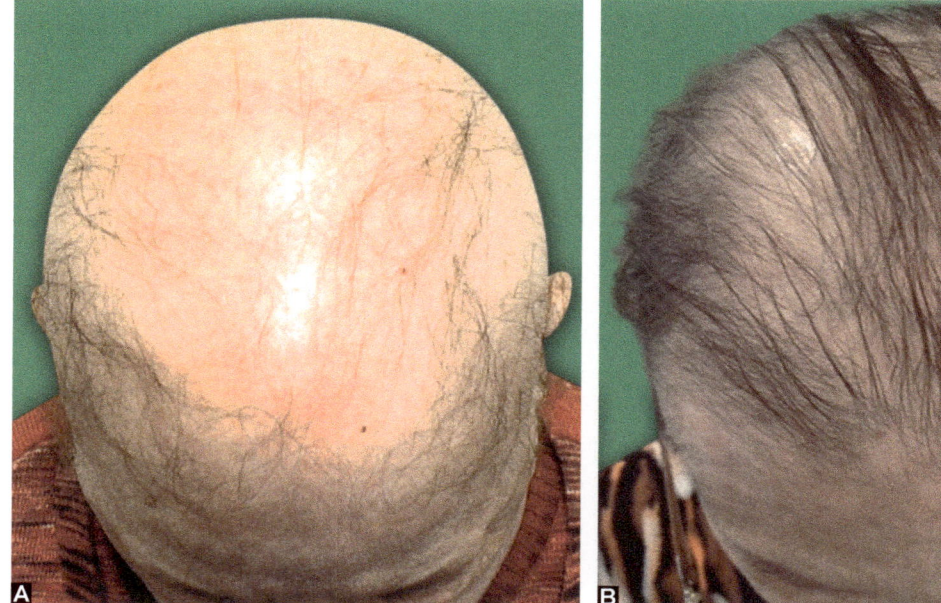

Figs. 4.9.1A and B: Chemotherapy-induced alopecia. (A) Anagen effluvium with diffuse and acute scalp and eyebrow hair shedding. (B) Permanent alopecia. Long-lasting diffuse hair thinning and decreased hair density, mostly on the vertex scalp area.

Nonscarring Alopecias

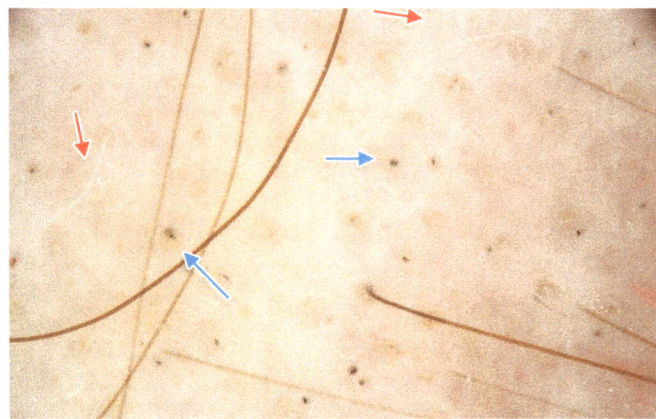

Fig. 4.9.2: Chemotherapy-induced alopecia. Note the same findings from an anagen effluvium: black dots, yellow dots (some containing black dots—blue arrows), empty follicles, and thinner hairs. Note some hypopigmented hair shafts (red arrows).

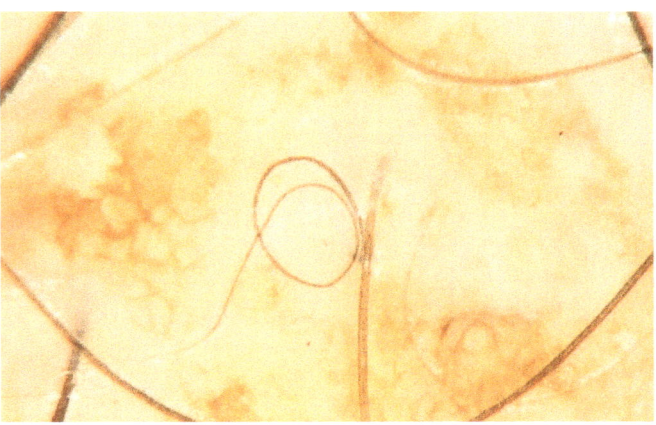

Fig. 4.9.3: Chemotherapy-induced alopecia. Partial hair regrowth can show pigtail or circle hairs.

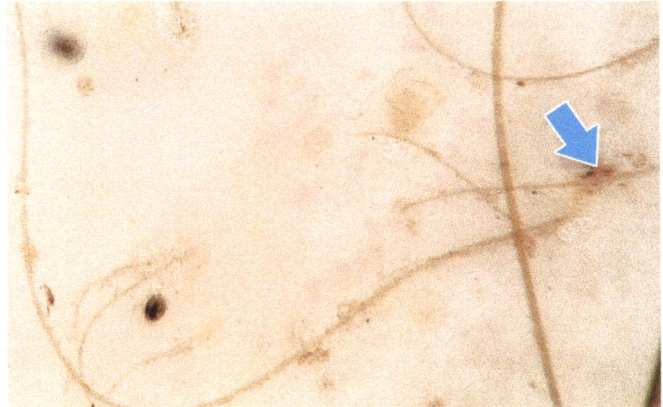

Fig. 4.9.4: Chemotherapy-induced alopecia. Some grain-like structures can be found surrounding defective regrowing hair shafts (thick blue arrow).

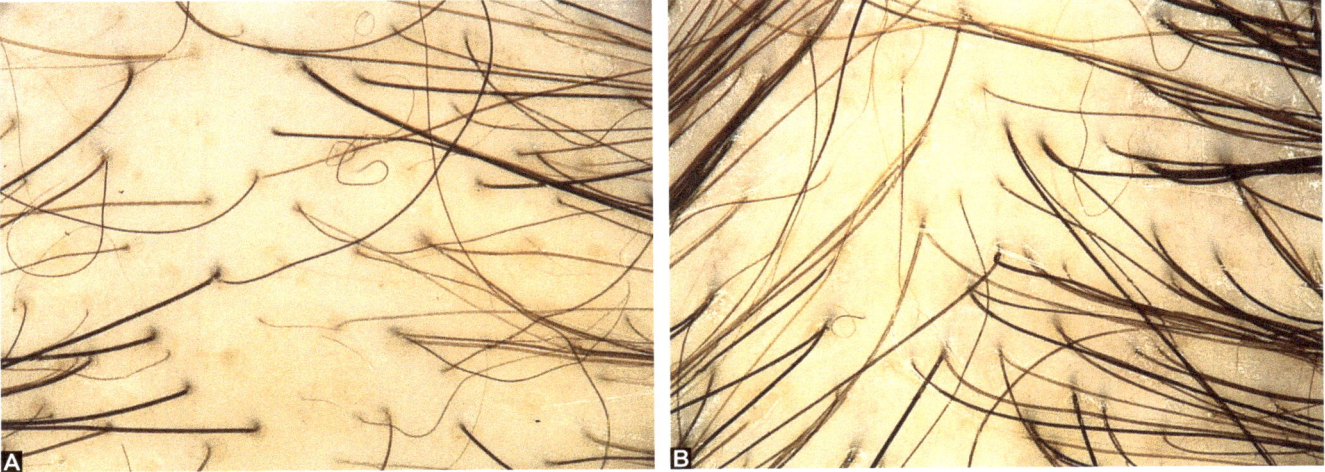

Figs. 4.9.5A and B: Chemotherapy-induced permanent alopecia. (A) Vertex scalp shows decreased hair density, yellow dots, vellus hairs, circle or pigtail hairs, and increased hair diameter variability. (B) The occipital area shows similar features, although less prominent.

> **Take-Home Message**
> - Chemotherapy-induced alopecia usually causes acute and severe anagen effluvium.
> - Permanent alopecia is rare and may occur with specific drug regimens.
> - Dermoscopy of anagen effluvium shows similar features to alopecia areata, such as broken hairs, black dots, yellow dots and dystrophic hairs.
> - Permanent alopecia shows a nonscarring process with diffuse hair thinning mostly on androgenic scalp areas.

SUGGESTED READING

1. Basilio FM, Mulinari-Brenner F, Werner B, et al. Clinical and histological study of permanent alopecia after bone marrow transplantation. An Bras Dermatol. 2015;90(6):814-21.
2. Hershman DL. Scalp cooling to prevent chemotherapy-induced alopecia: the time has come. JAMA. 2017;317(6):587-8.
3. Miteva M, Misciali C, Fanti PA, et al. Permanent alopecia after systemic chemotherapy: a clinicopathological study of 10 cases. Am J Dermatopathol. 2011;33(4):345-50.
4. Nangia J, Wang T, Osborne C, et al. Effect of a scalp cooling device on alopecia in women undergoing chemotherapy for breast cancer: the SCALP randomized clinical trial. JAMA. 2017;317(6):596-605.
5. Palamaras I, Misciali C, Vincenzi C, et al. Permanent chemotherapy-induced alopecia: a review. J Am Acad Dermatol. 2011;64(3):604-6.
6. Prevezas C, Matard B, Pinquier L, et al. Irreversible and severe alopecia following docetaxel or paclitaxel cytotoxic therapy for breast cancer. Br J Dermatol. 2009;160(4):883-5.
7. Tallon B, Blanchard E, Goldberg LJ. Permanent chemotherapy-induced alopecia: histopathologic criteria still to be defined. 2013. J Am Acad Dermatol. 2013;68(5):e151-2.
8. Tosti A, Piraccini BM, Vincenzi C, et al. Permanent alopecia after busulfan chemotherapy. Br J Dermatol. 2005;152(5):1056-8.
9. West HJ. Chemotherapu-induced hair loss (alopecia). JAMA Oncol. 2017;3(8):1147.
10. Yeager CE, Olsen EA. Treatment of chemotherapy-induced alopecia. Dermatol Ther. 2011;24(4):432-42.

4.10 Radiotherapy-induced Alopecia

Giselle Martins, Patricia Damasco, Isabella Doche

RADIATION-INDUCED ALOPECIA

Radiation-induced alopecia involves acute damage to the matrix cells of anagen follicles. Acute hair loss occurs approximately 1–3 weeks after radiation exposure and completely regrowth is usually seen 2–4 months after completion of radiotherapy. Additionally, a great number of drugs have also been reported to increase radiosensitivity.

Scalp alopecia results from immediate loss of dystrophic anagen hairs, followed by telogen shedding due to the premature catagen entry of follicles in late anagen. Patients present with an irregular nonscarring alopecic patch on the treated area or diffuse hair loss. The occipital, parietal, and temporal areas are the most commonly affected (Fig. 4.10.1). In some cases, depending on treatment dosages and duration, permanent diffuse and cicatricial alopecia may occur (Fig. 4.10.2).

Dermoscopic features are specific and include yellow dots, black dots, vellus hair, broken hairs, and variable dystrophic hairs (Figs. 4.10.3A to D). The main differential diagnoses are alopecia areata and other causes of anagen effluvium, such as chemotherapy. Dermoscopy of radiotherapy-induced permanent alopecia shows similar findings to androgenetic alopecia and chemotherapy-induced permanent alopecia, such as decreased hair density, vellus hairs, single hair units (follicle with one hair shaft), and yellow dots (Figs. 4.10.4A and B).

Although the condition is benign and self-limiting in most cases, awareness, monitoring, and limitation of radiation exposure to the patient are important strategies to prevent hair loss.

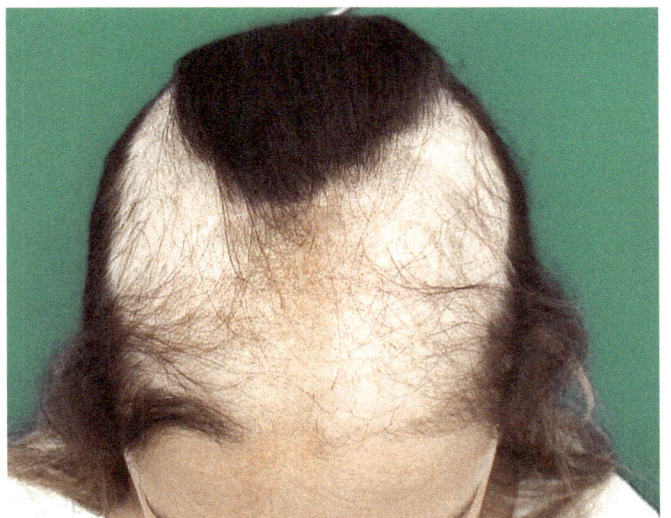

Fig. 4.10.1: Radiotherapy-induced alopecia. Acute nonscarring irregular patch alopecia over the frontal and lateral scalp areas that occurred after a meningioma radiation therapy.
Source: Dr Gabriel Sampaio.

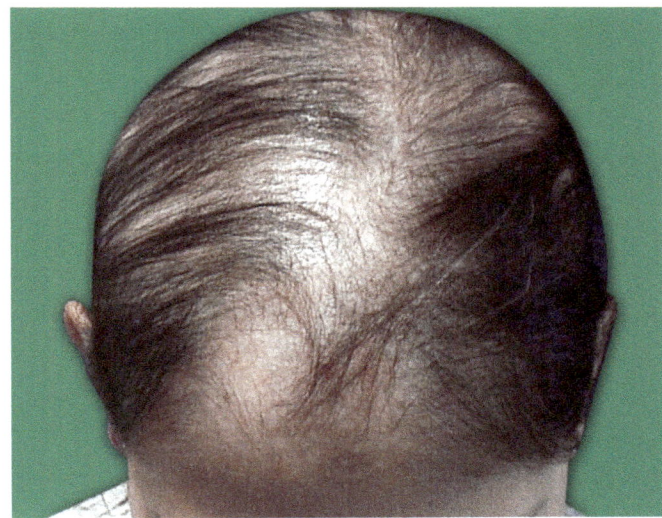

Fig. 4.10.2: Radiotherapy-induced permanent alopecia. Permanent and diffuse hair loss. Note some scarring areas and hair thinning mostly on the central scalp.

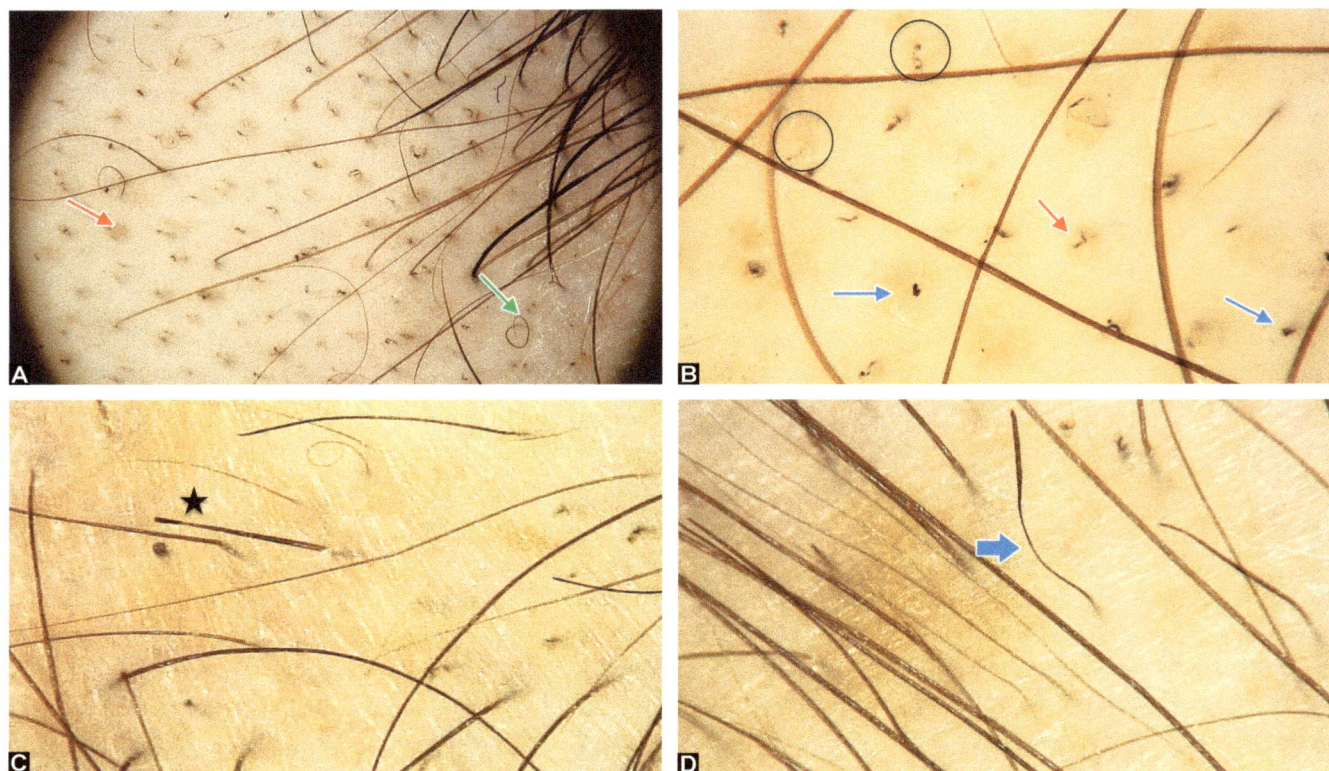

Figs. 4.10.3A to D: Radiotherapy-induced alopecia. (A and B) Note the findings from an anagen effluvium: black dots or cadaverized hairs (blue arrows), yellow dots, some containing cadaverized and dystrophic hair (red arrows), flame hairs (circles), circle hairs or pigtail hairs (green arrow), vellus hairs and short regrowing hairs. (C) Exclamation mark hair with a darker tip (star). (D) Pseudomonilethrix with irregular constrictions on the hair shaft (thick arrow).

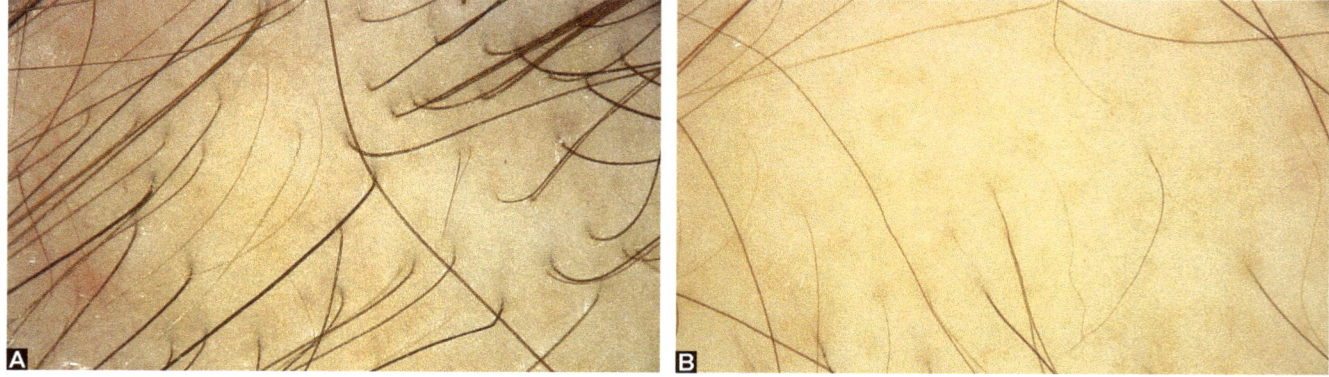

Figs. 4.10.4A and B: Permanent diffuse alopecia. (A) Decreased hair density, follicular units with only one hair shaft, thin hairs, and vellus hairs on the frontal scalp area. (B) Note multiple vellus hairs and empty follicles.

> **Take-Home Message**
> - Radiotherapy can cause anagen effluvium characterized by an irregular patch of nonscarring alopecia or diffuse hair loss.
> - Depending on the treatment dosages and duration, permanent diffuse and secondary cicatricial alopecia can occur.
> - Dermoscopy of anagen effluvium shows similar features to alopecia areata, such as black dots, yellow dots, vellus hair, broken hair, and variable dystrophic hairs.
> - Dermoscopy of permanent diffuse alopecia shows decreased hair density, follicular unit with only one hair shaft, thin hairs, vellus hairs, and empty follicles, similar to androgenetic alopecia and post-chemotherapy permanent alopecia.

SUGGESTED READING

1. Cho S, Choi MJ, Lee JS, et al. Dermoscopic findings in radiation-induced alopecia after angioembolization. Dermatology. 2014;229(2):141-5.
2. Kawano M, Umeda S, Yasuda T, et al. FGF18 signaling in the hair cycle resting phase determines radioresistance of hair follicles by arresting hair cycling. Adv Radiat Oncol. 2016;1(3):170-81.
3. Lawenda BD, Gagne HM, Gierga DP, et al. Permanent alopecia after cranial irradiation: dose–response relationship. Int J Radiat Oncol Biol Phys. 2004;60(3):879-87.
4. Podlipnik S, Giavedoni P, San-Román L, et al. Square alopecia: a new type of transient alopecia of the scalp following fluoroscopically endovascular embolization. Int J Trichol. 2013;5(4):201-3.
5. Rogers S, Donachie P, Suqden E, et al. Comparison of permanent hair loss in children with standard risk PNETS of the posterior fossa following radiotherapy alone or chemotherapy and radiotherapy after surgical resection. Pediatr Blood Cancer. 2011;57(6):1074-6.
6. Severs GA, Griffin T, Werner-Wasik M. Cicatricial alopecia secondary to radiation therapy: case report and review of the literature. Cutis. 2008;81(2):147-53.
7. Soref CM, Fahl WE. A new strategy to prevent chemotherapy and radiotherapy-induced alopecia using topically applied vasoconstrictor. Int J Cancer. 2015;136(1):195-203.
8. Vaccaro M, Guarneri F, Brianti P, et al. Temporary radiation-induced alopecia after embolization of a cerebral arteriovenous malformation. Clin Exp Dermatol. 2015;40(1):88-90.
9. Verma S, Srinivas CR, Thomas M. Radiation-induced temporary alopecia after embolization of cerebral aneurysm. Indian J Dermatol. 2014;59(6):633.

4.11 Traction Alopecia (Initial Stage)

Patricia Damasco, Giselle Martins, Isabella Doche

TRACTION ALOPECIA

Traction alopecia (TA) usually occurs as a result of repetitive tension in the hair shaft. TA is most prevalent in black patients, mainly attributed to hairstyle habits such as tight ponytails, buns, hair weaves, cornrows, chignons, braids, and others.

Initially, patients may report sudden-onset or gradual, patchy, symmetric hair loss along the marginal scalp. When the temporal and frontal areas are affected, there is a preservation of hairs at the hairline, forming a "fringe sign" (Figs. 4.11.1A and B). Sometimes, small associated perifollicular papules and pustules could be noted (Fig. 4.11.2). Patients may also report symptoms of scalp tenderness, stinging, headaches, and itching, which should alert the clinician to the possibility of high-risk hairstyling practices (Fig. 4.11.3).

Dermoscopy of early lesions shows persistence of vellus hairs and follicular openings and decreased terminal hair shafts, which are more easily pulled out by traction. The presence of hair casts is a sign of active traction. Perifollicular erythema, perifollicular scale, yellow dots, broken hairs, and black dots may also be present (Figs. 4.11.4 to 4.11.7).

Although early stages of TA are reversible, it is important to educate the patients about haircare and hairstyle practices. Topical and intralesional corticosteroids, antibiotics, and topical minoxidil may also be used to suppress perifollicular inflammation and increase hair density.

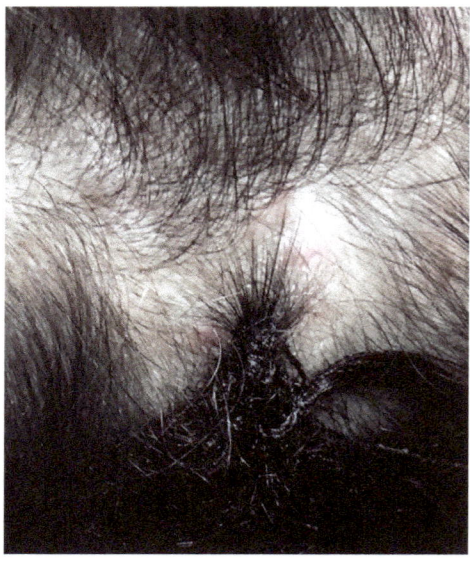

Fig. 4.11.2: Traction alopecia, initial stage. Perifollicular erythema and telogen roots entrapped by the glue can be seen in this patient with hair extensions.

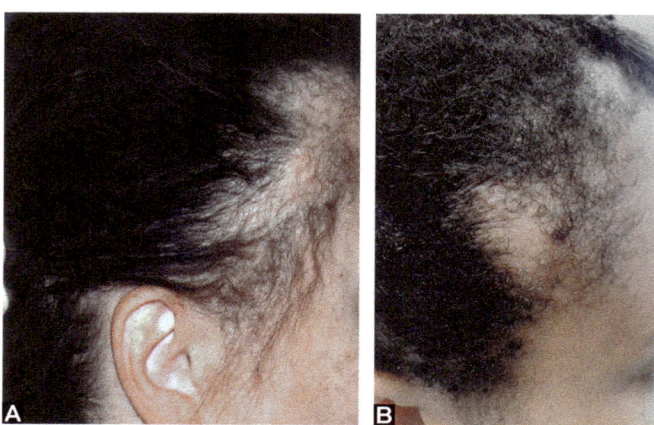

Figs. 4.11.1A and B: Traction alopecia, initial stage. (A) Fringe sign in a Caucasian woman using tight ponytails. (B) Round alopecic patches and fringe sign in an African-descent girl.
Source: Division of Dermatology, Hospital das Clínicas, University of São Paulo Medical School.

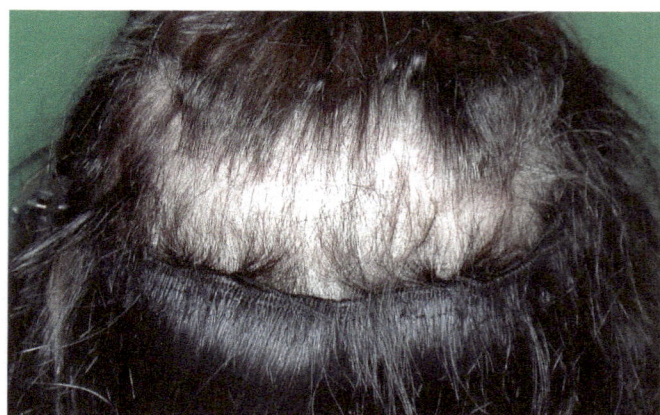

Fig. 4.11.3: Traction alopecia, initial stage. Note the linear patch of alopecia in this patient using the traction hairstyle.

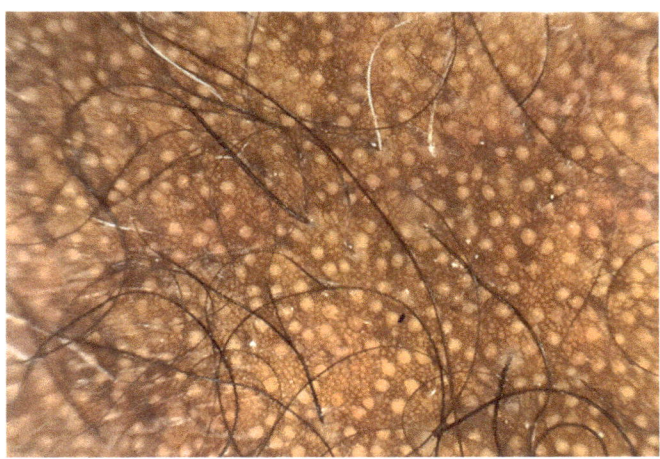

Fig. 4.11.4: Traction alopecia, initial stage. Vellus hairs, mild perifollicular scales and regularly distributed pinpoint white dots, indicating preserved follicular openings in the scalp from an African-descent patient. Perifollicular erythema is hardly seen in dark skinned patients.
Source: Division of Dermatology, Hospital das Clínicas, University of São Paulo Medical School.

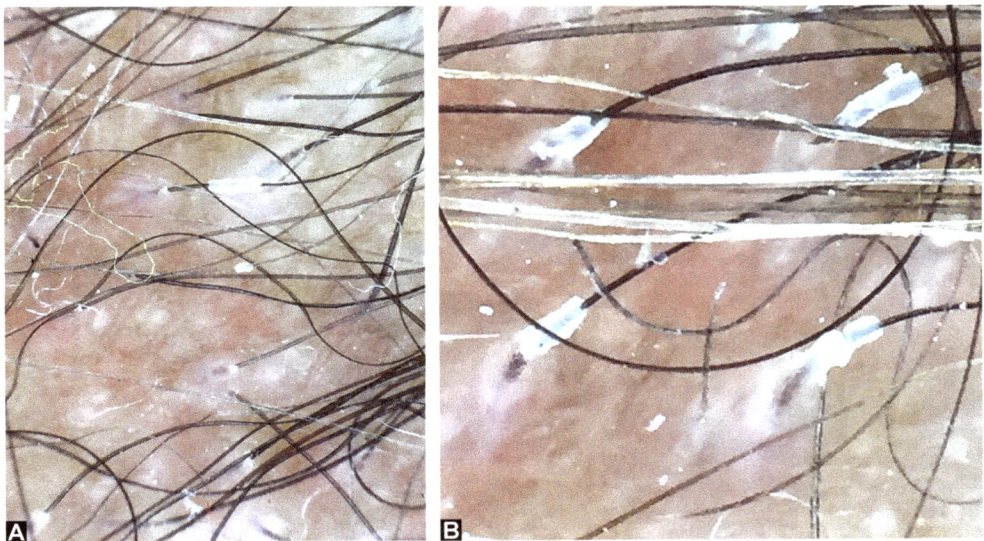

Figs. 4.11.5A and B: Hair casts, cylindrical whitish masses of keratin cells encircling the hair shafts, indicate active traction alopecia in a patient with central centrifugal alopecia.

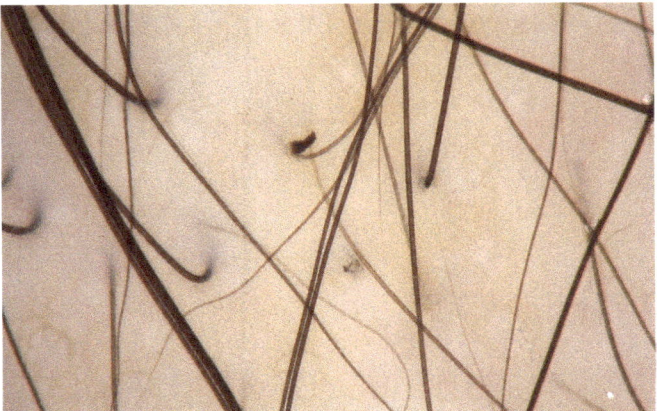

Fig. 4.11.6: Traction alopecia—initial stage. Note few broken hairs. Vellus hairs are preserved as they are too short to be pulled.

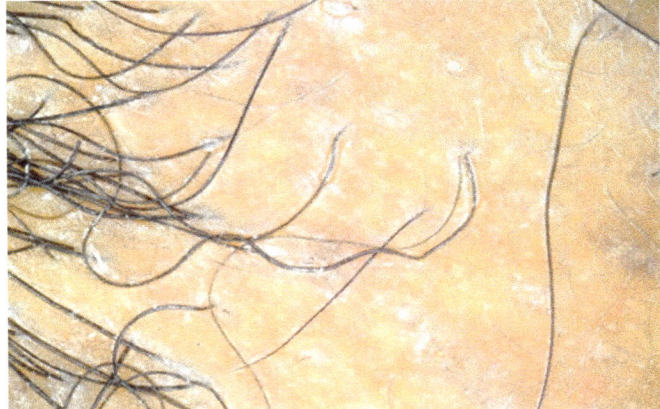

Fig. 4.11.7: Traction alopecia—initial stage. Hair casts and preserved follicular openings. Note a mild erythema and perifollicular hyperpigmentation in the scalp of a dark skinned girl.

Take-Home Message

- Traction alopecia is more common in African descents due to the repetitive tension on the hair shaft in some hair practices.
- Initially nonscarring and potentially reversible alopecia if early treated.
- Dermoscopy of early lesions shows the persistence of follicular openings, vellus hairs and decreased terminal hairs. Yellow dots, broken hairs, black dots, perifollicular erythema and scale may be present and alopecia areata has to be ruled out.
- Hair casts indicate active traction.
- Stopping the traction is important to prevent disease progression.

SUGGESTED READING

1. Haskin A, Aguh C. All hairstyles are not created equal: What the dermatologist needs to know about black hairstyling practices and the risk of traction alopecia (TA). J Am Acad Dermatol. 2016;75(3):606-11.
2. Lawson CN, Hollinger J, Sethi S, et al. Updates in the understanding and treatments of skin and hair disorders in women of color. Int J Womens Dermatol. 2017;16:3(1 Suppl):S21-37.
3. Lindsey SF, Tosti A. Ethnic hair disorders. Curr Probl Dermatol. 2015;47:139-49.
4. Mirmirani P, Khumalo NP. Traction alopecia: how to translate study data for public education—closing the KAP gap? Dermatol Clin. 2014;32(2):153-61.
5. Polat M. Evaluation of clinical signs and early and late trichoscopy findings in traction alopecia patients with Fitzpatrick skin type II and III: a single-center, clinical study. Int J Dermatol. 2017;56(8):850-5.
6. Semble AL, McMichael AJ. Hair Loss in patients with skin of color. Semin Cutan Med Surg. 2015;34(2):81-8.
7. Tanus A, Oliveira CC, Villarreal DJ, et al. Black women's hair: the main scalp dermatoses and aesthetic practices in women of African ethnicity. An Bras Dermatol. 2015;90(4):450-65.
8. Tosti A, Miteva M, Torres F, et al. Hair casts are a dermoscopic clue for the diagnosis of traction alopecia. Br J Dermatol. 2010;163(6):1353-5.
9. Yang A, Iorizzo M, Vincenzi C, et al. Hair extensions: a concerning cause of hair disorders. Br J Dermatol. 2009;160(1):207-9.

4.12 Pressure-induced Alopecia

Isabella Doche

PRESSURE-INDUCED ALOPECIA

Pressure-induced alopecia is a patchy alopecia that occurs after local traumas or a prolonged immobile state of the scalp. Although most cases are nonscarring and complete hair regrowth occurs, some may lead to scarring lesions. Hair loss is due to hypoxia changes in certain areas of the scalp, caused by pressure. It is often presented as a discrete, skin-colored and hairless patch area (Figs. 4.12.1A and B).

Pressure-induced alopecia usually occurs in the occiput as a rare and preventable complication after a surgical procedure under general anesthesia or after a prolonged period of lying in an intensive care unit.

Dermoscopy of acute lesions shows features similar to alopecia areata, with broken hairs, black dots, and exclamation mark hairs (Fig. 4.12.2). Most cases resolve spontaneously after a few months.

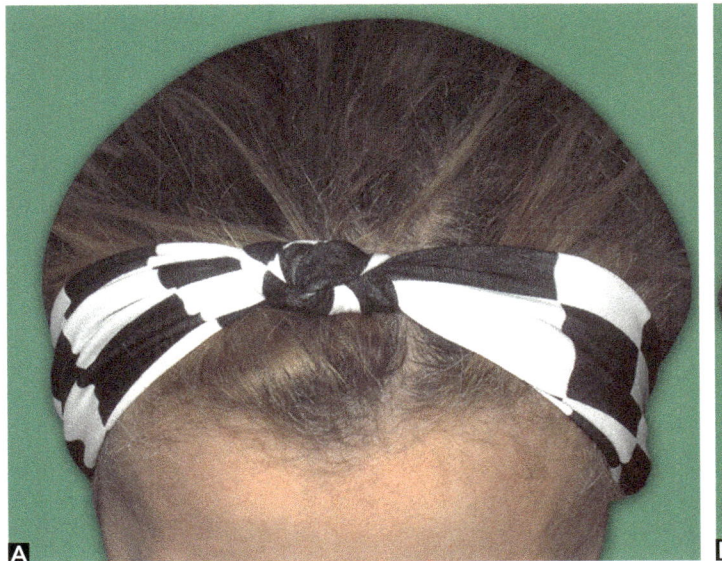 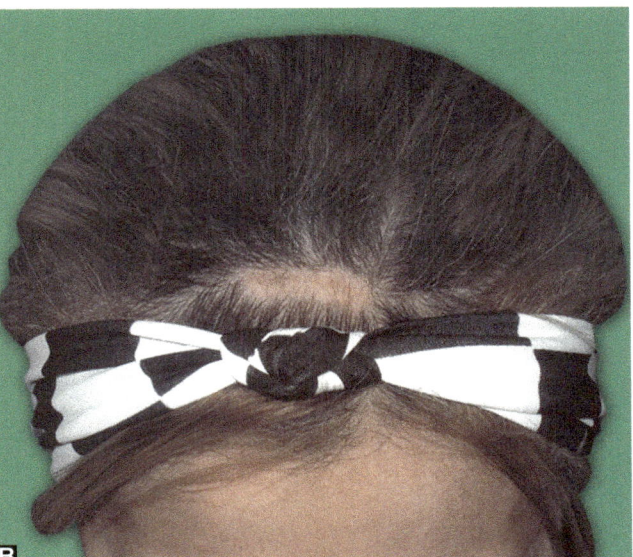

Figs. 4.12.1A and B: (A and B) Pressure-induced alopecia. Localized patchy alopecia after the chronic use of a very tight headwrap on the frontal area of the scalp.
Source: Division of Dermatology, Hospital das Clínicas, University of São Paulo Medical School

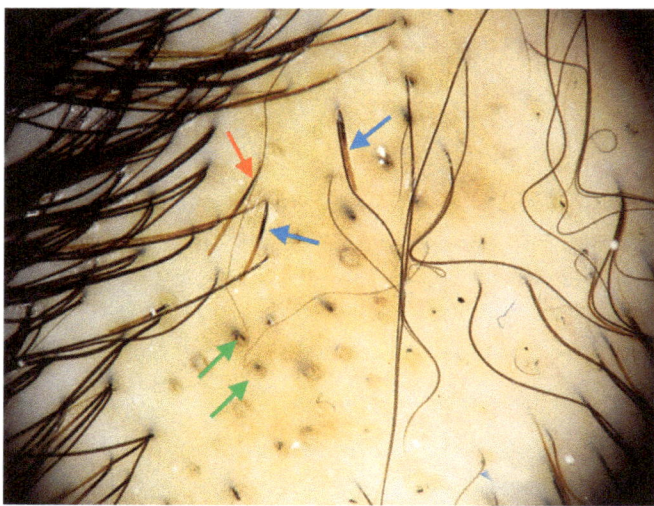

Fig. 4.12.2: Pressure alopecia. Acute lesions show broken hairs (blue arrows), black dots (green arrows), and exclamation mark hair (red arrow), similar to alopecia areata.

Source: Division of Dermatology, Hospital das Clínicas, University of São Paulo Medical School

Take-Home Message

- Pressure-induced alopecia can be nonscarring (most cases) or scarring depending on the duration of scalp injury.
- Dermoscopy of acute lesions shows features similar to alopecia areata.

SUGGESTED READING

1. Chang ZY, Ngian J, Chong C, et al. Postoperative permanent pressure alopecia. J Anesth. 2016;30(2):349-51.
2. Davies, KE, Yesudian, P. Pressure alopecia. Int J Trichology. 2012;4(2):64-8.
3. Dominguez-Aunon, JD, Garcia-Arpa, M, Perez-Suarez, B, et al. Pressure alopecia. Int J Dermatol. 2004;43:928-30.
4. Khokhar RS, Baaj J, Alhazmi HH, et al. Pressure-induced alopecia in pediatric patients following prolonged urological surgeries: the case reports and a review of literature. Anesth Essays Res. 2015;9(3):430-2.
5. Lencaste A, Tosti A. Role of trichoscopy in children's scalp and hair disorders. Pediatr Dermatol. 2013;30(6):674-82.
6. Papaiordanou F, da Silveira BR, Piñeiro-Maceira J, et al. Trichoscopy of noncicatricial pressure-induced alopecia resembling alopecia areata. Int J Trichology. 2016;8(2):89-90.

CHAPTER 5

Scarring Alopecias

*Isabella Doche, Giselle Martins, Patricia Damasco, Laura N Uwakwe,
Amy McMichael, Lidia Rudnicka, Maria Cecília da Matta Rivitti Machado*

INTRODUCTION

Primary scarring or cicatricial alopecias are a group of disorders affecting the scalp that destroy permanently the hair follicle and the stem cells. During the 2001 North American Hair Research Society Workshop on Cicatricial Alopecia held at the Duke University Medical Center, a useful and practical classification system for cicatricial alopecia was developed, based on the prominent inflammatory infiltrate on a representative biopsy of an area of active loss.

Primary cicatricial alopecias are divided into lymphocytic, neutrophilic, and mixed groups (Table 5.1). Although some cases may still remain unclassifiable, this division is important to choose the best treatment for the patient, since it is likely that medications will not be effective on both lymphocytic and neutrophilic predominant cases of cicatricial alopecia.

Table 5.1: Primary scarring alopecias.

Inflammatory infiltrate	Disease

Lymphocytic	Chronic cutaneous lupus erythematosus
	Lichen planopilaris
	    Classic lichen planopilaris
	    Frontal fibrosing alopecia
	    Graham-Little syndrome
	Classic pseudopelade of Brocq
	Central centrifugal cicatricial alopecia
	Alopecia mucinosa
	Keratosis follicularis spinulosa decalvans

Neutrophilic	Folliculitis decalvans Dissecting cellulitis/folliculitis (*perifolliculitis abscedens et suffodiens*)
Mixed	Folliculitis (acne) keloidalis Folliculitis (acne) necrotica Erosive pustular dermatosis
Nonspecific (end stage)	

Source: Olsen EA, Bergfeld WF, Cotsarelis G, et al. Summary of North American Hair Research Society (NAHRS)-sponsored Workshop on Cicatricial Alopecia, Duke University Medical Center, February 10 and 11, 2001. J Am Acad Dermatol. 2003;48(1):103-10.

5.1 Lichen Planopilaris

Isabella Doche

Lichen planopilaris is a chronic and progressive lymphocytic scarring alopecia. This disease affects middle-aged Caucasian men and women with few case reports in children.

Usually, clinical lesions start on the vertex area of the scalp with erythema and scaling and symptoms as itching, burning, and pain may be present. Although this disease shows a slow progression, some cases may spread very quickly all over the scalp and be very devastating (Figs. 5.1.1 to 5.1.4).

On dermoscopy, the most important features are the absence of follicular ostia, the absence of vellus hairs, white scarring areas/dots, perifollicular scale/cast, perifollicular erythema, and diffuse erythema. Pili torti, broken hairs, black dots, and pigment incontinence (in dark-skinned patients) may also be noted (Figs. 5.1.5 to 5.1.13).

Treatment options include topical and intralesional steroids, hydroxychloroquine, doxycycline, isotretinoin, peroxisome proliferator-activated receptor-γ agonists, methotrexate, mycophenolate mofetil, and biological medications. Main differentials include other lymphocytic and neutrophilic scarring types of alopecias.

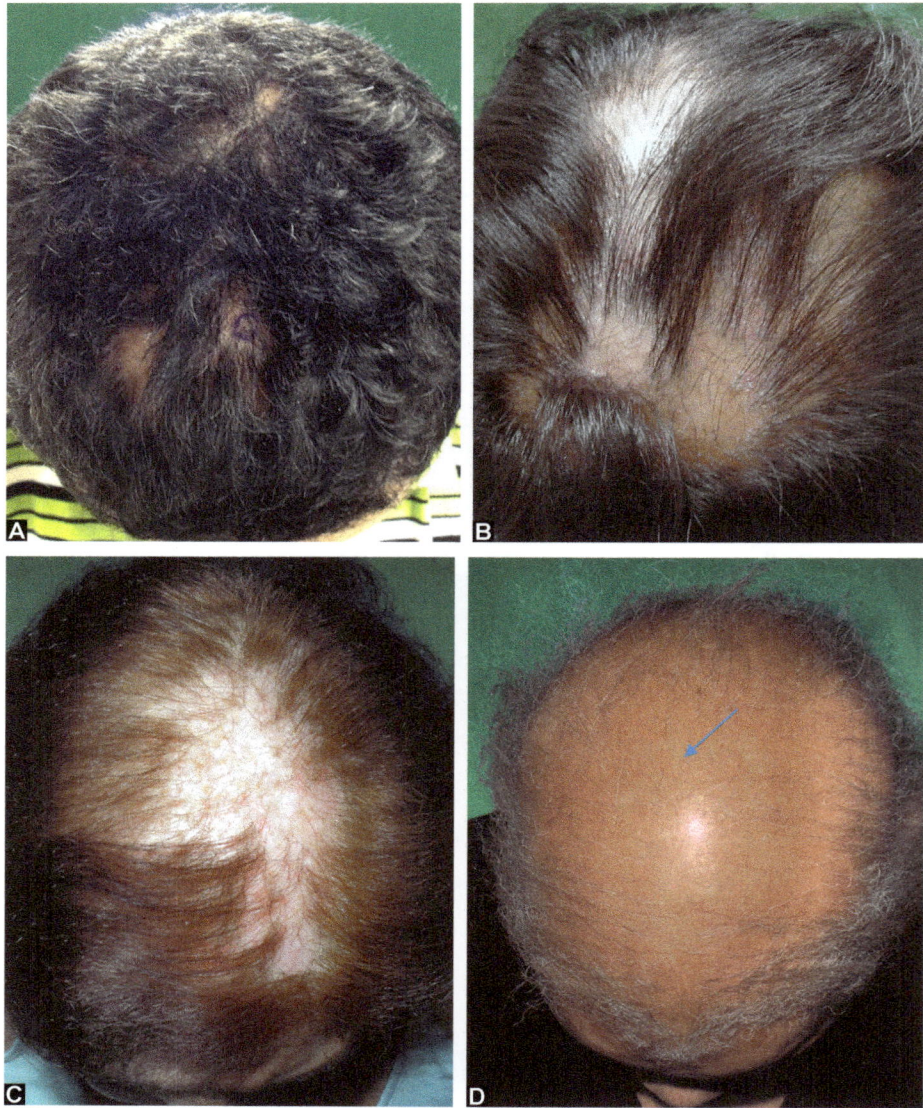

Figs. 5.1.1A to D: Lichen planopilaris. Clinical presentation may vary from (A) multiple, (B) unique, (C) localized, or (D) diffuse scarring alopecic patches, mostly on the vertex scalp. Active lesions present with erythema and scaling (A and B).
Source: Division of Dermatology, Hospital das Clínicas, University of São Paulo Medical School

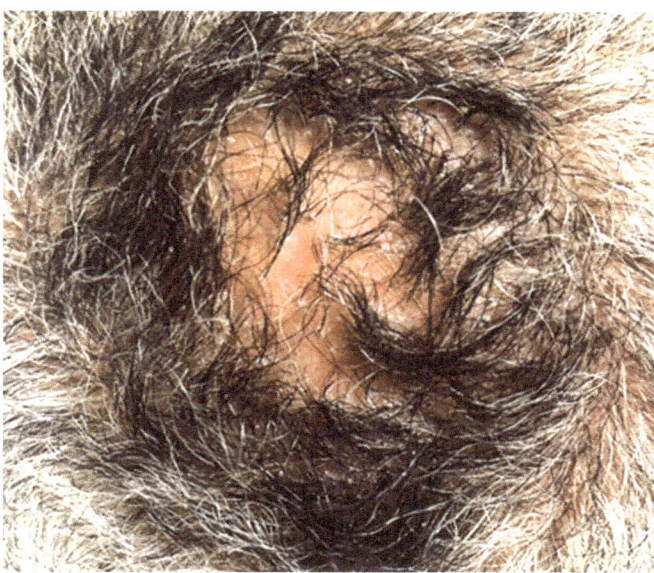

Fig. 5.1.2: Lichen planopilaris. Although some lesions may clinically resemble folliculitis decalvans due to white-porcelain scalp surface, the absence of big hair tuftings and less pronounced peripilar scales suggest the diagnosis of lichen planopilaris.

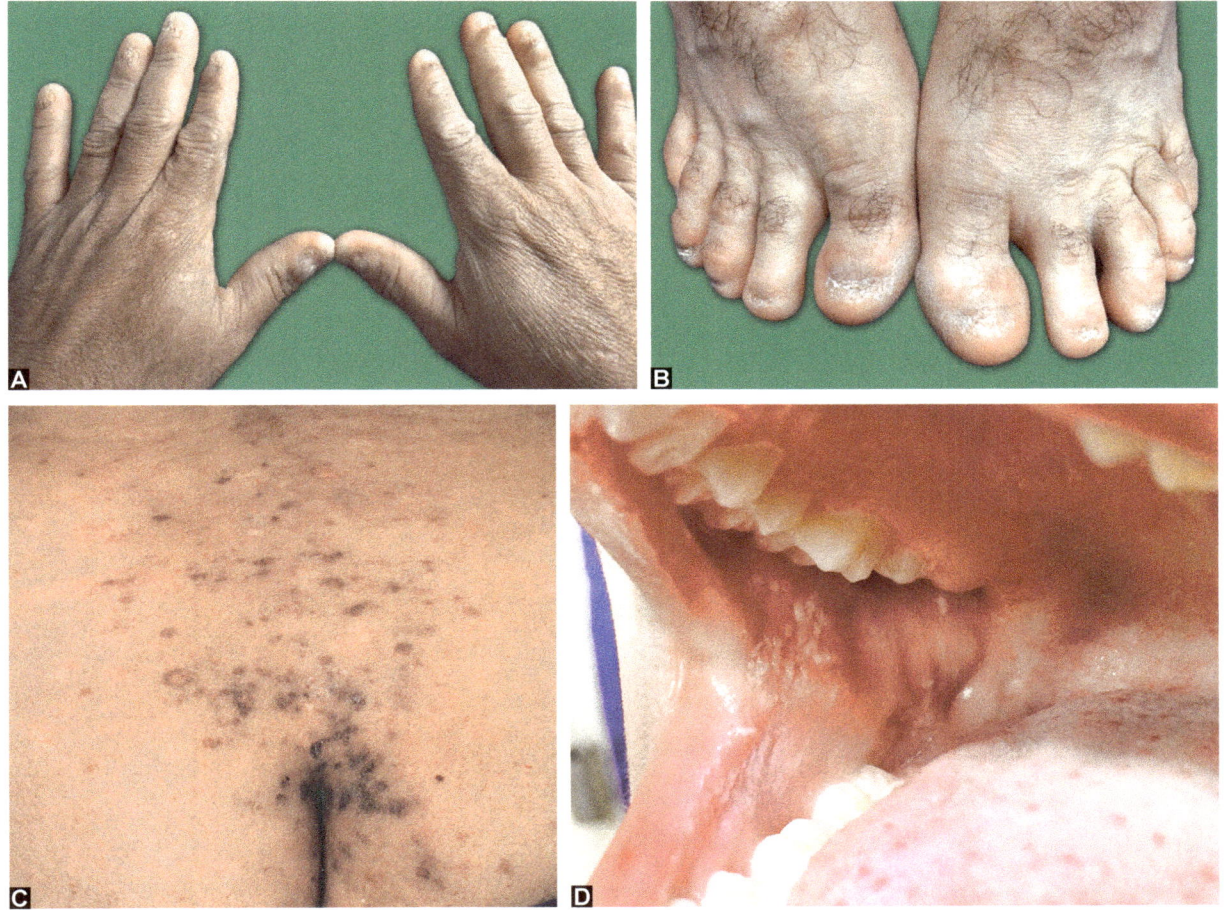

Figs. 5.1.3A to D: (A and B) Nail lichen planus. (C) Cutaneous lichen planus. (D) Oral lichen planus. Lesions on the nails, skin, and mucosa may be associated with scalp alopecia.

Source: Division of Dermatology, Hospital das Clínicas, University of São Paulo Medical School.

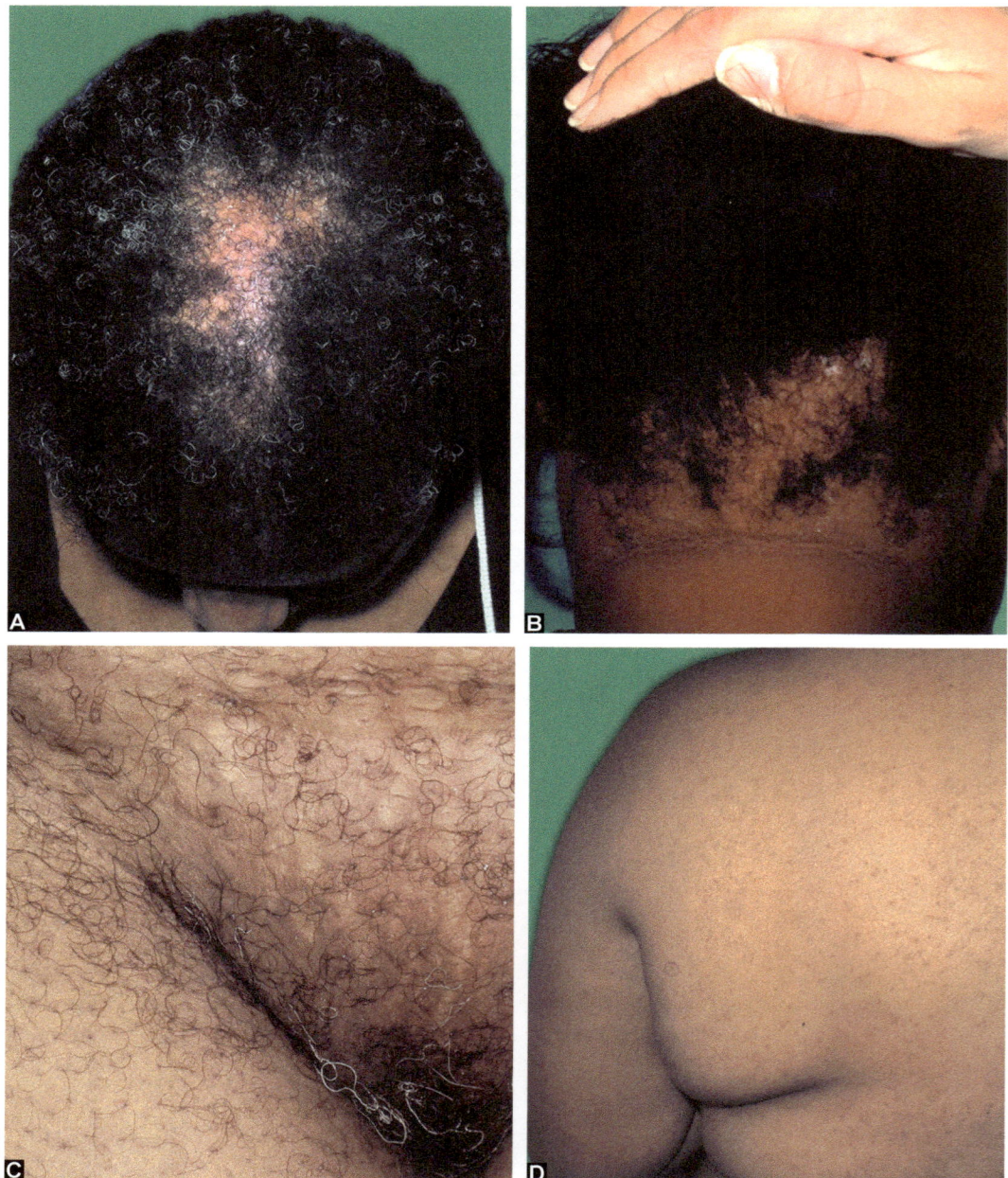

Figs. 5.1.4A to D: Graham-Little syndrome. (A) Lichen planopilaris on the vertex (B) On the occipital scalp. (C) Pubic hair loss. (D) Keratosis pilaris on the back.

Source: Division of Dermatology, Hospital das Clínicas, University of São Paulo Medical School.

Scarring Alopecias

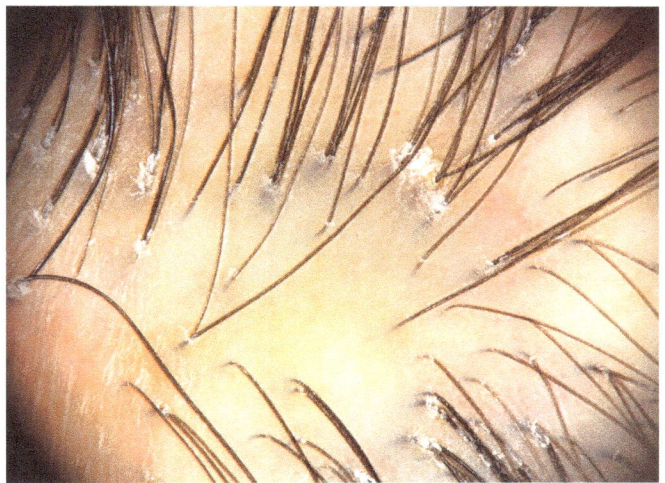

Fig. 5.1.5: Lichen planopilaris. Perifollicular scale/cast, absence of follicular ostia, absence of vellus hairs, and small tufts of hairs (less than 6). Scaling is a sign of active disease.
Source: Division of Dermatology, Hospital das Clínicas, University of São Paulo Medical School.

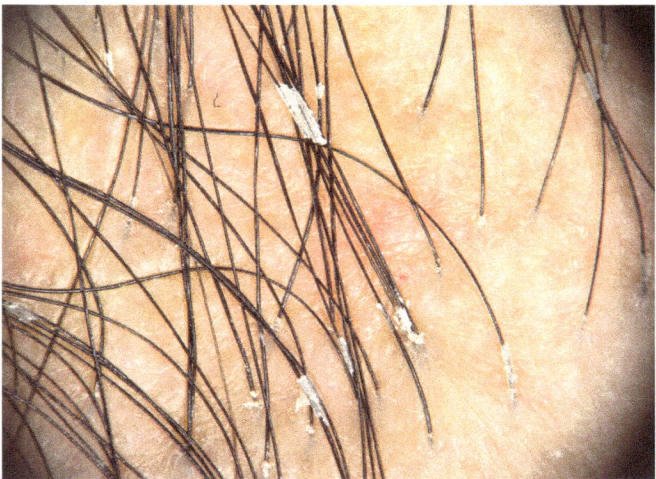

Fig. 5.1.6: Lichen planopilaris. Note tubular whitish structures (casts) surrounding the hair shafts.
Source: Division of Dermatology, Hospital das Clínicas, University of São Paulo Medical School.

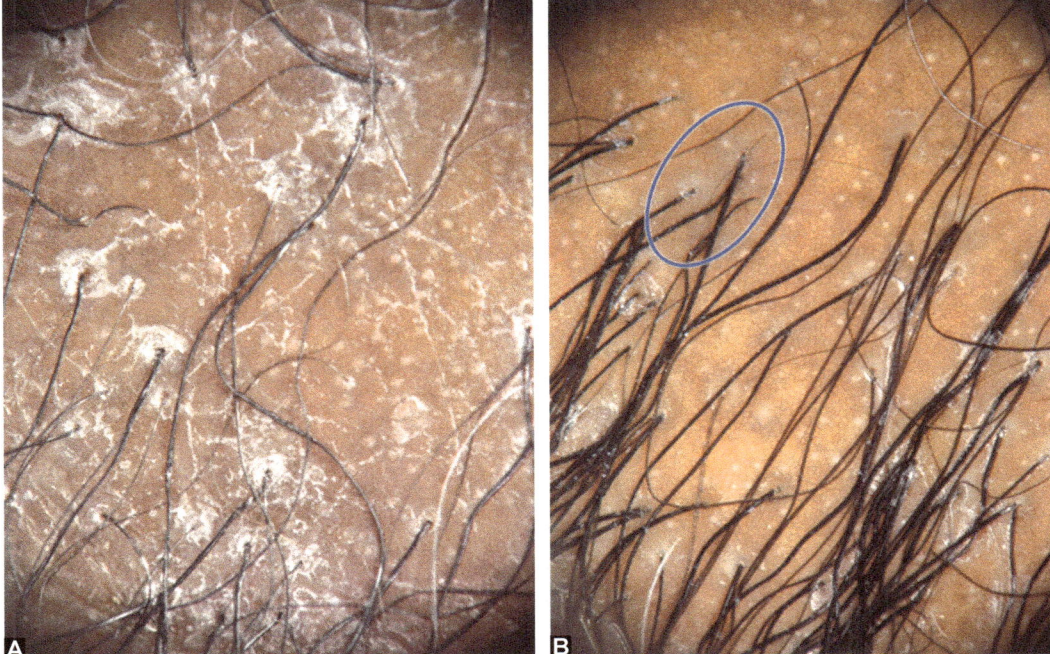

Figs. 5.1.7A and B: Lichen planopilaris in dark-skinned patient. (A) On dry dermoscopy, note perifollicular and mild interfollicular scales. (B) In the same patient, dermoscopy with immersion fluid shows the absence of follicular openings, pinpoint white dots irregularly distributed, and gray-white peripilar halos surrounded by a bluish discoloration (blue circle).
Source: Division of Dermatology, Hospital das Clínicas, University of São Paulo Medical School.

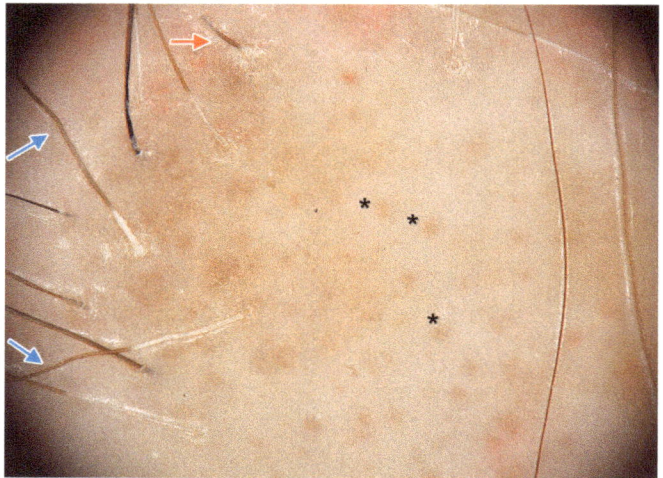

Fig. 5.1.8: Lichen planopilaris. Peripilar scale, pili torti (blue arrows), broken hair (red arrow), and multiple red dots (*). Red dots are uncommon in lichen planopilaris and indicate early disease. Red dots are more frequent in glabellar lesions from patients with frontal fibrosing alopecia and in early lesions of discoid lupus erythematosus.

Source: Division of Dermatology, Hospital das Clínicas, University of São Paulo Medical School.

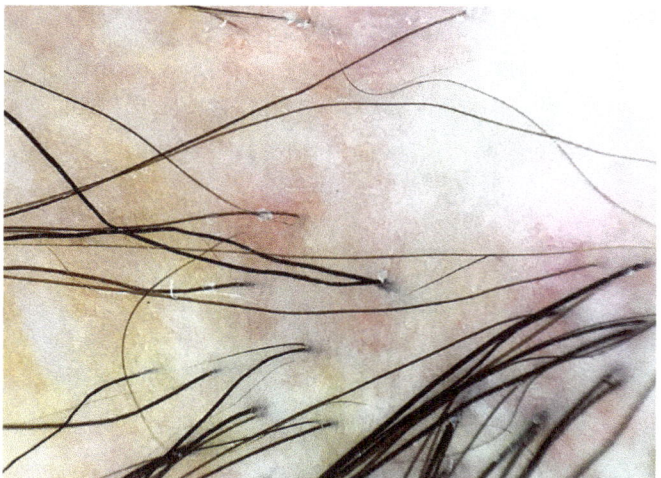

Fig. 5.1.9: Lichen planopilaris. White scarring patches, white dots, pili torti, and areas with skin brownish discoloration. Note some short regrowing hairs.

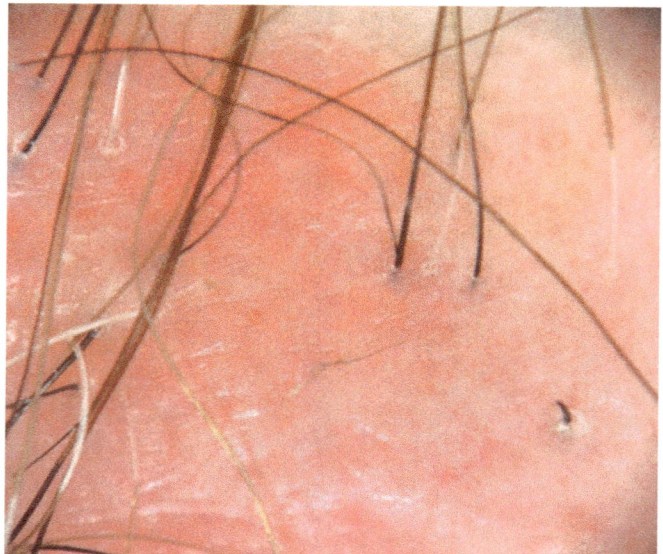

Fig. 5.1.10: Lichen planopilaris. Milky-red (strawberry ice cream pattern) areas lacking follicular openings may be present in an early fibrotic phase of the disease. Note also peripilar scales and one broken hair.

Source: Division of Dermatology, Hospital das Clínicas, University of São Paulo Medical School.

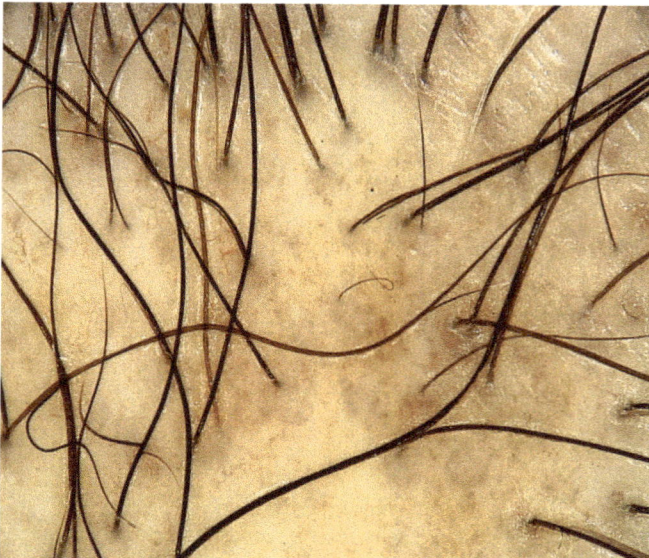

Fig. 5.1.11: Lichen planopilaris in dark-skinned patient. Note a skin brown discoloration with blue-gray peripilar halos (target pattern) resultant of pigment incontinence. Scattered brown discoloration is more frequently seen in lesions of discoid lupus erythematosus.

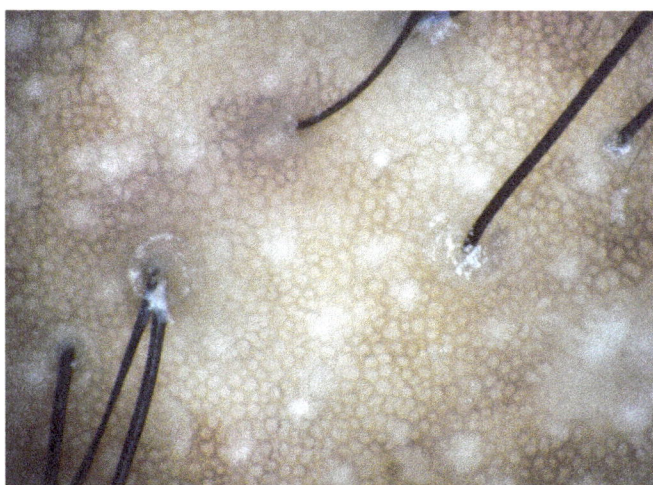

Fig. 5.1.12: Lichen planopilaris in a dark-skinned patient. Note white patches, and violaceous peripilar halo due to pigment incontinence.

Source: Division of Dermatology, Hospital das Clínicas, University of São Paulo Medical School.

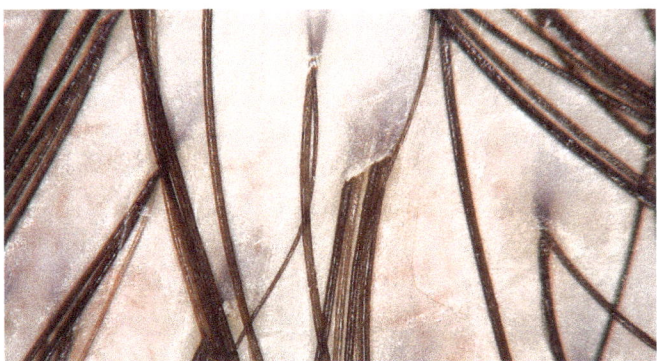

Fig. 5.1.13: Lichen planopilaris. Note mild peripilar scaling and small hair tufts in the occipital "normal-appearing" scalp. Mild dermoscopic features of inflammation may be seen all over the scalp in patients with scarring alopecias, despite the absence of evident clinical lesions.

Take-Home Message

- Lichen planopilaris is the most common type of scarring alopecia.
- Usually, it starts with scalp itching on the vertex area of the scalp.
- Skin, nails, vulvar, and gingival mucosa can show typical associated lesions.
- Scalp dermoscopy shows absence of follicular ostia and vellus hairs, peripilar erythema, peripilar scale, and diffuse erythema. Broken hairs, pili torti, and pigment incontinence may also be present.
- Peripilar scale indicates disease activity.
- "Normal-appearing" scalp areas may also show mild dermoscopic features, irrespective of evident clinical lesions.
- Treatment should be started as soon as possible to prevent disease progression.

SUGGESTED READING

1. Baibergenova A, Donovan J. Lichen planopilaris: update on pathogenesis and treatment. Skinmed. 2013;11(3):161-5.
2. Bolduc C, Sperling LC, Shapiro J. Primary cicatricial alopecia: Lymphocytic primary cicatricial alopecias, including lichen planopilaris, frontal fibrosing alopecia, and Graham-Little syndrome. J Am Acad Dermatol. 2016;75(6):1081-99.
3. Chiang C, Sah D, Cho BK, et al. Hydroxychloroquine and lichen planopilaris: efficacy and introduction of Lichen PlanopilarisActivity Index scoring system. J Am Acad Dermatol. 2010;62(3):387-92.
4. Christensen KN, Lehman JS, Tollefson MM. Pediatric lichen planopilaris: clinicopathologic study of four new cases and a review of the literature. Pediatr Dermatol. 2015;32(5):621-7.
5. Harries MJ, Messenger A. Treatment of frontal fibrosing alopecia and lichen planopilaris. J Eur Acad Dermatol Venereol. 2014;28(10):1404-5.
6. Meinhard J, Stroux A, Lünnemann L, et al. Lichen planopilaris: epidemiology and prevalence of subtypes—a retrospective analysis in 104 patients. J Dtsch Dermatol Ges. 2014;12(3):229-35, 229-36.
7. Mesinkovska NA, Tellez A, Dawes D, et al. The use of oral pioglitazone in the treatment of lichen planopilaris. J Am Acad Dermatol. 2015;72(2):355-6.
8. Misiak-Galazka M, Olszewska M, Rudnicka L. Lichen planopilaris in three generations: grandmother, mother, and daughter—a genetic link? Int J Dermatol. 2016;55(8):913-5.
9. Miteva M, Tosti A. Dermoscopy guided scalp biopsy in cicatricial alopecia. J Eur Acad Dermatol Venereol. 2013;27(10):1299-303.
10. Mubki T, Rudnicka L, Olszewska M, et al. Evaluation and diagnosis of the hair loss patient: part II. Trichoscopic and laboratory evaluations. J Am Acad Dermatol. 2014;71(3):431.
11. Naeini FF, Saber M, Asilian A, Hosseini SM. Clinical Efficacy and Safety of Methotrexate versus Hydroxychloroquine in Preventing LichenPlanopilaris Progress: A Randomized Clinical Trial. Int J Prev Med. 2017;8:37.
12. Olszewska M, Banka-Wrona A, Skrok A, et al. Vulvovaginal-gingival lichen planus: association with lichen planopilaris and stratified epithelium-specific antinuclear antibodies. Acta Derm Venereol. 2016;96(1):92-6.
13. Rakowska A, Slowinska M, Kowalska-Oledzka E, et al. Trichoscopy of cicatricial alopecia. J Drugs Dermatol. 2012;11(6):753-8.
14. Spano F, Donovan JC. Efficacy of oral retinoids in treatment-resistant lichen planopilaris. J Am Acad Dermatol. 2014;71(5):1016-8.
15. Vendramini DL, Silveira BR, Duque-Estrada B, et al. Isolated body hair loss: an unusual presentation of lichen planopilaris. Skin Appendage Disord. 2017;2(3-4):97-9.

5.2 Frontal Fibrosing Alopecia

Isabella Doche

Frontal fibrosing alopecia is a slowly progressive lymphocytic scarring alopecia. First considered as a subtype of lichen planopilaris in postmenopausal Caucasian women, this intriguing condition has become widespread worldwide in the last decade and appears to have different clinical lesions and responses to treatment.

Usually, this disease starts with eyebrow alopecia that progresses to frontotemporal band-like recession. Sometimes, areas of alopecia on the vertex and occipital scalp, facial papules, and lichen planus pigmentosum can be associated (Figs. 5.2.1A to D, 5.2.2A and B, 5.2.3, and 5.2.4A to C). Patients may refer symptoms as burning, pain, and itching.

On dermoscopy, the features are very similar, but milder to those in lichen planopilaris. The most common findings are the absence of follicular ostia, and of vellus hairs, peripilar erythema, peripilar scale, isolated and few black dots, pili torti, and occasional broken hairs (Figs. 5.2.5 to 5.2.10A to D, 5.2.11, and 5.2.12A and B).

Treatment options include finasteride/dutasteride, hydroxychloroquine, doxycycline, topical steroids, topical tacrolimus, and isotretinoin.

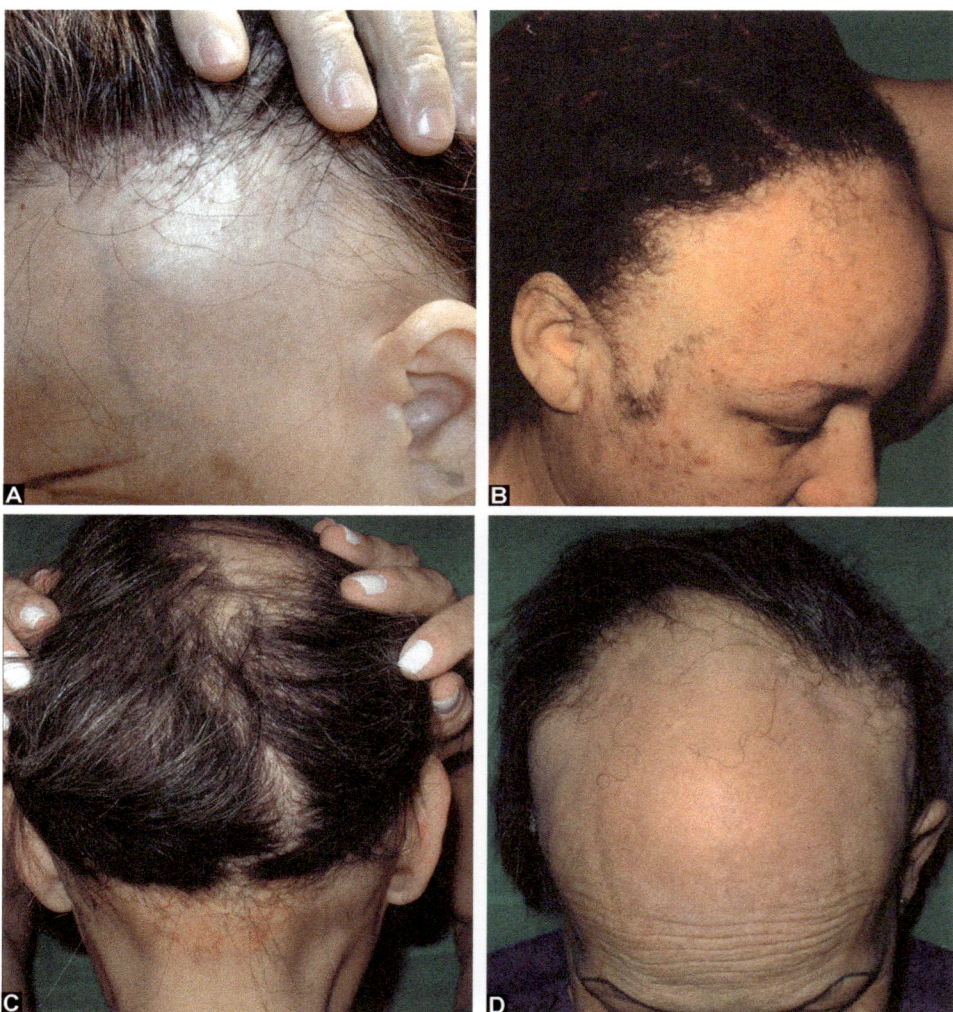

Figs. 5.2.1A to D: Frontal fibrosing alopecia. (A) Frontotemporal alopecia, mild peripilar erythema, single terminal hairs, scalp atrophy, and prominent frontal blood vessels. (B) "Pseudofringe" sign (unusual retention of the hairline), mimicking traction alopecia. (C) Vertex and occipital patches of scarring alopecia. (D) Extensive hairline recession.
Source: Division of Dermatology, Hospital das Clínicas, University of São Paulo Medical School.

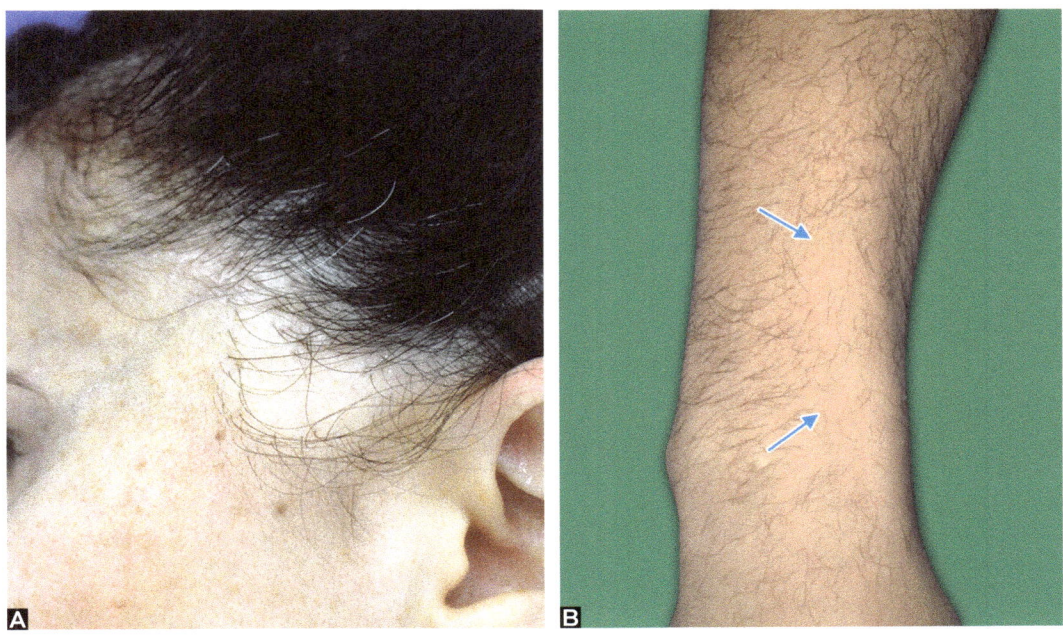

Figs. 5.2.2A and B: Frontal fibrosing alopecia (early disease). Early presentations may show localized areas of hair loss (blue arrows), mimicking alopecia areata.

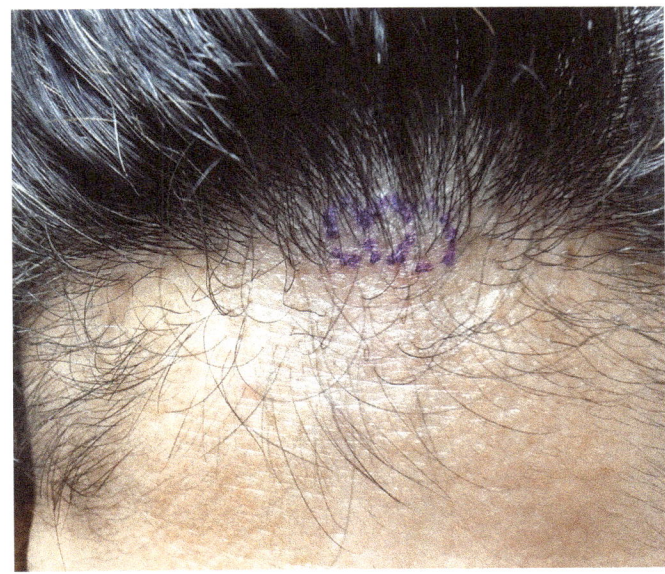

Fig. 5.2.3: Early frontal fibrosing alopecia. Patients may keep vellus hairs in early lesions. The irregular area of hair loss on the hairline made us suspect of the diagnosis which was later confirmed by the biopsy (marked areas).

Source: Division of Dermatology, Hospital das Clínicas, University of São Paulo Medical School.

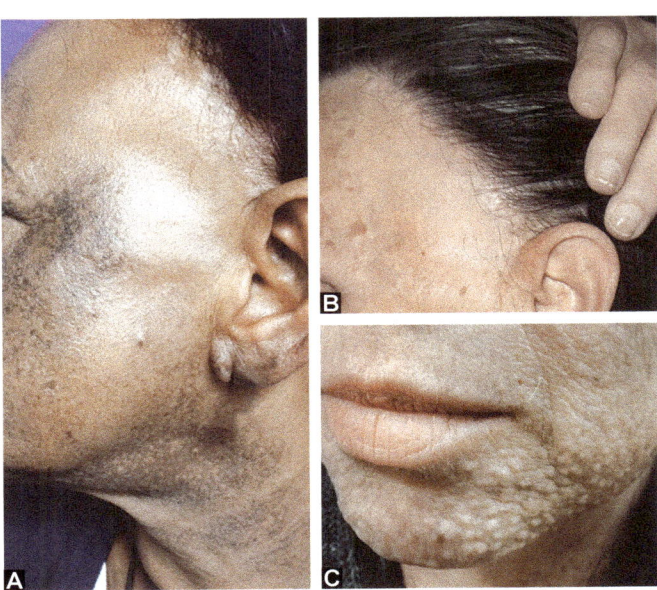

Figs. 5.2.4A to C: Frontal fibrosing alopecia. (A) Lichen planus pigmentosum on the face and neck. (B) Hypopigmented areas associated with temporal scarring alopecia. (C) Extensive facial papules.

Source: Division of Dermatology, Hospital das Clínicas, University of São Paulo Medical School.

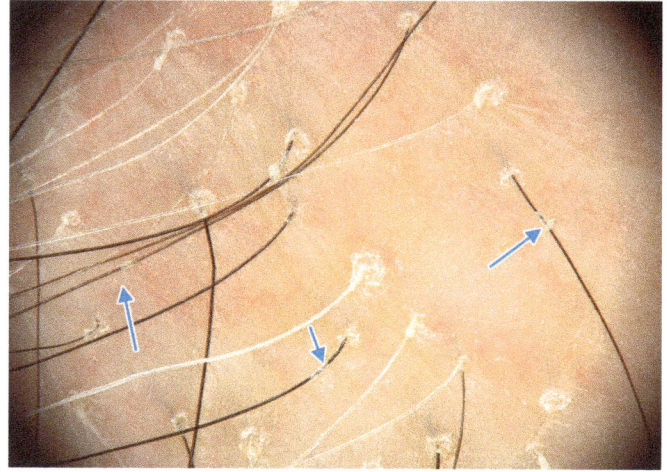

Fig. 5.2.5: Frontal fibrosing alopecia. Peripilar scale, absence of follicular ostia, and of vellus hairs. Note hair casts (blue arrows). Peripilar scales indicate active disease.

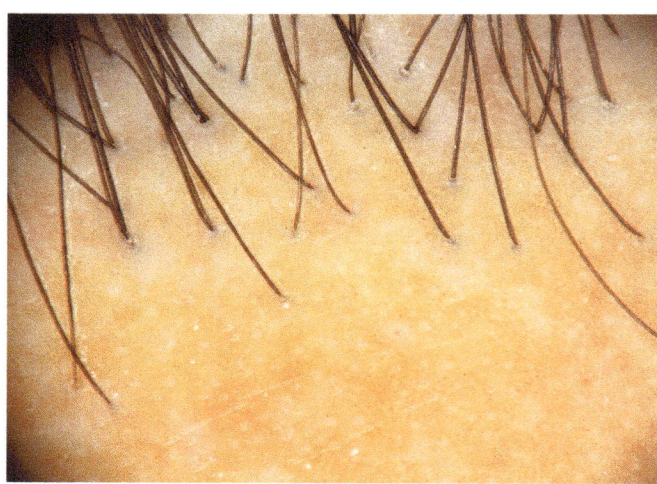

Fig. 5.2.6: Frontal fibrosing alopecia. Note the reduction of peripilar scale after the treatment (dry dermoscopy).

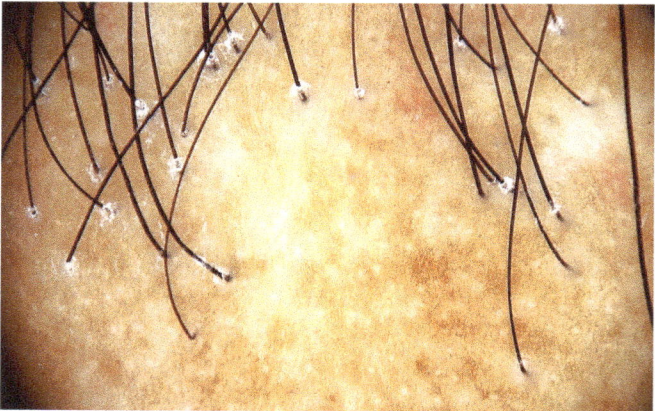

Fig. 5.2.7: Frontal fibrosing alopecia in dark-skinned patient. Note peripilar scale, white patches, and disruption of honeycomb pattern.

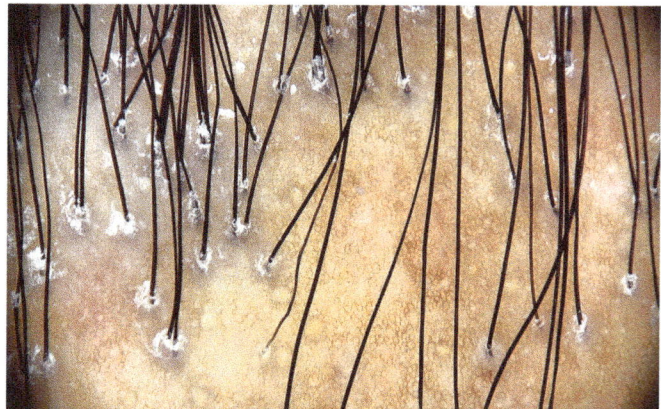

Fig. 5.2.8: Frontal fibrosing alopecia in dark-skinned patient. Note blue-gray peripilar halos and one pili torti.

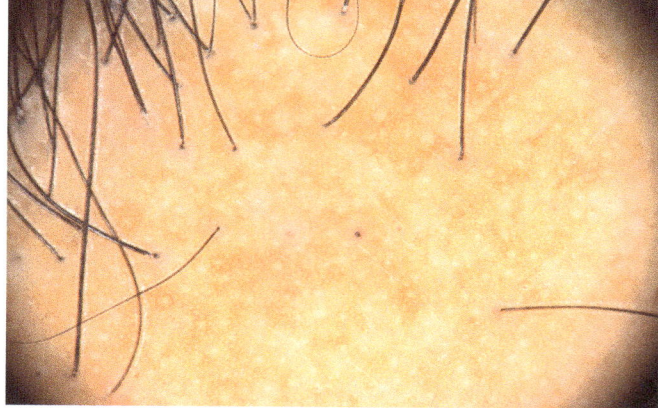

Fig. 5.2.9: Frontal fibrosing alopecia. Note isolated black dots.
Source: Division of Dermatology, Hospital das Clínicas, University of São Paulo Medical School.

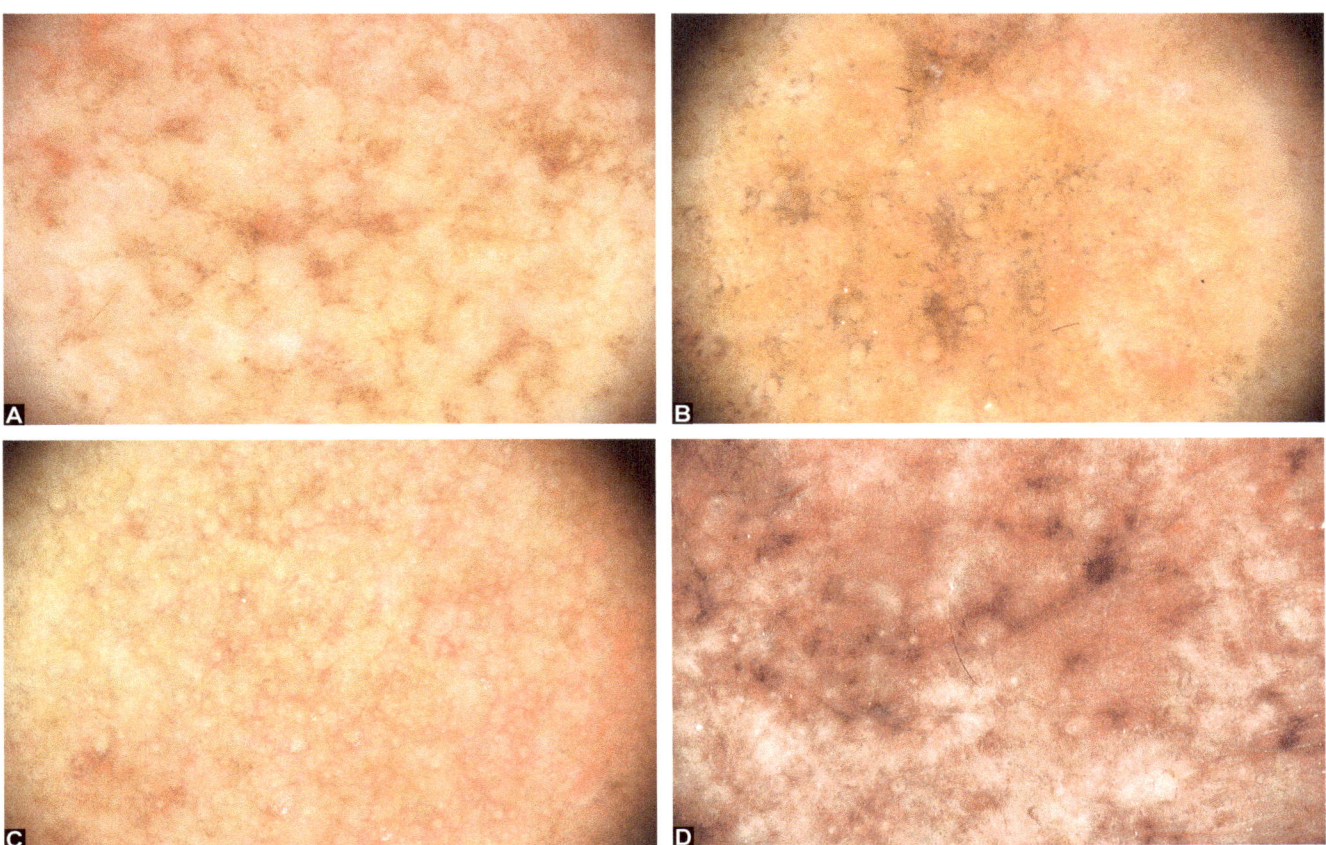

Figs. 5.2.10A to D: Lichen planus pigmentosum. Different dermoscopy presentations. Note (A) Speckled, (B) Mixed; and (C) Target, (D) Patterns of granular dots ranging from gray-brown to violaceus colors.
Source: Division of Dermatology, Hospital das Clínicas, University of São Paulo Medical School.

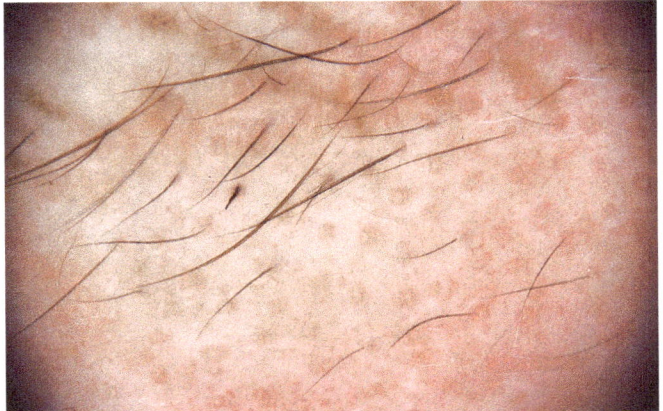

Fig. 5.2.11: Frontal fibrosing alopecia. Follicular red dots in the glabella and eyebrow areas. Note also yellow keratin plugs.
Source: Division of Dermatology, Hospital das Clínicas, University of São Paulo Medical School.

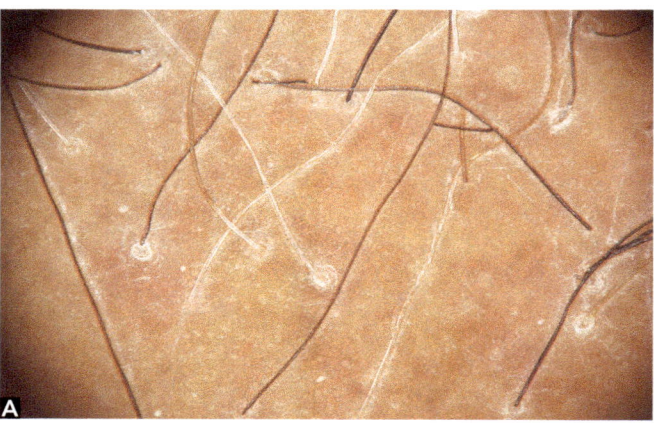 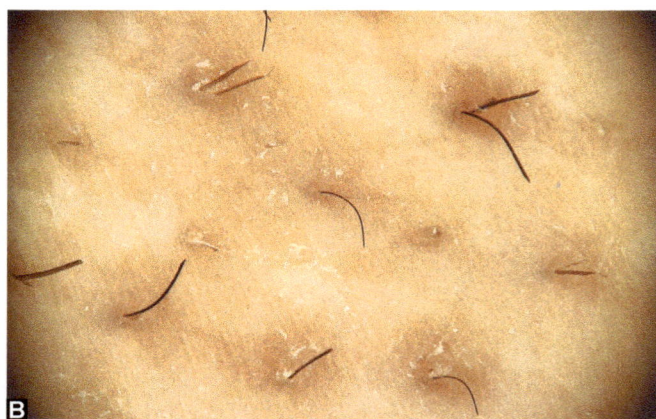

Figs. 5.2.12A and B: Frontal fibrosing alopecia. (A) Peripilar scale, broken hairs, and pili torti in the pubic skin area. (B) Mild peripilar scale, broken hairs, and hyperpigmented peripilar halos in the axillae.

Source: Division of Dermatology, Hospital das Clínicas, University of São Paulo Medical School.

Take-Home Message

- Frontal fibrosing alopecia is a scarring alopecia that usually presents with frontotemporal band-like recession, and eyebrow alopecia.
- Clinically, lesions are less inflamed than in lichen planopilaris, and patients may refer pain, burning, and itching.
- Lichen planus pigmentosum, "pseudofringe" sign, hypopigmented lesions, facial papules, and extremity alopecia may be associated.
- Dermoscopy shows absence of follicular ostia, and of vellus hairs, peripilar scale, and hair casts. Pili torti, broken hairs, black dots and glabellar red dots may often be present.
- "Normal-appearing" scalp and body areas may also show peripilar scale and mild erythema, irrespective of evident clinical lesions.

SUGGESTED READING

1. Alegre-Sánchez A, Saceda-Corralo D, Bernárdez C, et al. Frontal fibrosing alopecia in male patients: a report of 12 cases. J Eur Acad Dermatol Venereol. 2017;31(2):e112-4.
2. Anzai A, Donati A, Valente NY, et al. Isolated eyebrow loss in frontal fibrosing alopecia: relevance of early diagnosis and treatment. Br J Dermatol. 2016;175(5):1099-101.
3. Bolduc C, Sperling LC, Shapiro J. Primary cicatricial alopecia: lymphocytic primary cicatricial alopecias, including chronic cutaneous lúpus erythematosus, lichen planopilaris, frontal fibrosing alopecia, and Graham-Little syndrome. J Am Acad Dermatol. 2016;75(6):1081-99.
4. Bomar L, McMichael A. Frontal fibrosing alopecia: a research letter. Br J Dermatol. 2017;177(3):e58-9.
5. Dlova NC, Dadzie OE. Frontal fibrosing alopecia severity index (FFASI): a call for a more inclusive and globally relevant severity index for frontal fibrosing alopecia. Br J Dermatol. 2017;177(3):883-4.
6. Donati A, Molina L, Doche I, et al. Facial papules in frontal fibrosing alopecia: evidence of vellus follicle involvement. Arch Dermatol. 2011;147(12):1424-7.
7. Fertig R, Tosti A. Frontal fibrosing alopecia treatment options. Intractable Rare Dis Res. 2016;5(4):314-5.
8. Harries MJ, Wong S, Farrant P. Frontal fibrosing alopecia and increased scalp sweating: Is neurogenic inflammation a common link? Skin Appendage Disord. 2016;1(4):179-84.
9. Jimenez F, Harries M, Poblet E. Frontal fibrosing alopecia: a disease fascinating for the researcher, disappointing for the clinician and distressing for the patients. Exp Dermatol. 2016;25(11):853-4.
10. Lin J, Valdebran M, Bergfeld W, et al. Hypopigmentation in frontal fibrosing alopecia. J Am Acad Dermatol. 2017;76(6):1184-6.
11. Moreno-Arrones OM, Saceda-Corralo D, Fonda-Pascual P, et al. Frontal fibrosing alopecia: clinical and prognostic classification. J Eur Acad Dermatol Venereol. 2017;31(10):1739-45.
12. Pirmez R, Duque-Estrada B, Barreto T, et al. Successful treatment of facial papules in frontal fibrosing alopecia with oral isotretinoin. Skin Appendage Disord. 2017;3(2):111-3.
13. Pirmez R, Duque-Estrada B, Donati A, et al. Clinical and dermoscopic features of licehn planus pigmentosum in 37 patients with frontal fibrosing alopecia. Br J Dermatol. 2016;175(6):1387-90.

14. Pirmez R, Duque-Estrada B, Abraham LS, et al. It's not all traction: the pseudo 'fringe sign' in frontal fibrosing alopecia. Br J Dermatol. 2015;173(5):1336-8.
15. Rakowska A, Slowinska M, Kowalska-Oledzka E, et al. Trichoscopy of cicatricial alopecia. J Drugs Dermatol. 2012;11(6):753-8.
16. Romiti R, Biancardi Gavioli CF, Anzai A, et al. Clinical and histopathological findings of frontal fibrosing alopecia-associated lichen planus pigmentosum. Skin Appendage Disord. 2017;3(2):59-63.
17. Rossi A, Grassi S, Fortuna MC, et al. Unusual patterns of presentation of frontal fibrosing alopecia: a clinical and trichoscopic analysis of 98 patients. J Am Acad Dermatol. 2017;77(1):172-4.
18. Tziotzios C, Stefanato CM, Fenton DA, et al. Frontal fibrosing alopecia: reflections and hypotheses on aetiology and pathogenesis. Exp Dermatol. 2016;25(11):847-52.
19. Vañó-Galván S, Molina-Ruiz AM, Serrano-Falcón AC, et al. Frontal fibrosing alopecia: a multicenter review of 355 patients. J Am Acad Dermatol. 2014;70(4):670-8.
20. Yin NC, Tosti A. A systematic approach to Afro-textured hair disorders: dermatoscopy and when to biopsy. Dermatol Clin. 2014;32(2):145-51.

5.3 Fibrosing Alopecia in a Pattern Distribution

Giselle Martins, Patricia Damasco, Isabella Doche

Fibrosing alopecia in a pattern distribution (FAPD) is a distinct type of cicatricial alopecia characterized by inflammation and fibrosis limited to the area of androgenetic hair loss. It remains unclear whether FAPD represents a variant of lichen planopilaris (LPP) or an unusual manifestation of androgenetic alopecia (AGA) with reactive, lichenoid inflammation on histopathology.

The striking differences between AGA and FAPD include perifollicular erythema, perifollicular scale, and areas without follicular orifices in the central scalp in FAPD (Figs. 5.3.1A and B). Compared with LPP, patients with FAPD usually present a milder inflammation with a partial hair loss in the central area of the scalp, without areas of frank alopecia (Fig. 5.3.1C)

Dermoscopy shows increased variability of hair shaft diameter, vellus hairs, perifollicular scale, and erythema, due to follicular inflammation and fibrosis. Usually, follicular ostia are preserved, but, in some cases, focal absence of follicular openings can be seen, suggesting a scarring process (Figs. 5.3.2 and 5.3.3A and B). Small tufted hairs with two to four hair shafts emerging from the same ostium, known as compound hairs, associated with peripilar scales in an area of hair thinning may be present (Fig. 5.3.4A). As in LPP, "normal-appearing" scalp areas may also show a mild peripilar scale and erythema in FAPD lesions (Figs. 5.3.4B and C).

Independent from the given name FAPD or subtle LPP associated with AGA, the clinician should be aware of this condition and proceed with scalp biopsies for the diagnosis in patients with hair thinning and concomitant redness and scaling. This is particularly true for patients who do not improve with standard treatment and those requesting hair transplantation.

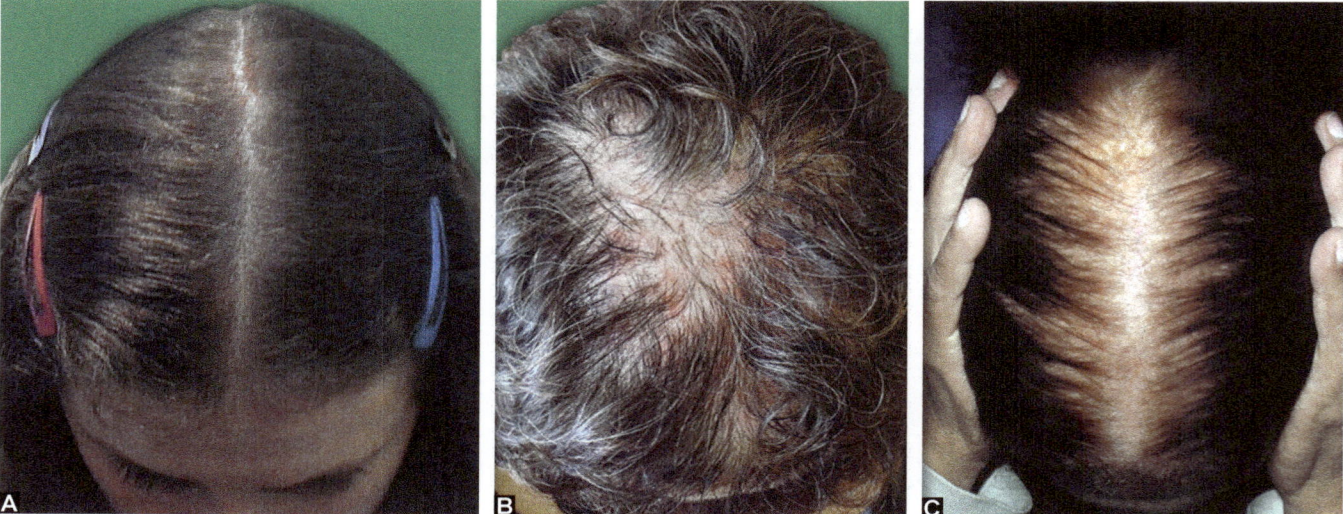

Figs. 5.3.1A to C: Fibrosing alopecia in a pattern distribution. (A) Early case with mild erythema and scale over the central region of the scalp. (B) Moderate hair thinning, partial hair loss, and erythema in the vertex scalp. (C) Severe hair loss with scarring areas in the anterior midline of the scalp.
Source: (C) Division of Dermatology, Hospital das Clínicas, University of São Paulo Medical School.

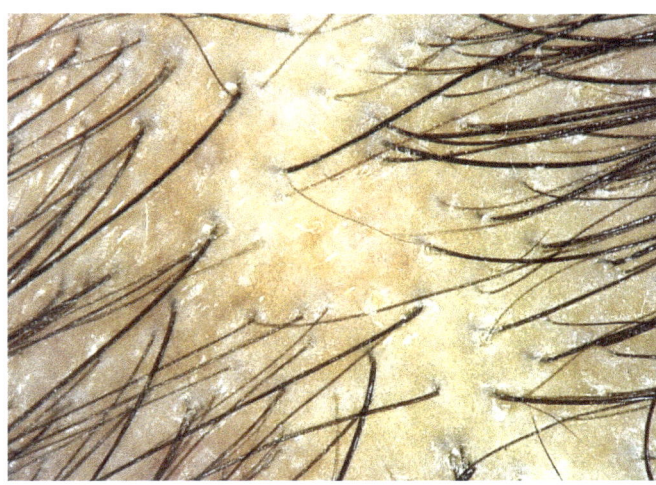

Fig. 5.3.2: Fibrosing alopecia in a pattern distribution. Dry dermoscopy shows hair thickness variability, peripilar scale, and some whitish areas devoid of hair follicles in the vertex area of the scalp from a patient with early disease.

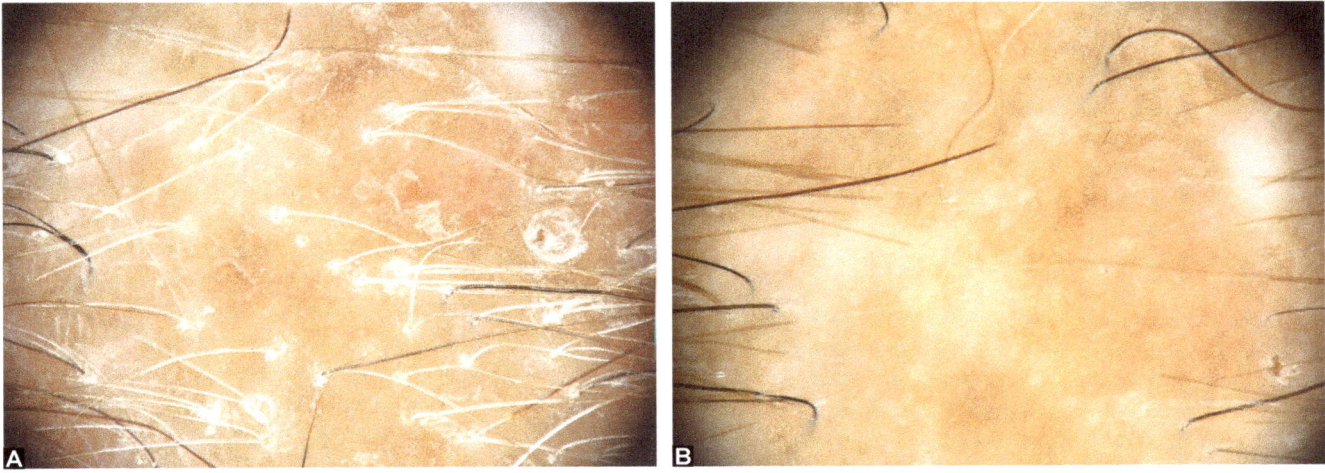

Figs. 5.3.3A and B: Fibrosing alopecia in a pattern distribution. (A) Dry dermoscopy can better detect peripilar scales surrounding white hair shafts. (B) Dermoscopy with immersion fluid shows white scarring patches devoid of follicular openings. Note that the visualization of white hair shafts is impaired by the immersion fluid.
Source: Division of Dermatology, Hospital das Clínicas, University of São Paulo Medical School.

There is no cure for FAPD and treatments are proposed to control symptoms or halt disease progression. Treatment options include topical minoxidil, oral finasteride or dutasteride, and systemic antiinflammatory treatment (corticosteroids, topical calcineurin inhibitors, oral doxycycline, and hydroxychloroquine).

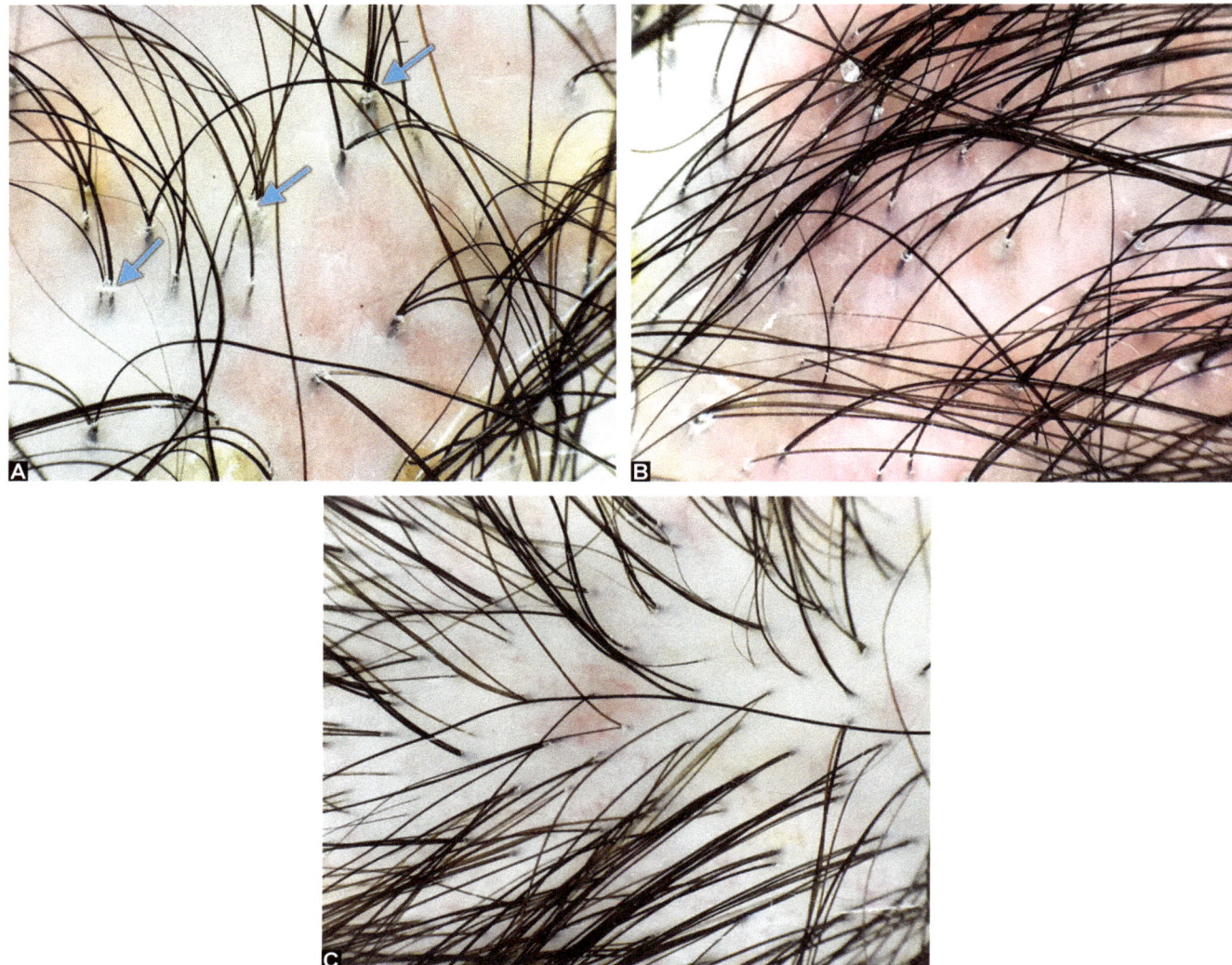

Figs. 5.3.4A to C: Fibrosing alopecia in a pattern distribution. (A) Dermoscopy from the vertex scalp shows hair thinning, peripilar scale, white scarring areas with the absence of follicular openings, and milky-red areas. Note the small tufts or "compound hairs," surrounded by a peripilar scale (blue arrows). (B) Perilesional peripilar scales and diffuse erythema. (C) "Normal-appearing" area in the occipital scalp shows also mild peripilar scales, hair thinning, and a mild erythema, pointing that all the scalp may be compromised in this disease.

Take-Home Message
- Fibrosing alopecia in a pattern distribution is considered a subtype of lichen planopilaris.
- Hair thinning and partial hair loss are associated with scaling and erythema, mostly in the central areas of the scalp.
- Dermoscopy shows increased hair diameter variability, vellus hairs, peripilar scale, peripilar erythema, and some white scarring areas with lack of follicular openings.
- Small tufts or "compound hairs" structures may be present.
- "Normal-appearing" areas may also show mild dermoscopic features of inflammation.
- Treatment includes antiandrogenic and antiinflammatory drugs.

SUGGESTED READING

1. Amato L, Chiarini C, Berti S, et al. Case study: fibrosing alopecia in a pattern distribution localized on alopecia androgenetica areas and unaffected scalp. Skinmed. 2004;3(6):353-5.
2. Abbasi A, Kamyab-Hesari K, Rabbani R, et al. A new subtype of lichen planopilaris affecting vellus hairs and clinically mimicking androgenetic alopecia. Dermatol Surg. 2016;42(10):1174-80.
3. Baquerizo Nole KL, Nusbaum B, Pinto GM, et al. Lichen planopilaris in the androgenetic alopecia area: a pitfall for hair transplantation. Skin Appendage Disord. 2015;1(1):49-53.
4. Chiu HY, Lin SJ. Fibrosing alopecia in a pattern distribution. J Eur Acad Dermatol Venereol. 2010;24(9):1113-4.
5. Fergie B, Khaira G, Howard V, et al. Diffuse scarring alopecia in a female pattern hair loss distribution. Australas J Dermatol. 2017;[Epub ahead of print].
6. Olsen EA. Female pattern hair loss and its relationship to permanent/cicatricial alopecia: a new perspective. J Investig Dermatol Symp Proc. 2005;10(3):217-21.
7. Ramanauskaite A, Trüeb RM. Facial papules in fibrosing alopecia in a pattern distribution (cicatricial pattern hair loss). Int J Trichology. 2015;7(3):119-22.
8. Trémezavques L, Vogt T, Müller CS. Frontal fibrosing alopecia with androgenetic pattern. A diagnostic challenge—a therapeutic problem. Hautarzt. 2012;63(5):411-4.
9. Turegano MM, Sperling LC. Lichenoid folliculitis: a unifying concept. J Cutan Pathol. 2017;[Epub ahead of print].
10. Zinkernagel MS, Trüeb RM. Fibrosing alopecia in a pattern distribution: patterned lichen planopilaris or androgenetic alopecia with a lichenoid tissue reaction pattern? Arch Dermatol. 2000;136(2):205-11.

5.4 Discoid Lupus Erythematosus

Patricia Damasco, Giselle Martins, Isabella Doche

Discoid lupus erythematosus (DLE) is a chronic lymphocytic scarring alopecia. Although controversial, some authors do not consider DLE as a primary cicatricial alopecia, because both interfollicular and follicular epidermis are damaged and the hair follicle is secondarily affected. The onset of DLE typically occurs between the ages of 20 and 40 years old, predominantly in females (3:2 to 3:1). It may occur in patients with systemic lupus erythematosus; however, only 5–10% of patients with DLE develop systemic disease.

In early stages, patients may complain of scalp tenderness, pain, and itching. DLE lesions are characterized by erythematous and edematous scaly plaques, with follicular hyperkeratosis, atrophy, and telangiectasia, mostly in the scalp, face, and ear areas (Figs. 5.4.1A to C). Dermoscopy shows loss of follicular openings, follicular red dots, thick arborizing vessels, and multiple small keratin plugs (Figs. 5.4.2 to 5.4.5). The presence of follicular red dots indicates active disease and a good prognosis (Fig. 5.4.6). Red dots correspond to dilated follicular openings surrounded by dilated vessels. In dark-skinned patients, pigmentary changes are often present, such as scattered brown discoloration and blue-gray dots in a specked pattern, and correspond to pigment incontinence in histopathology. In late stages, lesions become depressed and depigmented (Fig. 5.4.7). Milky-red areas and large yellow dots with radial, thin arborizing vessels emerging from the dot ("red

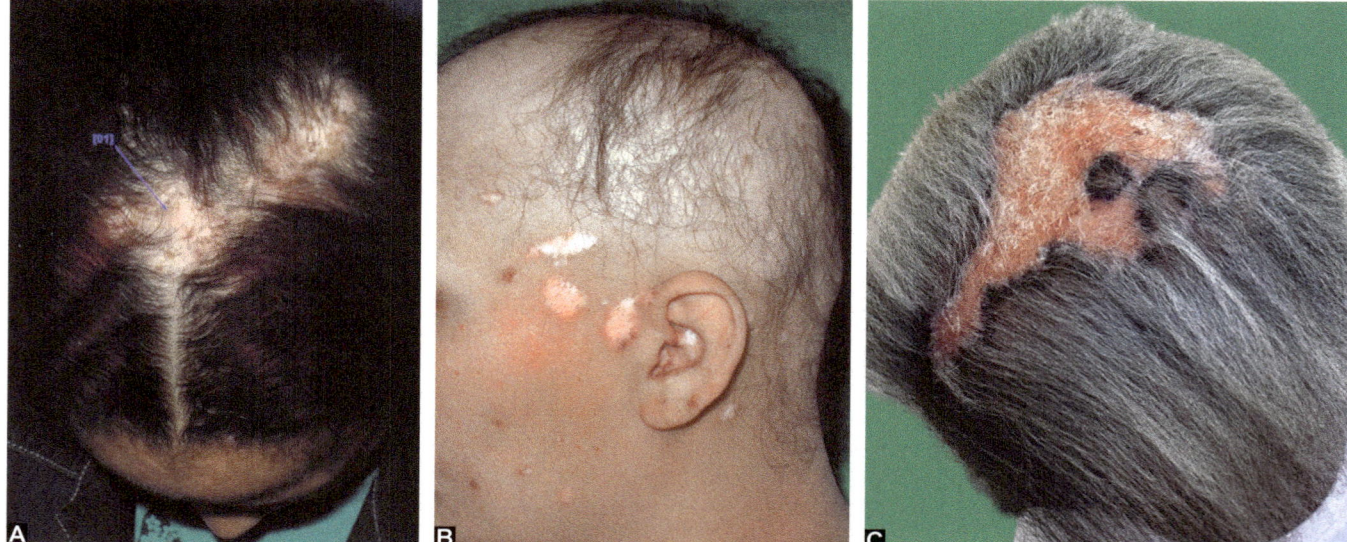

Figs. 5.4.1A to C: Discoid lupus erythematosus. (A) Scarring patches on the vertex scalp with pigmented areas. Loss of pigment (blue arrow) can also be seen and is a typical finding. (B) Multiple discoid erythematous lesions on the face and inside the ears in a patient with systemic lupus and diffuse hair loss. (C) Severe presentation of the disease with edematous and diffuse thick scaling areas of alopecia.
Source: (A and B) Division of Dermatology, Hospital das Clínicas, University of São Paulo Medical School.

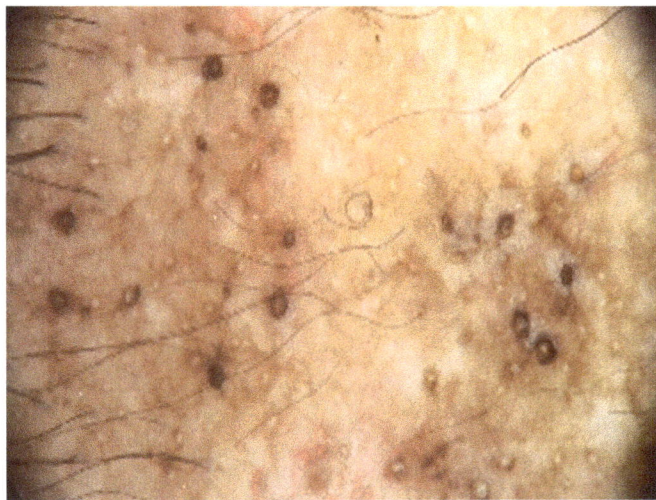

Fig. 5.4.2: Discoid lupus erythematosus. Multiple and small keratotic plugs are seen in active disease and correspond to keratin occluding the dilated infundibular openings. Note also a scattered brown discoloration as a result of pigment incontinence and loss of follicular openings.

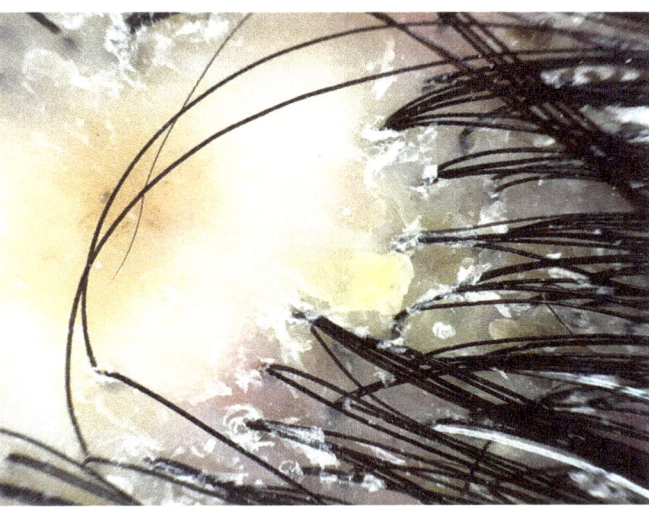

Fig. 5.4.3: Discoid lupus erythematosus. Scales at the periphery of the lesion, peripilar scales, and a white fibrotic central area devoid of follicular openings. Perifollicular scale may resemble lichen planopilaris lesions.

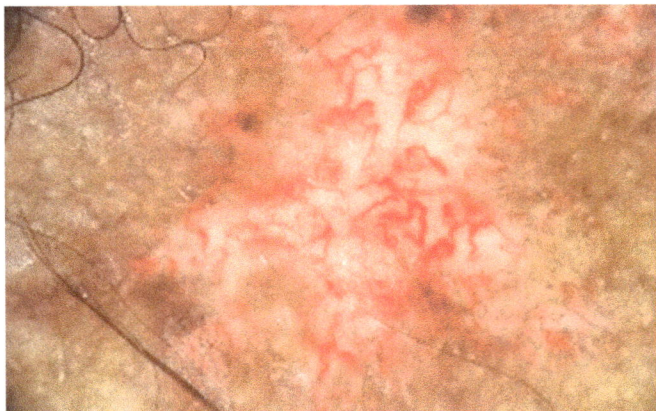

Fig. 5.4.4: Discoid lupus erythematosus. Enlarged branching vessels associated with pigmentary changes are highly suggestive for diagnosis of discoid lupus. Note the tortuous and irregular "bushy" capillaries.

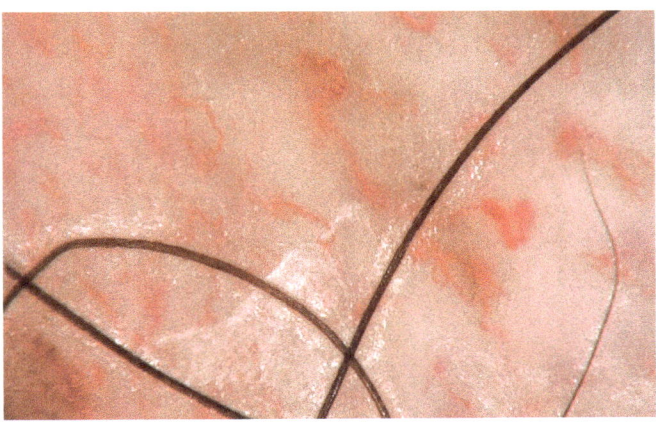

Fig. 5.4.5: Discoid lupus erythematosus. Thick arborizing vessels are thicker than the average of the hair shaft diameter. Note also speckled brown pigmentation.

spider" in a yellow dot) are considered highly characteristic of late, prefibrotic DLE lesions (Fig. 5.4.8).

Active discoid lupus should be early treated in order to prevent permanent and scarring alopecia. Localized disease can be treated with topical and/or intralesional steroids. Multiple and systemic presentations may require systemic steroids and antimalarials. Alternative options with variable efficacy include dapsone, mycophenolate mofetil, methotrexate, azathioprine, isotretinoin, clofazimine, and oral vitamin E.

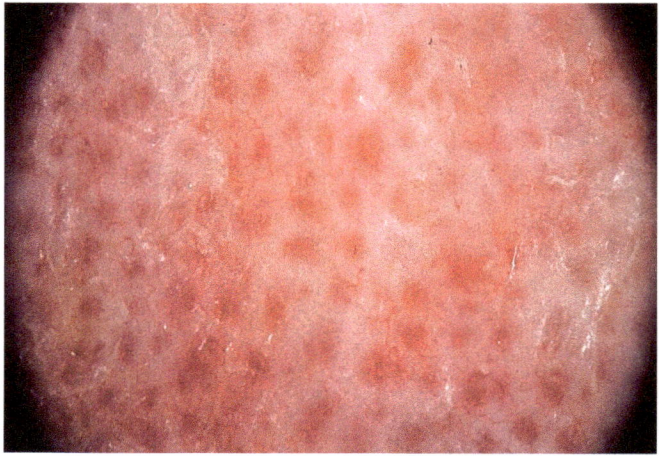

Fig. 5.4.6: Discoid lupus erythematosus. Red dots are indicative of active disease with the possibility of hair regrowth with treatment. They correspond to widened infundibula with dense perivascular infiltrate, dilated vessels, and extravasated erythrocytes.

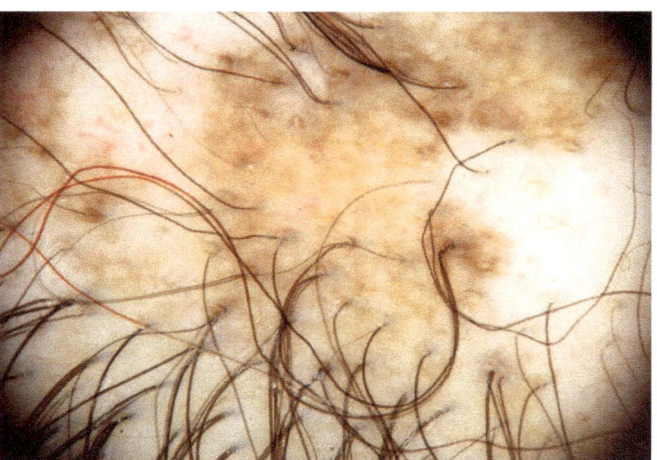

Fig. 5.4.7: Discoid lupus erythematosus. Loss of follicular openings, pili torti, loss of pigment, thick vessels, and scattered brown pigmentation.
Source: Division of Dermatology, Hospital das Clínicas, University of São Paulo Medical School.

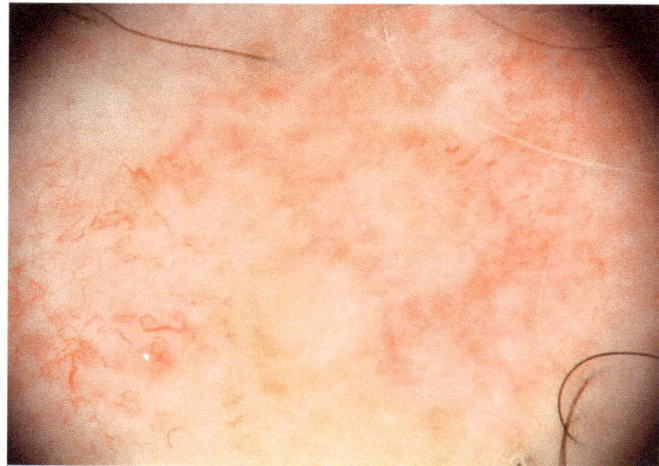

Fig. 5.4.8: Discoid lupus erythematosus. Milky-red areas, fibrotic scarring patches, with thin arborizing ("red spiders") and giant vessels surrounding large yellow dots (left) indicate late stage of the disease.
Source: Division of Dermatology, Hospital das Clínicas, University of São Paulo Medical School.

Take-Home Message
- Multiple oval-shaped scarring patches over the scalp (especially sun-exposed areas) are the main clinical presentation.
- Facial and ear lesions may be also present.
- Dermoscopy shows multiple and small keratotic plugs, follicular red dots, thick arborizing vessels, perifollicular scale, hair casts, loss of follicular openings, and white scarring patches.
- Dark-skinned patients usually show areas with loss of pigment, scattered brown pigmentation, and blue-gray dots in a speckled pattern.
- In longstanding disease, milky-red or white scarring areas are present.
- Follicular red dots indicate good prognosis with high chances of hair regrowth.
- Early treatment may prevent areas of permanent hair loss.

SUGGESTED READING

1. Duque-Estrada B, Tamler C, Sodre CT, et al. Dermatoscopy patterns of cicatricial alopecia resulting from discoid lupus erythematosus and lichen planopilaris. An Bras Dermatol. 2010;85(2):179-83.
2. Hordinsky M. Cicatricial alopecia: discoid lupus erythematosus. Dermatol Ther. 2008;21(4):245-8.
3. Lopez-Tintos BO, Garcia-Hidalgo L, Orozco-Topete R. Dermoscopy in active discoid lupus. Arch Dermatol. 2009;145(3):358.
4. Miteva M, Tosti A. Hair and scalp dermatoscopy. J Am Acad Dermatol. 2012;67(5):1040-8.
5. Moghadam-Kia S, Franks AG Jr. Autoimmune disease and hair loss. Dermatol Clin. 2013;31(1):75-91.
6. Rakowska A, Slowinska M, Kowalska-Oledzka E, et al. Trichoscopy of cicatricial alopecia. J Drugs Dermatol. 2012;11(6):753-8.
7. Rigopoulos D, Stamatios G, Ioannides D. Primary scarring alopecias. Curr Probl Dermatol. 2015;47:76-86.
8. Ross EK, Shapiro J. Primary cicatricial alopecia. In: Blume-Peytavi U, Tosti A, Whiting D, Trueb R, (Eds). Hair Growth and Disorders. Leipzig: Springer; 2008. pp. 293-4.
9. Rudnicka L, Rakowska A, Olszewska M. Trichoscopy. How it may help the clinician. Dermatol Clin. 2013;31(1):29-41.
10. Tosti A, Torres F, Misciali C, et al. Follicular red dots: a novel dermoscopic pattern observed in scalp discoid lupus erythematosus. Arch Dermatol. 2009;145(12):1406-9.

5.5 Traction Alopecia—Late Stage

Patricia Damasco, Giselle Martins, Isabella Doche

Traction alopecia (TA) is a form of alopecia that occurs as a result of chronic and excessive tension on the hair follicles. Although reversible if early treated, longstanding TA can lead to permanent hair loss. It is most prevalent in black patients, mainly attributed to the specific hair care practices (tight braids, hair weaves, and cornrows).

Usually, the areas of alopecia are symmetrical along the frontotemporal areas, as these areas bear the most tension. The presence of short hairs scattered along the frontotemporal line is a characteristic finding of TA and is called "fringe sign" (Fig. 5.5.1). The involvement of the occipital region is unusual, and the differential diagnosis with ophiasis alopecia is imperative (Fig. 5.5.2).

Thin and vellus hairs are typically preserved, as these are not traction bearing. In longstanding diseases, fibrosis occurs, and hair loss can be permanent. A similar clinical presentation, a "pseudofringe sign", can occur in patients with frontal fibrosing alopecia, despite the presence of associated TA. Some cases may require skin biopsies to rule out frontal fibrosing alopecia.

Dermoscopy of late stage lesions shows decreased hair density, thinned hairs, and lack of follicular openings with white irregular patches. Broken hairs and black dots may eventually be found (Figs. 5.5.3 and 5.5.4). Disrupted pigment network can be easily seen in dark-skinned patients (Fig. 5.5.5).

Treatment involves adopting hair practices that minimize traction and treating the inflammation if present. Stopping traction and use of topical minoxidil can help hair regrowth in early cases. Advanced cases may require surgical options as hair transplantation.

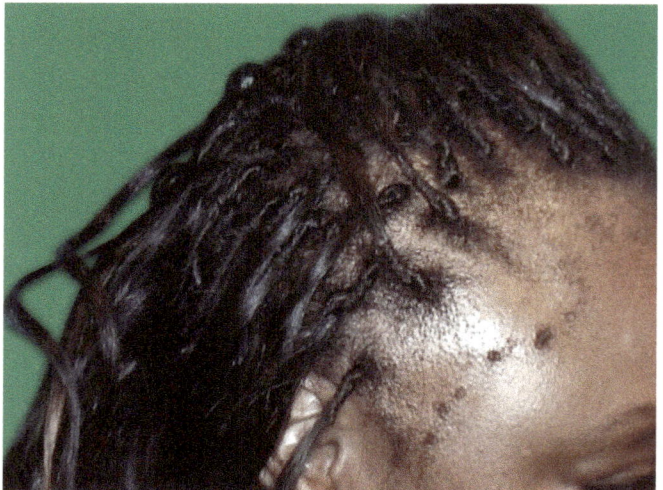

Fig. 5.5.1: Traction alopecia, late stage. Fringe sign, the presence of hairs along the frontal and/or terminal is highly suggestive. Note the shiny and atrophic scalp skin. A similar clinical presentation (pseudofringe sign) can occur in patients with frontal fibrosing alopecia, despite the presence of associated traction alopecia.

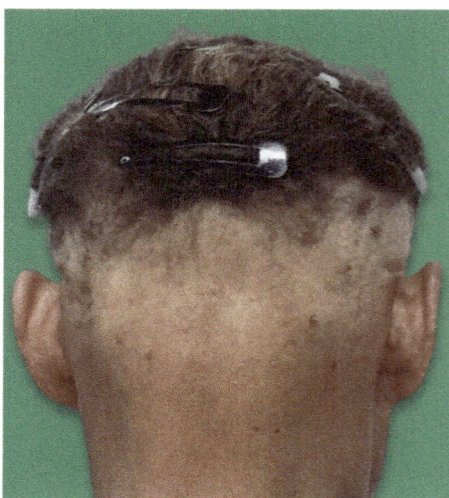

Fig. 5.5.2: Traction alopecia, late stage. Severe decrease of hair density in the occipital scalp.

Scarring Alopecias

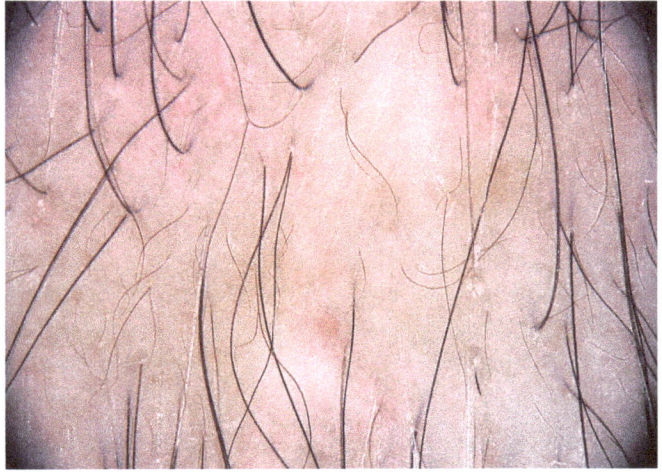

Fig. 5.5.3: Traction alopecia, late stage. Broken hairs, vellus hairs, and white scarring areas with loss of follicular openings in a Caucasian patient.

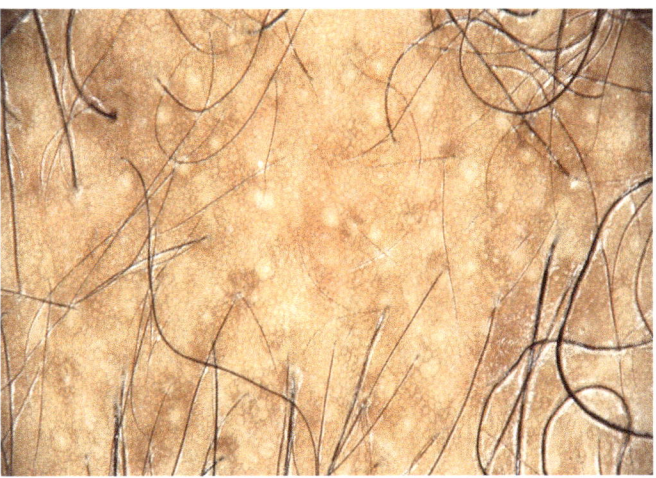

Fig. 5.5.4: Traction alopecia, late stage. Note the persistence of vellus hairs in a dark-skinned patient.

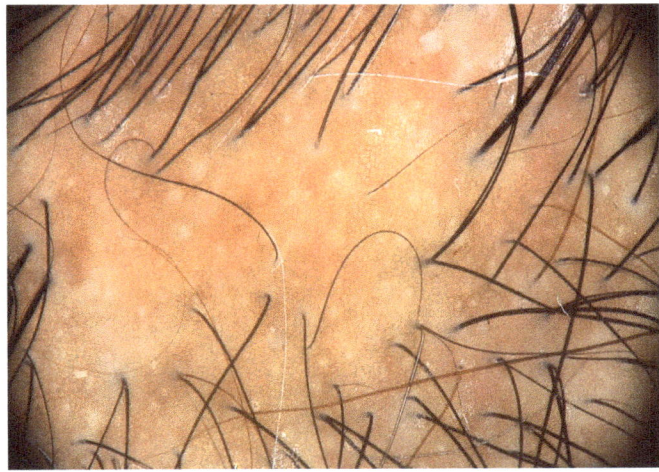

Fig. 5.5.5: Traction alopecia, late stage. Loss of follicular openings, disrupted honeycomb pattern, irregular pinpoint white dots and white patches in a dark-skinned patient.

Take-Home Message
- Traction alopecia is a hair loss secondary to repetitive tension on the hair.
- Longstanding traction alopecia can lead to permanent alopecia.
- The presence of retained hairs along the frontal and/or temporal rim known as "fringe sign" is highly suggestive.
- "Pseudofringe sign" can be present in frontal fibrosing alopecia, despite hair traction.
- Dermoscopy of late stage disease shows decreased hair density, thinned hairs, lack of follicular openings, white scarring patches. Broken hairs and black dots may eventually be present.
- Disrupted pigmented network may be easily seen in dark-skinned patients and may be a clue to the diagnosis.

SUGGESTED READING

1. Barbosa AB, Donati A, Valente NS, et al. Patchy alopecia mimicking areata. Int J Trichology. 2015;7(4):184-6.
2. Haskin A, Aguh C. All hairstyles are not created equal: what the dermatologist needs to know about black hairstyling practices and the risk of traction alopecia. J Am Acad Dermatol. 2016;75(3):606-11.
3. Heath CR, Taylor SC. Alopecia in an ophiasis pattern: traction alopecia versus alopecia areata. Cutis. 2012;89(5):213-6.
4. Lawson CN, Hollinger J, Sethi S, et al. Updates in the understanding and treatments of skin and hair disorders in women of color. Int J Womens Dermatol. 2017;3(1 Suppl):S21-37.
5. Lindsey SF, Tosti A. Ethnic hair disorders. Curr Probl Dermatol. 2015;47:139-49.
6. Pirmez R, Duque-Estrada B, Abraham LS, et al. It's not all traction: the pseudo 'fringe sign' in frontal fibrosing alopecia. Br J Dermatol. 2015;173(5):1336-8.
7. Polat M. Evaluation of clinical signs and early and late trichoscopy findings in traction alopecia patients with Fitzpatrick skin type II and III: a single-center, clinical study. Int J Dermatol. 2017;56(8):850-5.
8. Samrao A, Price VH, Zedek D, et al. The "Fringe Sign"—A useful clinical finding in traction alopecia of the marginal hair line. Dermatol Online J. 2011;17(11):1.
9. Xu L, Liu KX, Senna MM. A practical approach to the diagnosis and management of hair loss in children and adolescents. Front Med (Lausanne). 2017;4:112.

5.6 Central Centrifugal Cicatricial Alopecia

Laura N Uwakwe, Amy McMichael, Patricia Damasco, Isabella Doche

Central centrifugal cicatricial alopecia (CCCA) is a primary lymphocytic scarring disorder commonly seen in African American women. Its current name, created by the North American Hair Research Society, was coined to reflect the clinical features of this condition: a form of scarring hair loss (cicatricial alopecia) that typically begins at the vertex or crown of the scalp (central) and progresses outward (centrifugal). CCCA is the most common scarring alopecia among African American women, although rare in male patients.

The etiology of CCCA remains uncertain. First described as "hot comb alopecia," CCCA was previously believed to be the result of chronic inflammation caused by heated petrolatum making contact with the scalp, during the process of hair straightening with a heated metal comb or hot comb. This hypothesis was later debunked when several cases of CCCA were described in patients that had never used a hot comb to straighten their hair. Other hair grooming habits that result in physical stress or trauma to the hair follicle, such as the use of chemical hair straighteners making contact with the scalp, the uses of hooded hair dryers, or hair styles that pull tightly on the hair (e.g. braided extensions and weaves), may play a role. A genetic component may also contribute to the process, as two studies indicated a likely autosomal dominant pattern with partial penetrance.

Patients typically present with complaints of balding at the vertex or crown of their scalp. Scalp tenderness, erythema, and itching may occur. Hair breakage in the crown region may also be an early sign of CCCA. Physical findings include symmetrical hair loss confined to the vertex of the scalp that is most pronounced in the center of the affected area that may coalesce to scarring patches (Fig. 5.6.1A). Traction alopecia is usually associated (Fig. 5.6.1B). Early cases can mimic androgenetic alopecia. In long-standing and inflamed lesions, lichen planopilaris should be ruled out.

Dermoscopy shows perifollicular scale with a peripilar gray-white halo which corresponds to the lamellar fibrosis surrounding the outer root sheath on pathology (Fig. 5.6.2). A blue-gray perifollicular color can also be present in more inflamed lesions due to pigment incontinence in dark-skinned patients. Other findings include preserved honeycomb pattern, irregular pinpoint white dots distribution, some vellus hairs with sparse terminal hairs, and irregular white scarring areas with the absence of follicular openings (Fig. 5.6.3). Broken hairs and black dots may also be present. Perifollicular erythema may be difficult to notice in dark-skinned patients. The main differential diagnosis is lichen planopilaris, which usually presents with more inflamed lesions and variable associated body lesions.

Treatment is typically centered in halting the inflammatory process from progressing and preserving the hair follicles that have not been destroyed. Varied combinations of daily topical steroid use serial intralesional steroid injections, and oral tetracycline antibiotics are used as first-line therapy, and hydroxychloroquine or immunosuppressants may be considered for refractory cases. Avoiding any hair care practice that may put any stress on the hair follicle and early intervention are the keys, as hair follicles that have been destroyed cannot be recovered.

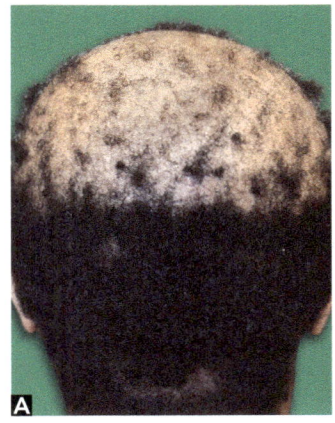 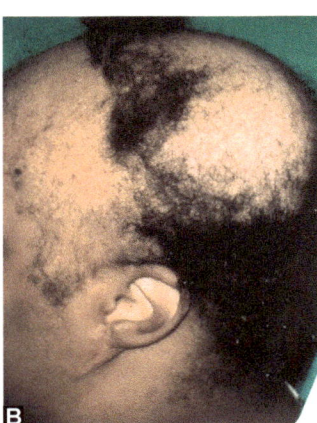

Figs. 5.6.1A and B: Central centrifugal cicatricial alopecia. (A) Diffuse alopecic patch sparing some areas of terminal hair shafts on the vertex and lateral scalp. Note that the patches are not completely bald. (B) Associated traction alopecia. Note the "fringe sign", some hairs retained on the frontotemporal line.

Source: Division of Dermatology, Hospital das Clínicas, University of São Paulo Medical School.

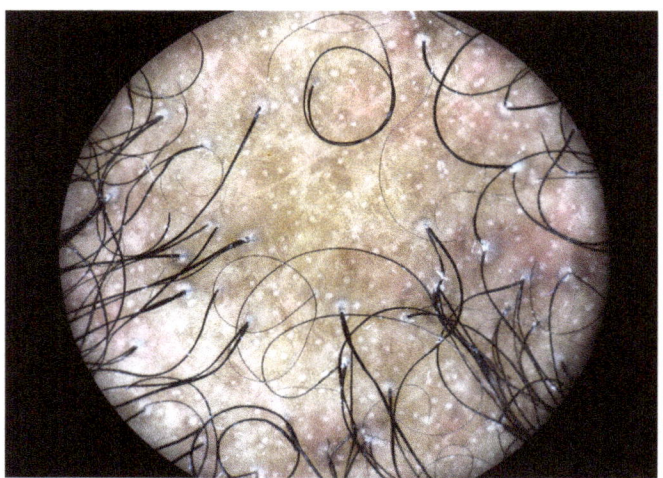

Fig. 5.6.2: Central centrifugal cicatricial alopecia. Perifollicular scale and gray-white halo in the occipital scalp from an African descent patient. Note also a mild erythema and white scarring dots.

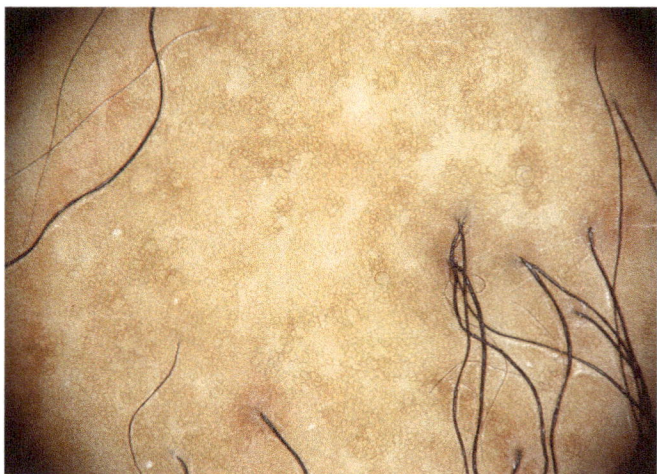

Fig. 5.6.3: Central centrifugal cicatricial alopecia. Irregular distribution of pinpoint white dots, irregular white scarring areas, decreased hair density with few vellus hairs, and scarce terminal hairs with hyperpigmented perifollicular halo in an African descent patient.

Source: Division of Dermatology, Hospital das Clínicas, University of São Paulo Medical School.

> **Take-Home Message**
> - Central centrifugal cicatricial alopecia is the most common type of scarring alopecia in African descent women.
> - Usually, it affects the vertex of the scalp with a centrifugal spread pattern.
> - Scalp itching and tenderness may be present.
> - Dermoscopy shows gray-white perifollicular halo, perifollicular discoloration, irregular white patch areas, absence of follicular ostia, irregular distribution of pinpoint white dots, few vellus hairs, perifollicular scale, and broken hairs.
> - Androgenetic alopecia and lichen planopilaris are the main differential diagnoses.

SUGGESTED READING

1. Callender VD, Onwudiwe O. Prevalence and etiology of central centrifugal cicatricial alopecia. Arch Dermatol. 2011;147:972-4.
2. Callender VD, Wright DR, Davis EC, et al. Hair breakage as a presenting sign of early or occult central centrifugal cicatricial alopecia: clinicopathologic findings in 9 patients. Arch Dermatol. 2012;148:1047-52.
3. Callender VD, McMichael AJ, Cohen GF. Medical and surgical therapies for alopecias in black women. Dermatol Ther. 2004;17:164-76.
4. Dlova NC, Forder M. Central centrifugal cicatricial alopecia: possible familial aetiology in two African families from South Africa. Int J Dermatol. 2012;51(Suppl 1):17-20.
5. Dlova NC, Jordaan FH, Sarig O, et al. Autosomal dominant inheritance of central centrifugal cicatricial alopecia in black South Africans. J Am Acad Dermatol. 2014;70:679-82.e1.
6. Gathers RC. Central centrifugal cicatricial alopecia: past, present, and future. J Am Acad Dermatol. 2009;60:660-8.
7. Gathers RC, Jankowski M, Eide M, et al. Hair grooming practices and central centrifugal cicatricial alopecia. J Am Acad Dermatol. 2009;60:574-8.
8. Horenstein MG, Simon J. Investigation of the hair follicle inner root sheath in scarring and non-scarring alopecia. J Cutan Pathol. 2007;34:762-8.
9. Khumalo NP, Pillay K, Ngwanya RM. Acute 'relaxer'-associated scarring alopecia: a report of five cases. Br J Dermatol. 2007;156:1394-7.
10. LoPresti P, Papa CM, Kligman AM. Hot comb alopecia. Arch Dermatol. 1968;98:234-8.
11. Miteva M, Tosti A. Dermatoscopic features of central centrifugal cicatricial alopecia. J Am Acad Dermatol. 2014;71:443-9.
12. Nnoruka EN, Nnoruka NE. Hair loss: is there a relationship with hair care practices in Nigeria? Int J Dermatol. 2005;44(Suppl 1):13-7.
13. Olsen EA, Bergfeld WF, Cotsarelis G, et al. Summary of North American Hair Research Society (NAHRS)-sponsored Workshop on Cicatricial Alopecia, Duke University Medical Center, February 10 and 11, 2001. J Am Acad Dermatol. 2003;48:103-10.
14. Olsen EA, Callender V, McMichael A, et al. Central hair loss in African American women: incidence and potential risk factors. J Am Acad Dermatol. 2011;64:245-52.
15. Suchonwanit P, Hector CE, Bin Saif GA, et al. Factors affecting the severity of central centrifugal cicatricial alopecia. Int J Dermatol. 2016;55:e338-43.
16. Summers P, Kyei A, Bergfeld W. Central centrifugal cicatricial alopecia—an approach to diagnosis and management. Int J Dermatol. 2011;50:1457-64.
17. Whiting DA, Olsen EA. Central centrifugal cicatricial alopecia. Dermatol Ther. 2008;21:268-78.

5.7 Pseudopelade of Brocq

Isabella Doche

Pseudopelade of Brocq is a primary lymphocytic scarring alopecia characterized by asymptomatic, noninflamed white porcelain or flesh-colored patches of scalp alopecia. Lesions can form multiple small round areas or large irregular patches with a smooth cicatricial surface, remembering "footprints in the snow" (Figs. 5.7.1 and 5.7.2). This is a slow progressive disease that usually affects the vertex or parietal scalp from middle-aged patients.

Most authors believe that pseudopelade of Brocq is a distinct entity, although some still consider it as a final stage of a scarring process. A recent research using microarray technique identified different gene expression patterns in pseudopelade of Brocq compared with lichen planopilaris, suggesting diverse etiopathogenic mechanisms for both diseases.

Dermoscopy features are inespecific, with the absence of follicular openings, white patches, and few dystrophic hairs. No peripilar scale, erythema, and black or red dots can be noted (Figs. 5.7.3 and 5.7.4). Therapeutic drugs are scarce and there is no standard treatment for this condition. Main differential diagnoses are late-stage cicatricial alopecias of other origin and longstanding alopecia areata.

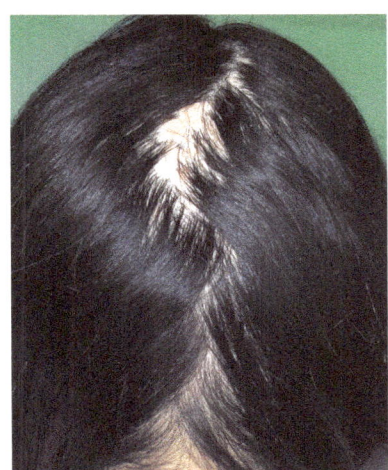

Fig. 5.7.1: Pseudopelade of Brocq. Lesions coalesced to form an irregular, atrophic scarring patch with a porcelain-white color, as "footprints in the snow." Note the lesions are slightly depressed, and may mimic a longstanding alopecia areata.

Source: Division of Dermatology, Hospital das Clínicas, University of São Paulo Medical School.

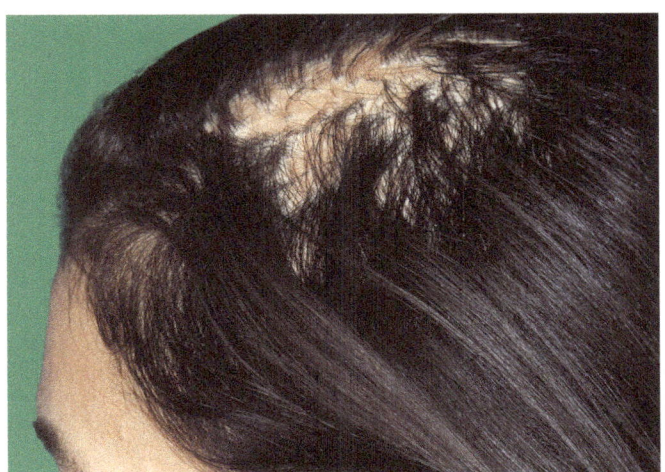

Fig. 5.7.2: Pseudopelade of Brocq. Lesions with flesh-colored appearance on the parietal scalp area. The color of the lesions may range from white to red, depending on the thickness of epidermis, disease duration, or sun exposure.

Source: Division of Dermatology, Hospital das Clínicas, University of São Paulo Medical School.

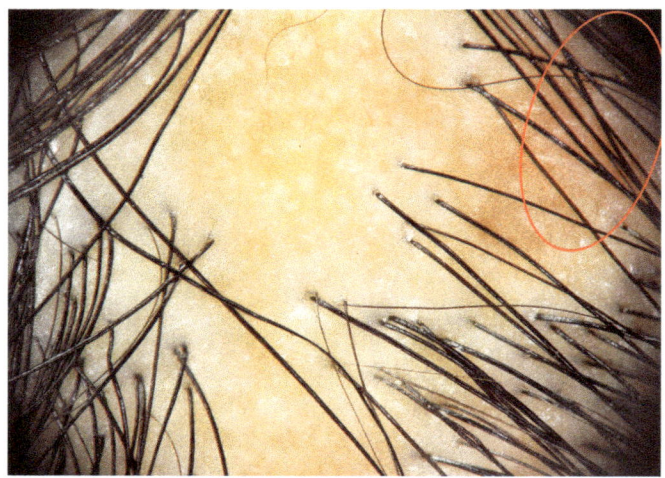 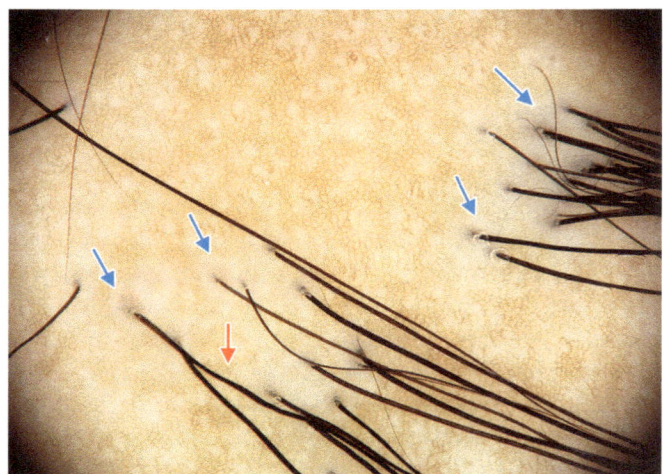

Fig. 5.7.3: Pseudopelade of Brocq. Absence of follicular openings and white scarring patches. Even with dry dermoscopy, no sign of typical peripilar scale can be noted. A subtle erythema can be occasionally present (red ring).
Source: Division of Dermatology, Hospital das Clínicas, University of São Paulo Medical School.

Fig. 5.7.4: Pseudopelade of Brocq. Honeycomb pattern and peripilar whitish halos (blue arrows) that correspond to dermal fibrosis in high skin types. Note one pili torti (red arrow).
Source: Dermatology, Hospital das Clínicas, University of São Paulo Medical School.

Take-Home Message

- Pseudopelade of Brocq is a primary lymphocytic scarring alopecia.
- First thought to be a final stage of many scarring processes, nowadays this entity is considered a separate disease with an unknown etiology.
- This disease may be suspected based on the presence of small smooth hairless areas lacking follicular openings when no other specific features of scarring alopecias are present.
- Clinically, some lesions may mimic longstanding alopecia areata.
- Dermoscopy shows scarring areas devoid of signs of inflammation.

SUGGESTED READING

1. Bolduc C, Sperling LC, Shapiro J. Primary cicatricial alopecia: other lymphocytic primary cicatricial alopecias and neutrophilic and mixed primary cicatricial alopecias. J Am Acad Dermatol. 2016;75(6):1101-17.
2. Kittridge A, Haught JM, English JC III. Alopecia areata mimicking pseudopelade of Brocq. Cutis. 2010;86(4):187-9.
3. Moure ER, Romiti R, Machado MC, et al. Primary cicatricial alopecias: a review of histopathologic findings in 38 patients from a clinical university hospital in São Paulo, Brazil. Clinics. 2008;63(6):747-52.
4. Ramos-e-Silva M, Pirmez R. Disorders of hair growth and the pilosebaceous unit: facts and controversies. Clin Dermatol. 2013;31(6):759-63.
5. Rigopoulos D, Stamatios G, Ioannides D. Primary scarring alopecias. Curr Probl Dermatol. 2015;47:76-86.
6. Singh S, De D, Saikia UN, et al. Pseudopelade of Brocq in two Brothers: possible role of hereditary factors in the pathogenesis. Indian J Dermatol Venereol Leprol. 2012;78(5):637-40.
7. Stefanato CM. Histopathology of alopecia: a clinicopathological approach to diagnosis. Histopathology. 2010;56(1):24-38.
8. Yu M, Bell RH, Ross EK, et al. Lichen planopilaris and pseudopelade of Brocq envolve distinct disease associated gene expression patterns by microarray. J Dermatol Sci. 2010;57(1):27-36.

5.8 Alopecia Mucinosa and Folliculotropic Mycosis Fungoides

Lidia Rudnicka

"Alopecia mucinosa" refers to hair loss associated with a histological pattern characterized by the accumulation of mucin in the infundibular, follicular, or sebaceous epithelium. The term is being differently understood by different authors. Three types of alopecia mucinosa have been distinguished: idiopathic, chronic benign associated with inflammatory conditions, and associated with lymphoma. Some authors indicate that any type of alopecia mucinosa can progress to cutaneous T-cell lymphoma, while others believe that alopecia mucinosa always represents variants of mycosis fungoides with follicular mucinosis in histopathology. Up to now, over 30 different subtypes of mycosis fungoides have been described. From the point of view of hair and scalp disorders, the folliculotropic form of mycosis fungoides may be a significant diagnostic challenge. Folliculotropic mycosis fungoides of the scalp can be associated with follicular mucinosis (alopecia mucinosa), but this is not a constant finding.

Folliculotropic mycosis fungoides is characterized histologically preferential infiltration of the follicular epithelium by T-cells (folliculotropism). The interfollicular epidermis is usually spared. There seems to be no clinical or trichoscopy difference between folliculotropic mycosis fungoides with or without associated follicular mucinosis.

Clinically, the lesions of folliculotropic mycosis fungoides are follicular papules, alopecic plaques, acneiform or comedo-like lesions, nodules, pustules, xanthomatous changes, and rarely erythema (Fig. 5.8.1). The patients are usually younger than patients with the classic form of mycosis fungoides (mean age at diagnosis 46.5 ± 12.2 years). Alopecia may be the first manifestation of the disease and may clinically mimic alopecia areata. A single biopsy may be not sufficient to confirm the diagnosis.

Trichoscopy of alopecia mucionosa and/or folliculotropic mycosis fungoides has been described only in a limited number of cases and clear-cut criteria for the trichoscopy diagnosis are still not available. In the described cases, the prominent trichoscopy features were spacious follicular openings that were the most characteristic of alopecia mucinosa (Fig. 5.8.2). Other features include milky-white globules, red and red-yellowish dots with/without centrally located black dots, trichoptilosis, short broken hairs, and pigtail hairs. Features of late-stage cicatricial alopecia may coexist. Scaling may be present.

No specific treatment has been proved to be effective for alopecia mucinosa. Treatments include topical, intralesional, and systemic corticosteroids. In addition, topical and systemic psoralen plus ultraviolet A light therapy, topical nitrogen mustard, and radiation therapy have been used with variable success. Primary and acute cases affecting children tend to resolve spontaneously. For other forms, the therapy does not seem to affect the poor prognosis and the course of the disease.

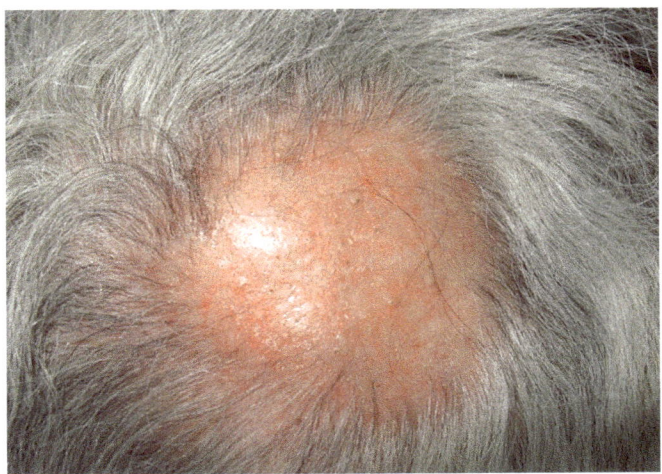

Fig. 5.8.1: Alopecia mucinosa associated with folliculotropic mycosis fungoides. Clinical features showing a hairless patch requiring differential diagnosis with alopecia areata, cicatricial alopecia, and metastates of malignant tumors to the scalp.

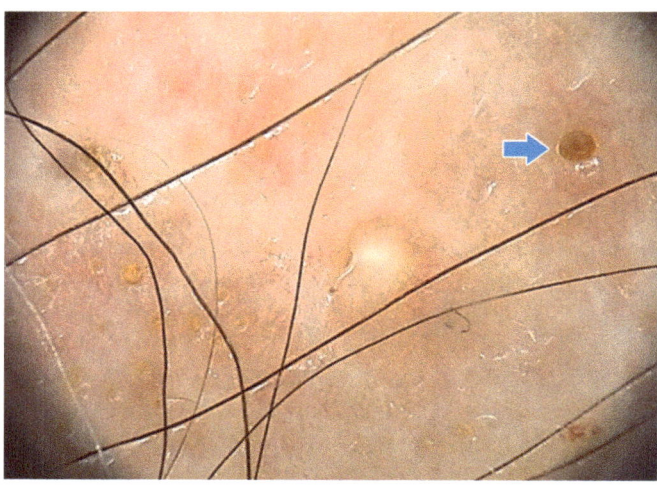

Fig. 5.8.2: Alopecia mucinosa associated with folliculotropic mycosis fungoides. Trichoscopy showing prominent spacious follicular openings (blue thick arrow).

Take-Home Message

- Folliculotropic form of mycosis fungoides of the scalp can be associated with follicular mucinosis (alopecia mucinosa).
- Alopecia areata is the main differential diagnosis.
- Spacious follicular openings are the prominent trichoscopy features.

SUGGESTED READING

1. Borgia F, Giuffrida R, Lentini M, et al. Follicular mucinosis with diffuse scalp alopecia treated with narrow-band UVB phototherapy: the role of trichoscopy in monitoring therapeutic outcomes. G Ital Dermatol Venereol. 2016;151(2):212-5.
2. Qi S, Zhao Y, Zhang X, et al. Clinical features of primary cicatricial alopecia in Chinese patients. Indian J Dermatol Venereol Leprol. 2014;80(4):306-12.
3. Rudnicka L, Rakowska A, Olszewska M. Trichoscopy in General Medicine. In: Atlas of Trichoscopy. Rudnicka L, Olszewska M, Rakowska A (Eds). London: Springer;2012. pp. 483-3.
4. Sławińska M, Sobjanek M, Olszewska B, et al. Trichoscopic spectrum of folliculotropic mycosis fungoides. J Eur Acad Dermatol Venereol. 2017.
5. Wieser I, Wang C, Alberti-Violetti S, et al. Clinical characteristics, risk factors and long-term outcome of 114 patients with folliculotropic mycosis fungoides. Arch Dermatol Res. 2017;309(6):453-9.

5.9 Keratosis Follicularis Spinulosa Decalvans

Isabella Doche

Keratosis follicularis spinulosa decalvans is a rare X-linked or autosomal dominant disorder affecting most male children and young adults. The disease is characterized by progressive scarring alopecia of the scalp, eyebrows, eyelashes, diffuse keratosis pilaris, corneal dystrophy, and photophobia (Figs. 5.9.1A to C and 5.9.2A and B). Palmoplantar keratoderma, atopy, deafness, axillary alopecia, acne keloidalis nuchae, tufted folliculitis, and facial ulerythema ophryogenes may occur.

On dermoscopy, intense peripilar casts, hair casts, absence of follicular openings, white scarring patches, and erythema are noted (Figs. 5.9.3 to 5.9.6). Main differentials are ichthyosis follicularis alopecia photophobia syndrome, lichen planopilaris, and lichen spinulosus. Treatment options include topical keratolytics agents, topical steroids, oral retinoids, oral antibiotics, and lasers, but no effective treatment has shown effective results so far.

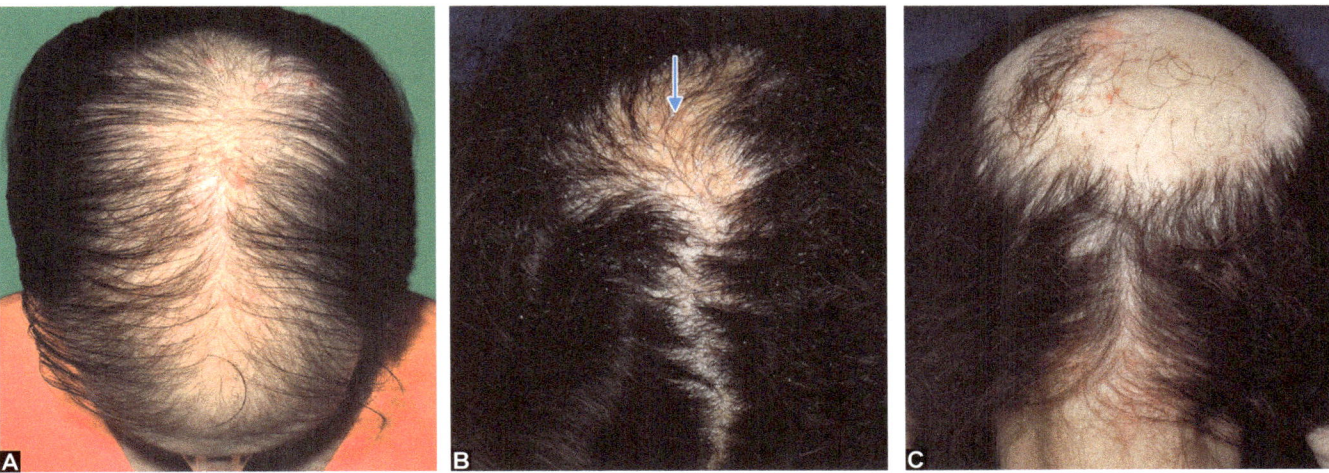

Figs. 5.9.1A to C: Keratosis follicularis spinulosa decalvans. (A) Scarring alopecia of the central scalp distributed in a diffuse pattern and (B) As a localized patch. (C) Extensive presentation of the disease in a female teenager. Note intense scaling and erythema (blue arrow).
Source: Division of Dermatology, Hospital das Clínicas, University of São Paulo Medical School.

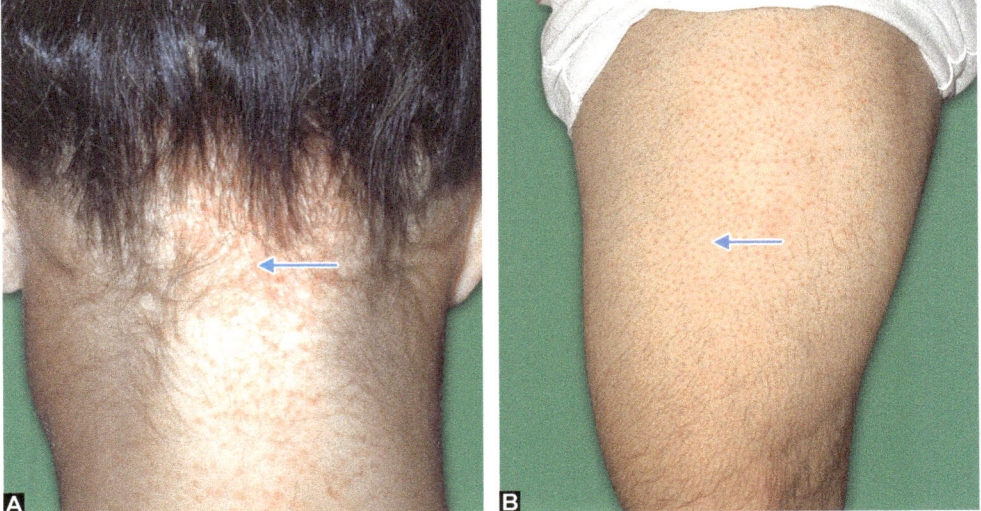

Figs. 5.9.2A and B: Keratosis follicularis spinulosa decalvans. Lesions of keratosis pilaris on the nuchae (A) and legs (B) (blue arrows).
Source: Division of Dermatology, Hospital das Clínicas, University of São Paulo Medical School.

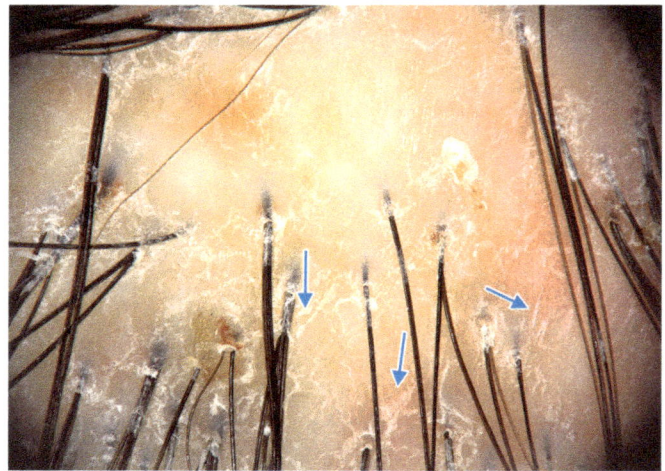

Fig. 5.9.3: Keratosis follicularis spinulosa decalvans. On dry dermoscopy, intense peripilar scaling with crusts and a centered white scarring area. Note fine parallel folds indicating a cicatricial process (→).
Source: Division of Dermatology, Hospital das Clínicas, University of São Paulo Medical School.

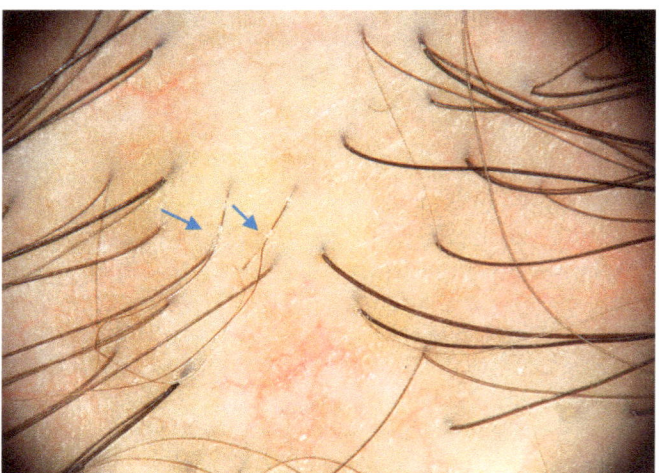

Fig. 5.9.4: Keratosis follicularis spinulosa decalvans. Absence of follicular openings and prominent arborizing blood vessels. Note hair casts (→).
Source: Division of Dermatology, Hospital das Clínicas, University of São Paulo Medical School.

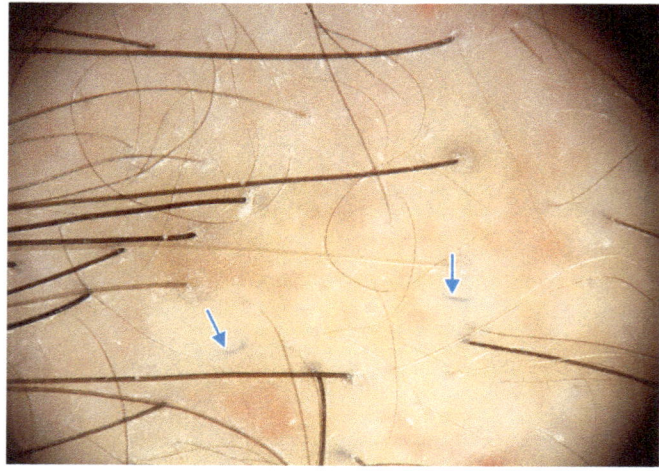

Fig. 5.9.5: Keratosis follicularis spinulosa decalvans. Ingrown hairs can be seen through the scalp due to scalp atrophy (→).
Source: Division of Dermatology, Hospital das Clínicas, University of São Paulo Medical School

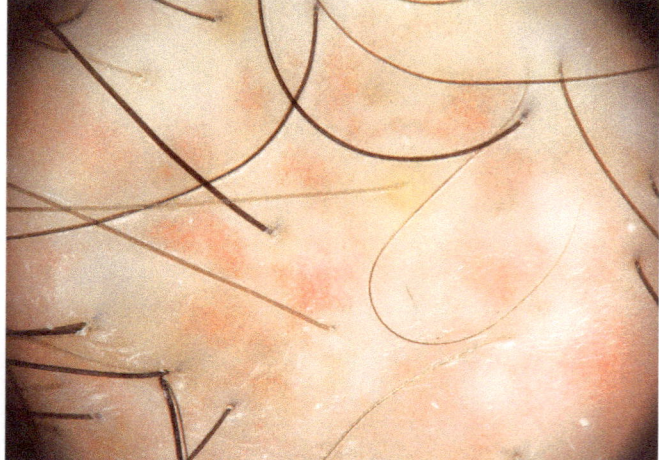

Fig. 5.9.6: Keratosis follicularis spinulosa decalvans. White patches and intense scalp erythema. Note the blood vessels spare perifollicular scarring areas.
Source: Division of Dermatology, Hospital das Clínicas, University of São Paulo Medical School.

Take-Home Message

- Keratosis follicularis spinulosa decalvans is a rare X-linked or autosomal dominant disorder.
- Usually, it affects children and young adults, who present with central scalp, eyebrows and eyelashes scarring alopecia, and keratosis pilaris.
- Vision and hearing examinations are strongly recommended.
- Dermoscopy shows intense peripilar scaling, absence of follicular openings, white scarring patches, scalp atrophy, and erythema.

SUGGESTED READING

1. Bellet JS, Kaplan AL, Selim MA, et al. Keratosis follicularis spinulosa decalvans in a family. J Am Acad Dermatol. 2008;58(3):499-502.
2. Bolduc C, Sperling LC, Shapiro J. Primary cicatricial alopecia: other lymphocytic primary cicatricial alopecias and neutrophilic and mixed cicatricial alopecias. J Am Acad Dermatol. 2016;75(6):1101-17.
3. Castori M, Covaciu C, Paradisi M, et al. Clinical and genetic heterogeneity in keratosis follicularis spinulosa decalvans. Eur J Med Genet. 2009;52(1):53-8.
4. Doche I, Hordinsky M, Wilcox GL, et al. Substance P in keratosis follicularis spinulosa decalvans. JAAD Case Rep. 2015;1(6):327-8.
5. Fong K, Takeichi T, Liu L, et al. Ichthyosis follicularis, atrichia, and photophobia syndrome associated with a new mutation in MBTPS2. Clin Exp Dermatol. 2015;40(5):529-32.
6. Gupta D, Kumari R, Bahunutula RK, et al. Keratosis follicularis spinulosa decalvans showing excelent response to isotretinoin. Indian J Dermatol Venereol Leprol. 2015;81(6):646-8.
7. Ramos-e-Silva M, Pirmez R. Red face revisited: Disorders of hair growth and the pilosebaceous unit. Clin Dermatol. 2014;32(6):784-99.
8. Turegano MM, Sperling LC. Lichenoid folliculitis: A unifying concept. J Cutan Pathol. 2017.
9. Verma R, Bhatnagar A, Vasudevan B, et al. Keratosis follicularis spinulosa decalvans. Indian J Dermatol Venereol Leprol. 2016;82(2):214-6.
10. Zhang J, Wang Y, Cheng R, et al. Novel MBTPS2 missense mutation causes a keratosis follicularis spinulosa decalvans phenotype: mutation update and review of literature. Clin Exp Dermatol. 2016;41(7):757-60.

5.10 Folliculitis Decalvans

Giselle Martins, Patricia Damasco, Isabella Doche

Folliculitis decalvans (FD) is a neutrophilic primary scarring alopecia that usually involves the vertex area of the scalp mostly from middle-aged men. There is no certainty about the cause of this disorder, but it is known that the bacterium *Staphylococcus aureus* has a central role. However, an abnormal host immune response may also be implicated in the development of this disease.

Clinically, FD starts with inflamed and pustular lesions that progress to scarring areas and follicular tuftings, with several hairs (more than 10) coming out of a single follicle, similar to doll's hair or bristles of a tooth brush or a broom (Figs. 5.10.1A and B). Crusts and symptoms as burning, itching, and pain sensations can be present. Sometimes, patients may present with associated acne or folliculitis keloidalis nuchae (Figs. 5.10.1C and D).

In early phase of the disease, dermoscopy shows tufts of several hair shafts emerging from a single follicular opening (polytrichia) and casts (Figs. 5.10.2A and B). Follicular pustules and pustular discharge are often present. Dry dermoscopy can show perifollicular scale forming a radiated appearance (Starburst-like pattern) (Fig. 5.10.3). Dermoscopy with immersion fluid helps to visualize coiled and elongated vessels arranged in loops (hairpin vessels), similar to scalp psoriasis (Figs. 5.10.4A and B). Late phase lesions show cutaneous clefts with multiple hairs shafts and ivory white scarring areas with very atrophic skin (Figs. 5.10.5 and 5.10.6). FD should be differentiated from lichen planopilaris with secondary infection. In this condition, tufts can also be present, but usually they show less than 6-10 hairs shafts emerging from the same follicular openings (Figs. 5.10.7A and B).

The treatment is quite challenging as the disease is progressive and relapses are frequent. Patients shoud be aware of the limited benefits of the treatment. Systemic antibiotics may be used alone or in combination with topical or intralesional corticosteroids. Other treatment options including isotretinoin, dapsone, biologics (infliximab and adalimumab), laser hair removal, and photodynamic therapy have been reported, with some success.

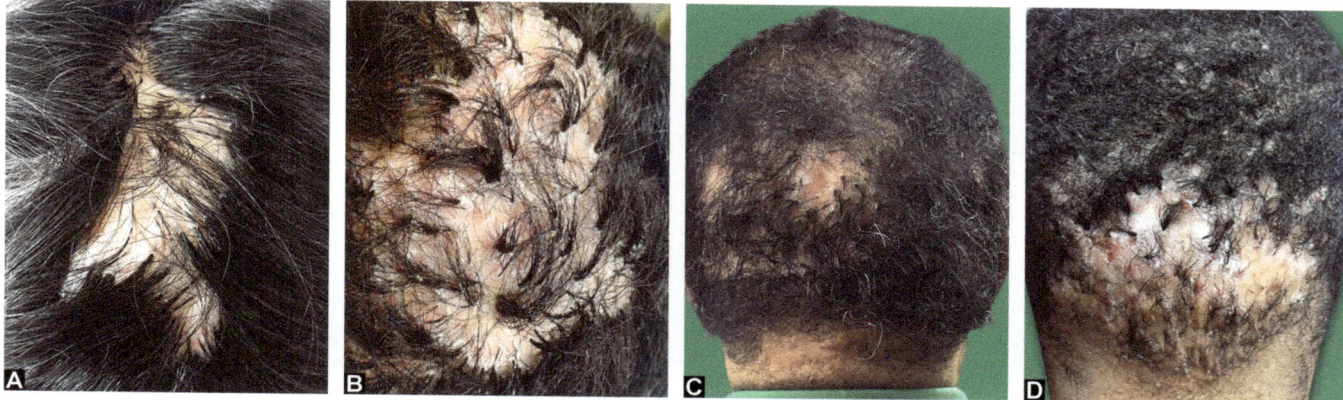

Figs. 5.10.1A to D: Folliculitis decalvans. (A) Scarring patch of alopecia with polyrtrichia on the vertex scalp area from a female patient. (B) Severe polytrichia. Note several hairs emerging from the same follicular opening, similar to doll's hair and bristles from a tooth brush or a broom. (C and D) Folliculitis decalvans lesions on the occipital scalp associated with acne or folliculitis keloidalis nuchae.
Source: (A,C and D) Division of Dermatology, Hospital das Clínicas, University of São Paulo Medical School.

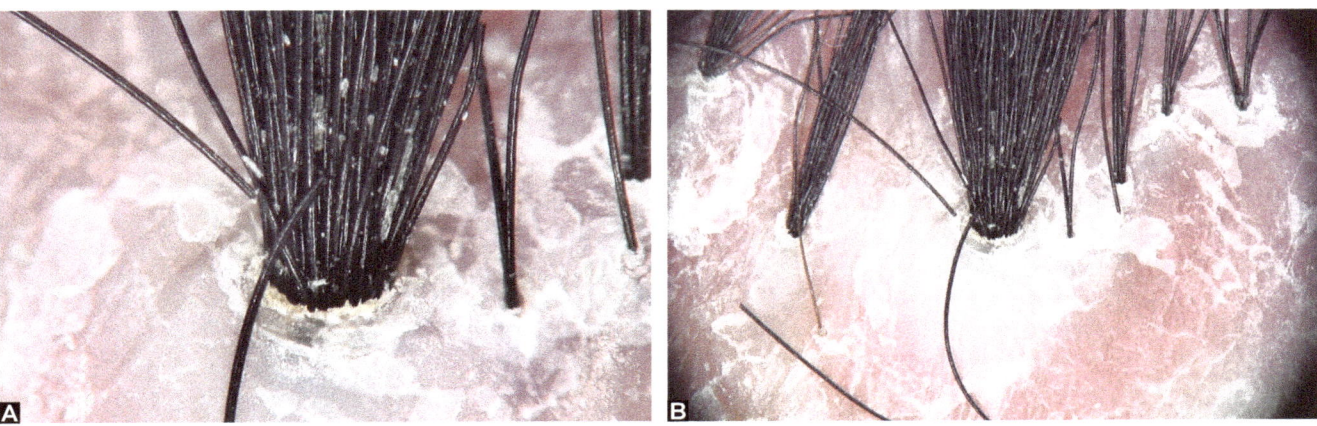

Figs. 5.10.2A and B: Folliculitis decalvans. Dry dermoscopy shows tufts containing more than 10 hairs, casts and perifollicular thick concentric scale. Interfollicular white scale may also be present in severe presentations.
Source: Hair Department, Division of Dermatology, Santa Casa de Misericórdia de Porto Alegre.

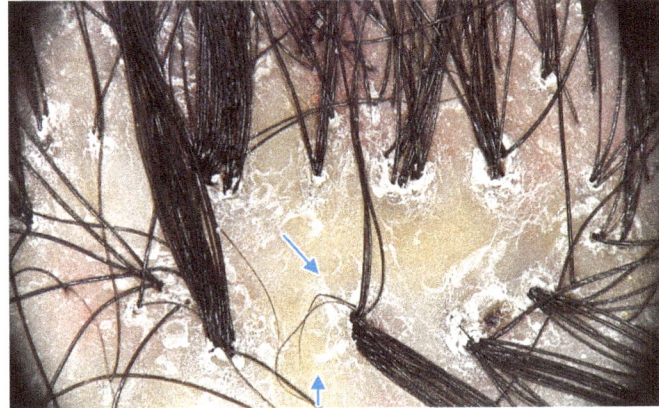

Fig. 5.10.3: Folliculitis decalvans. Starburst sign. Dry dermoscopy shows the presence of whitish scales with a radiated appearance (blue arrows) surrounding the hair tuftings.

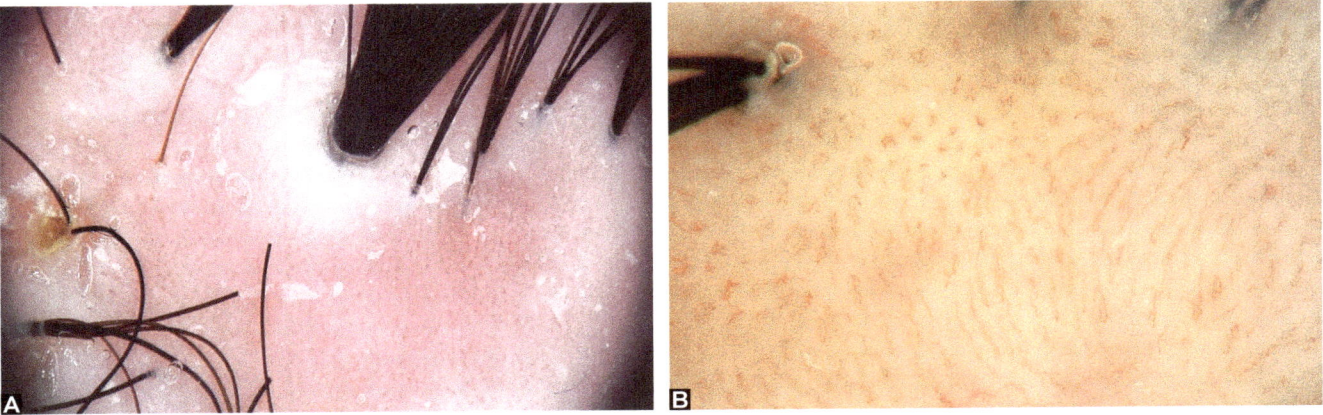

Figs. 5.10.4A and B: Folliculitis decalvans. Coiled vessels and elongated loops pointing mostly to hair follicles, very similar to scalp psoriasis.
Source: Hair Department, the Division of Dermatology, Santa Casa de Misericórdia de Porto Alegre.

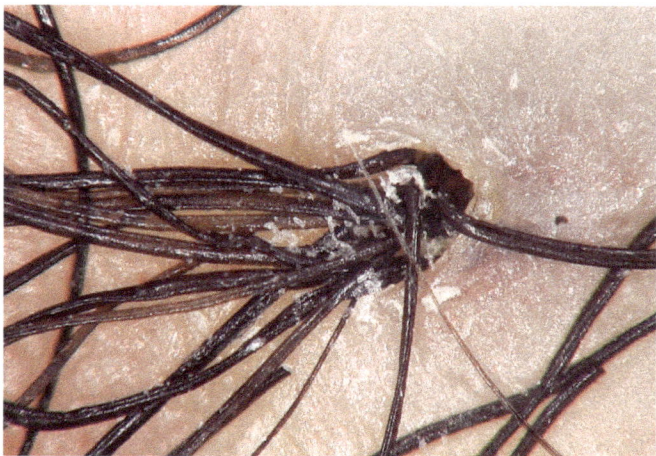

Fig. 5.10.5: Folliculitis decalvans. Cutaneous cleft containing multiple hair shafts may also be present.

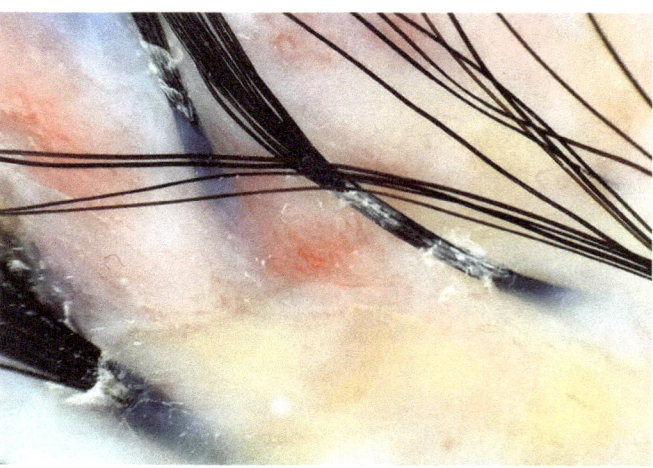

Fig. 5.10.6: Folliculitis decalvans. In late stage disease, hair shafts can be seen through the very atrophic skin.

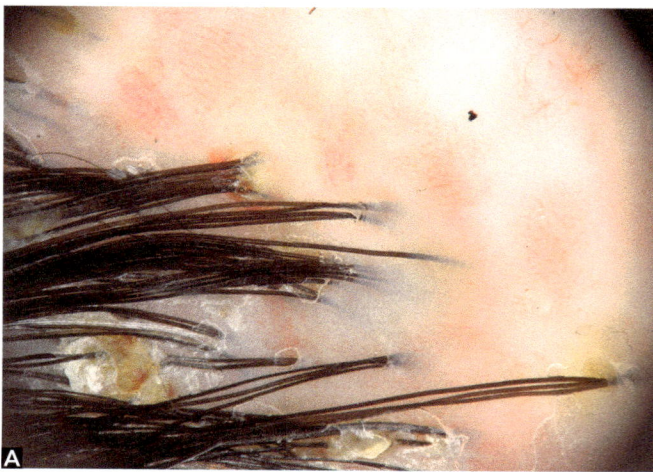

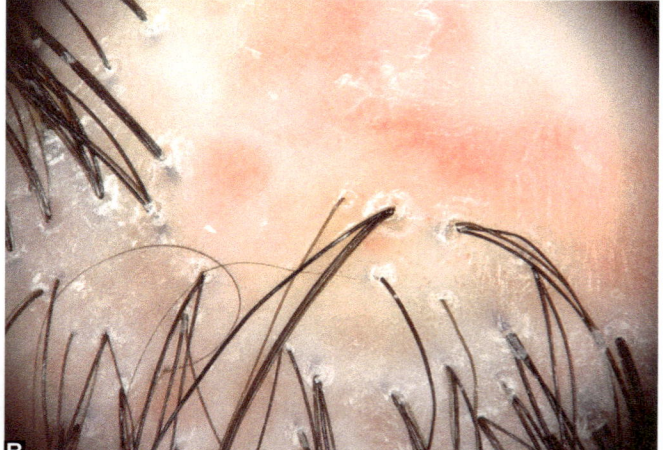

Figs. 5.10.7A and B: Lichen planopilaris with secondary infection. (A) Note tufts with less than 10 hairs, crusts, and follicular pustules. (B) After treatment, note the absence of large follicular tuftings, crusts and pustules. In this case, biopsies should be taken after a course of antibiotics to avoid the misdiagnosis of a neutrophilic, scarring process.
Source: Division of Dermatology, Hospital das Clínicas, University of São Paulo Medical School.

Take-Home Message
- Folliculitis decalvans is a chronic and severe inflammation of the vertex scalp.
- Usually, it starts with recurrent pustular and inflamed lesions that lead to a centrifugal hair loss.
- It is characterized by multiple hairs emerging from one single dilated follicular orifice (polytrichia) and intense scarring alopecia.
- Dermoscopy shows tufted hairs (more than 10), follicular pustules, and white concentric perifollicular scale, sometimes forming a Starburst-like appearance. Immersion fluid helps to visualize the coiled and elongated vessels, similar to scalp psoriasis.
- Folliculitis decalvans may mimic lichen planopilaris with secondary infection, on both clinical and dermoscopic examinations.

SUGGESTED READING

1. Bolduc C, Sperling LC, Shapiro J. Primary cicatricial alopecia: Other lymphocytic primary cicatrical alopecias and neutrophilic and mixed primary cicatricial alopecias. J Am Acad Dermatol. 2016;75(6):1101-17.
2. Bunagan MJ, Banka N, Shapiro J. Retrospective review of folliculitis decalvans in 23 patients with course and treatment analysis of long-standing cases. J Cut Med Surg. 2015;19(1):45-9.
3. Fabris MR, Melo CP, Melo DF. Folliculitis decalvans: the use of dermatoscopy as an auxiliary tool in clinical diagnosis. An Bras Dermatol. 2013;88(5):814-6.
4. Fernández-Crehuet P, Vaño-Galván S, Molina-Ruiz AM, et al. Trichoscopic features of folliculitis decalvans: results in 58 patients. Int J Trichology. 2017;9(3):140-1.
5. Miteva M, Tosti A. Dermoscopy guided scalp biopsy in cicatricial alopecia. J Eur Acad Dermatol Venereol. 2013;27(10):1299-303.
6. Morais KL, Martins CF, Anzai A, et al. Lichen planopilaris with pustules: a diagnostic challenge. Skin Appendage Disord. 2018;4(2):61-66.
7. Mubki T, Rudnicka L, Olszewska M, et al. Evaluation and diagnosis of the hair loss patient: part II. Trichoscopic and laboratory evaluations. J Am Acad Dermatol. 2014;71(3):431.e1-431.e11.
8. Rakowska A, Slowisnka M, Kowalska-Oledzka E, et al. Trichoscopy in cicatricial alopecia. J Drugs Dermatol. 2012;11(6):753-8.
9. Rigopoulos D, Stamatios G, Ioannides D. Primary scarring alopecias. Curr Probl Dermatol. 2015;47:76-86.
10. Vañó-Galván S, Molina-Ruiz AM, Fernández-Crehuet P, et al. Folliculitis decalvans: a multicentre review of 82 patients. J Eur Acad Dermatol Venereol. 2015;29(9):1750-7.

5.11 Dissecting Cellulitis (Late Stage)

Isabella Doche

Dissecting cellulitis is a chronic and progressive inflammatory scalp disorder that may lead to scarring alopecia. According to the North American Hair Research Society Classification in 2001, dissecting cellulitis was classified as a primary neutrophilic scarring alopecia. The initial stage of the disease is characterized by sterile pustules on the vertex and/or occipital scalp, painful, and boggy alopecic patches that are potentially reversible with treatment. However, longstanding lesions may progress to scarring hair loss and keloid lesions (Figs. 5.11.1A and B).

Dermoscopy of late stage lesions shows scarring alopecic patches with loss of follicular ostia, large keratin plugs, enlarged follicular openings (cutaneous clefts) containing small grouped hair shafts, and keloid lesions (Figs. 5.11.2 to 5.11.4).

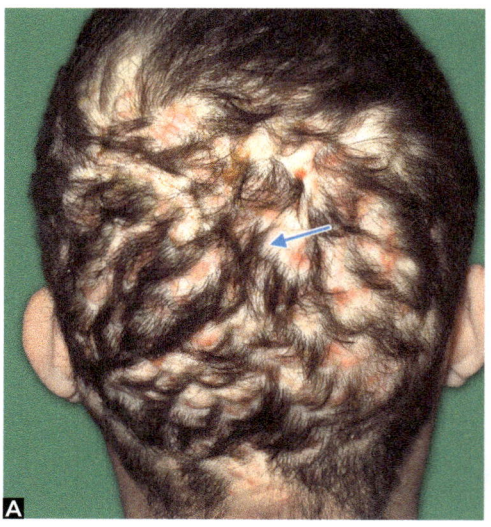
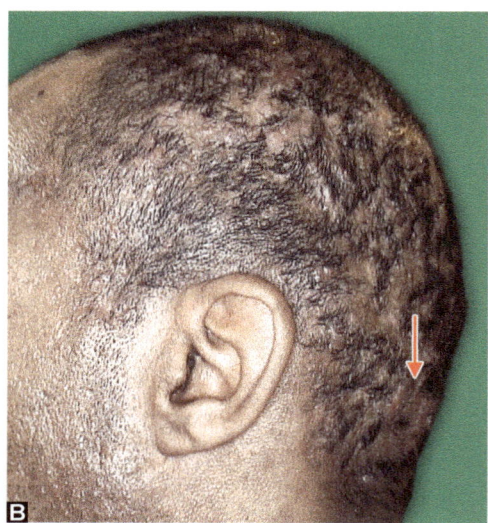

Figs. 5.11.1A and B: Dissecting cellulitis (late stage). Note multiple scarring alopecic patches (blue arrow) with keloid formation (red arrow).
Source: Division of Dermatology, Hospital das Clínicas, University of São Paulo Medical School.

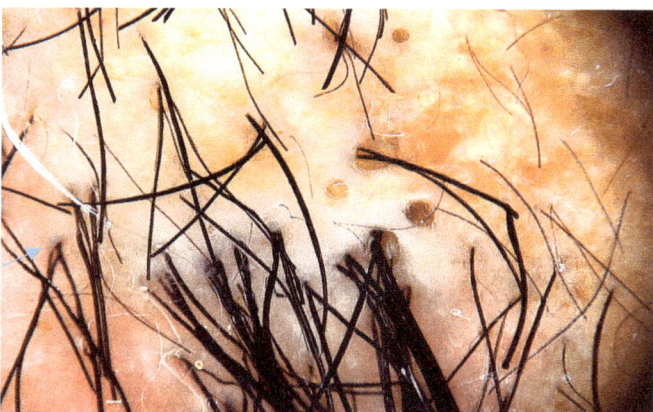

Fig. 5.11.2: Dissecting cellulitis (late stage). Note white fibrotic areas, large keratin plugs, and cutaneous cleft (arrow). Clefts are enlarged follicular openings containing keratin and emerging hairs or small tufts.
Source: Division of Dermatology, Hospital das Clínicas, University of São Paulo Medical School.

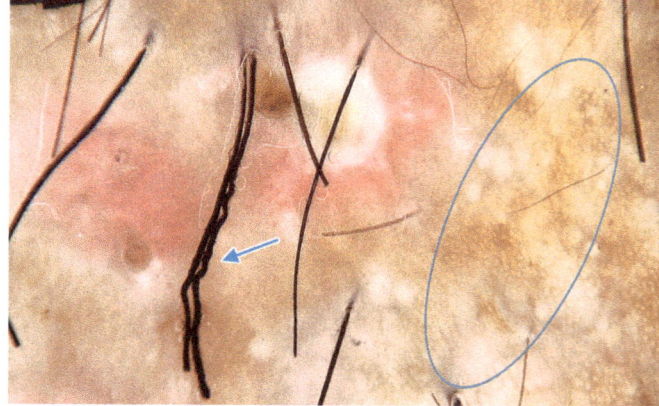

Fig. 5.11.3: Dissecting cellulitis (late stage). Acquired pili torti (→) may be present in all types of scarring alopecias. Note the disrupted honeycomb pattern in a dark-skinned patient (blue ring).
Source: Division of Dermatology, Hospital das Clínicas, University of São Paulo Medical School.

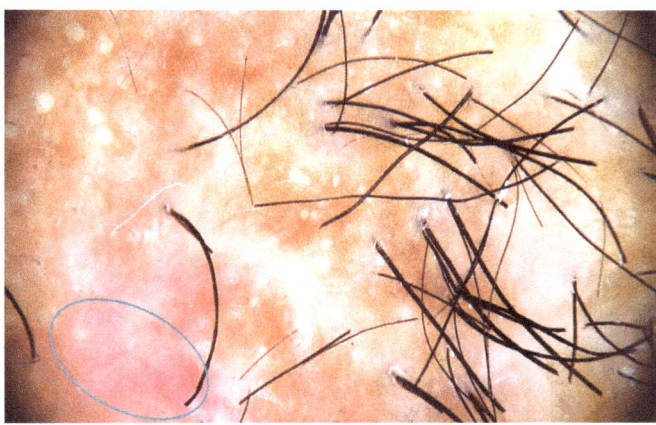

Fig. 5.11.4: Dissecting cellulitis (late stage). Note violaceous areas indicating a prefibrotic process (blue ring).

Source: Division of Dermatology, Hospital das Clínicas, University of São Paulo Medical School

Take-Home Message

- Late stages results in either atrophic or hypertrophic scarring alopecia, with keloid formation on the scalp, mostly seen in patients with dark skin types.
- Dermoscopy shows white fibrotic areas with loss of follicular ostia, large and few keratin plugs, cutaneous clefts, pili torti, and violaceous areas.
- Differentials are deep folliculitis, tinea capitis favosa, discoid lupus erythematosus, folliculitis decalvans, acne keloidalis nuchae, and alopecia mucinosa.

SUGGESTED READING

1. Badaoui A, Reygagne P, Cavelier-Balloy B, et al. Dissecting cellulitis of the scalp: a retrospective study of 51 patients and review of literature. Br J Dermatol. 2016;174(2):421-3.
2. Bolduc C, Sperling LC, Shapiro J. Primary cicatricial alopecia: other lymphocytic primary cicatricial alopecias and neutrophilic and mixed primary cicatricial alopecias. J Am Acad Dermatol. 2016;75(6):1101-17.
3. Gaopande VL, Kulkarni MM, Joshi AR, et al. Perifolliculitis capitis abscedens et suffodiens in a 7 years old male: a case report with review of literature. Int J Trichology. 2015;7(4):173-5.
4. Garelli V, Didona D, Paolino G, et al. Dissecting cellulitis: response to topical steroid and oral clindamycin. G Ital Dermatol Venereol. 2017;152(3):324-5.
5. Lacarrubba F, Micali G. Regarding trichoscopy of dissecting cellulitis of the scalp. J Am Acad Dermatol. 2017;76(6):e213.
6. Marquis K, Christensen LC, Rajpara A. Dissecting cellulitis of the scalp with excellent response to isotretinoin. Pediatr Dermatol. 2017;34(4):e210-1.
7. Martin-García RF, Rullán JM. Refractory dissecting cellulitis of the scalp successfully controlled with adalimumab. P R Health Sci J. 2015;34(2):102-4.
8. Mubki T, Rudnicka L, Olszewska M, et al. Evaluation and diagnosis of the hair loss patient: part II. Trichoscopic and laboratory evaluations. J Am Acad Dermatol. 2014;71(3):431.e1-431.e11.
9. Powers MC, Mehta D, Ozog D. Cutting out the tracts: staged excisions for dissecting cellulitis of the scalp. Dermatol Surg. 2017;43(5):738-40.
10. Scheinfeld N. Dissecting cellulitis (Perifolliculitis Capitis Abscedens et Suffodiens): a comprehensive review focusing on new treatments and findings of the last decade with commentary comparing the therapies and causes of dissecting cellulitis to hidradenitis suppurativa. Dermatol Online. 2014;20(5):22692.
11. Tosti A, Torres F, Miteva M. Dermoscopy of early dissecting cellulitis of the scalp simulates alopecia areata. Actas Dermosifiliogr. 2013;104(1):92-3.
12. Verzì AE, Lacarrubba F, Micali G. Heterogeneity of trichoscopy findings in dissecting cellulitis of the scalp: correlation to disease activity and duration. Br J Dermatol. 2017;177(6):e331–2.

5.12 Acne Keloidalis Nuchae

Maria Cecília da Matta Rivitti Machado, Isabella Doche

Acne keloidalis nuchae (AKN) or folliculitis keloidalis is a chronic inflammatory disease that commonly affects the occiput and/or the nape of the neck and develops almost exclusively in young, African descent male patients. Pathogenesis remains unknown, however, factors such as skin injury, aberrant immune reaction, and the characteristic curvature of afro-textured hair may be responsible for inciting the disease.

Clinically, AKN starts with small papular violaceous keloid-like lesions that coalesce over time forming tumors and scarring alopecic areas (Fig. 5.12.1). Although most cases are restricted to the occipital and neck areas, some lesions may spread over the scalp and be associated with other types of scarring alopecias, such as folliculitis decalvans, central centrifugal cicatricial alopecia, and dissecting cellulitis (Fig. 5.12.2). Patient may complain of pain and recurrent inflammation.

Dermoscopy shows broken hairs, peripilar scale, casts, small tuftings, and ingrown hairs. Crusts, pustules, and elongated vessels can be present. Perifollicular discoloration and disrupted honeycomb network and pinpoint white dots can be seen in dark-skinned patients (Figs. 5.12.3 to 5.12.5). "Normal-appearing" scalp areas may show peripilar scale, casts, small tuftings, and mild erythema (Fig. 5.12.6).

Treatment is challenging and relapses are common. Patients should avoid short haircuts or close shaves in order to prevent ingrown and inflamed hairs. Antibiotics, steroids, and retinoids can be used with partial results. Surgical excision and laser/light-based therapies can be tried in longstanding lesions.

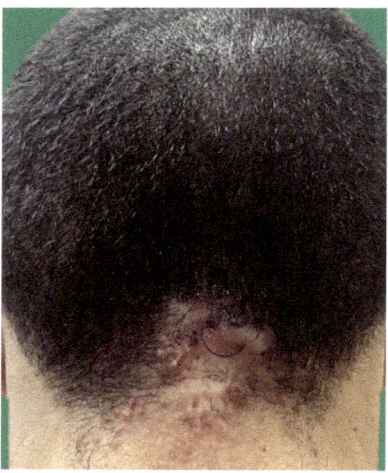

Fig. 5.12.1: Acne keloidalis nuchae. Note small violaceous keloid-like papules, cicatricial areas, and ingrown hairs in the occipital scalp.

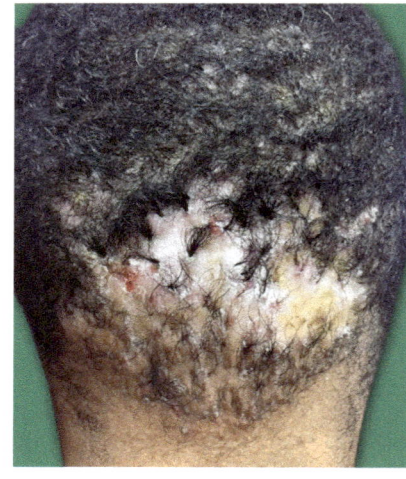

Fig. 5.12.2: Acne keloidalis nuchae associated with folliculitis decalvans. Note severe hair tuftings in an African descent patient.

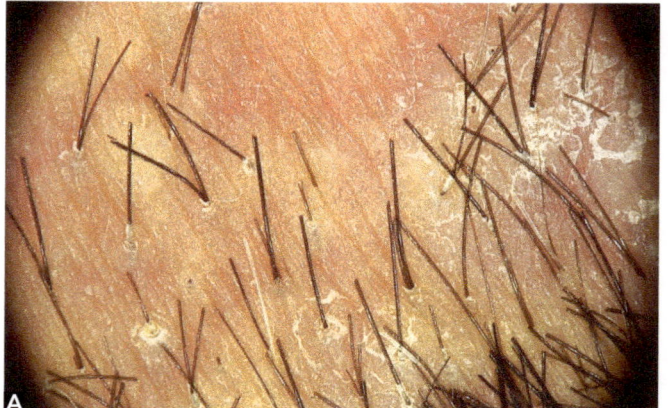

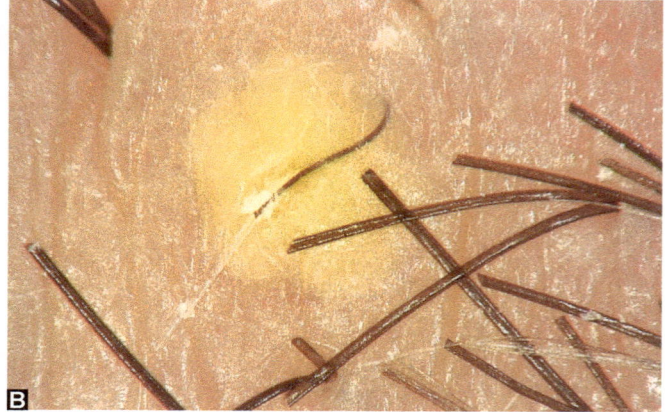

Figs. 5.12.3A and B: (A) Ache keloidalis nuchae. Broken hairs, black dots, peripilar scale, hair casts, and scarring areas with absence of follicular openings. (B) Ingrown hair within a pustule.

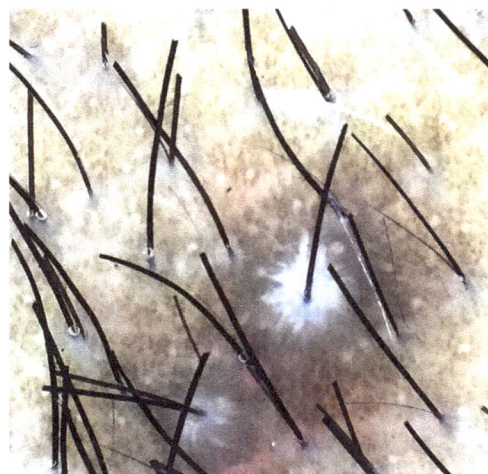

Fig. 5.12.4: Acne keloidalis nuchae. Peripilar discoloration and a whitish scarring halo can be seen in dark-skinned patients. Note the disrupted honeycomb network and the irregularly distributed pinpoint white dots.

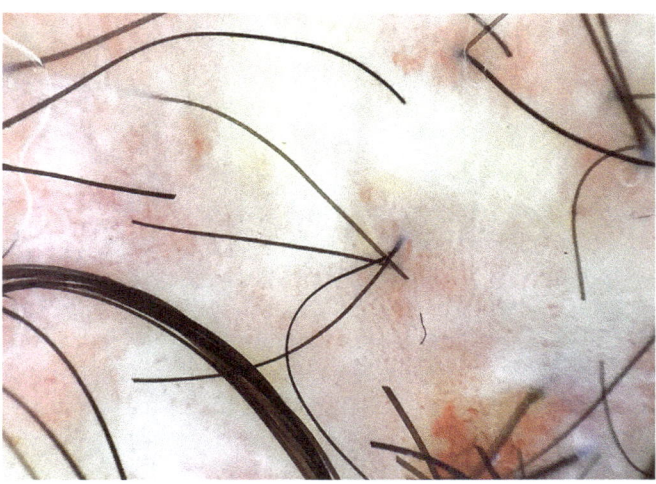

Fig. 5.12.5: Acne keloidalis nuchae. Note some glomerular, dotted, and elongated (hairpin) vessels within white scarring areas.

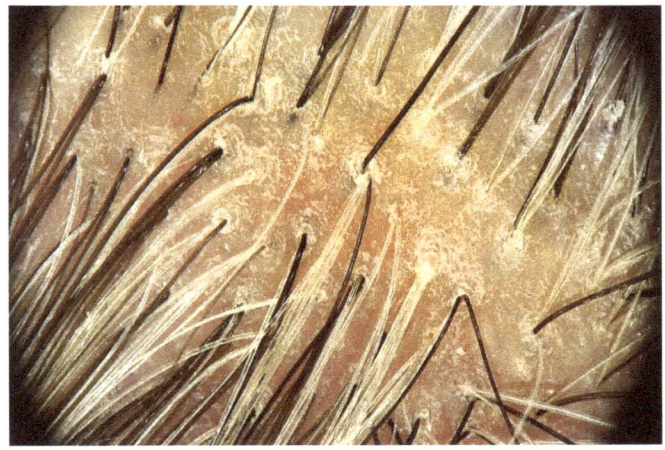

Fig. 5.12.6: Acne keloidalis nuchae. "Normal-appearing" scalp areas may show peripilar scale and small hair tuftings on dry dermoscopy.

Take-Home Message

- Acne keloidalis nuchae usually affects the occiput and nape of the neck from African descent male patients.
- Dermoscopy shows black dots, broken hairs, peripilar scale, casts, ingrown hairs, small tuftings, absence of follicular openings, and elongated vessels. Crusts and pustules may occur.
- Peripilar discoloration, whitish peripilar halo, disrupted honeycomb pattern, and pinpoint white dots irregularly distributed can be seen in dark-skinned patients.
- "Normal-appearing" scalp can also show peripilar scale, casts, small tuftings, and erythema.
- Treatment is challenging and relapses are common.

SUGGESTED READING

1. East-Innis ADC, Stylianou K, Paolino A, et al. Acne keloidalis nuchae: risk factors and associated disorders—a retrospective study. Int J Dermatol. 2017;56(8):828-32.
2. Lindsey SF, Tosti A. Ethnic hair disorders. Curr Probl Dermatol. 2015;47:139-49.
3. Maranda EL, Simmons BJ, Nguyen AH, et al. Treatment of acne keloidalis nuchae: a systematic review of the literature. Dermatol Ther. 2016;6(3):363-78.
4. Metin SA, Parish LC. Acne keloidalis nuchae—is the barber really to blame? Skinmed. 2017;15(4):247-9.
5. Ogunbiyi A. Acne keloidalis nuchae: prevalence, impact, and management challenges. Clin Cosmet Investig Dermatol. 2016;9:483-9.
6. Taylor SC, Barbosa V, Burgess C, et al. Hair and scalp disorders in adult and pediatric patients with skin of color. Cutis. 2017;100(1):31-5.

5.13. Erosive Pustular Dermatosis of the Scalp

Giselle Martins, Patricia Damasco, Isabella Doche

Erosive pustular dermatosis of the scalp (EPDS) is an uncommon chronic inflammatory disease affecting usually elderly people, with extensive pustular lesions, erosions, and crusting of the scalp. This condition usually leads to scarring alopecia of the affected areas. It typically develops in aged or sun-damaged skin and is most often accompanied by a history of local trauma. EPDS is reported after local injuries including burns, cryotherapy, radiotherapy, photodynamic therapy, skin grafts, contact dermatitis, and hair transplantation, as well as topical medication treatments including retinoids, imiquimod, and 5-fluorouracil. Although the pathogenesis of EPDS is still unknown, it seems that this condition is an autoimmune response toward the hair follicles induced by trauma with subsequent chronic inflammation and scarring. Cultures are generally negative, and laboratory and histopathological evaluations are not diagnostic.

Clinically, EPDS presents as chronic inflammatory patches associated with erythema, crusted erosions, multiple sterile pustules, early scarring alopecia, and skin atrophy (Figs. 5.13.1A to C). Several diseases must be considered in the differential diagnosis of EPDS, such as

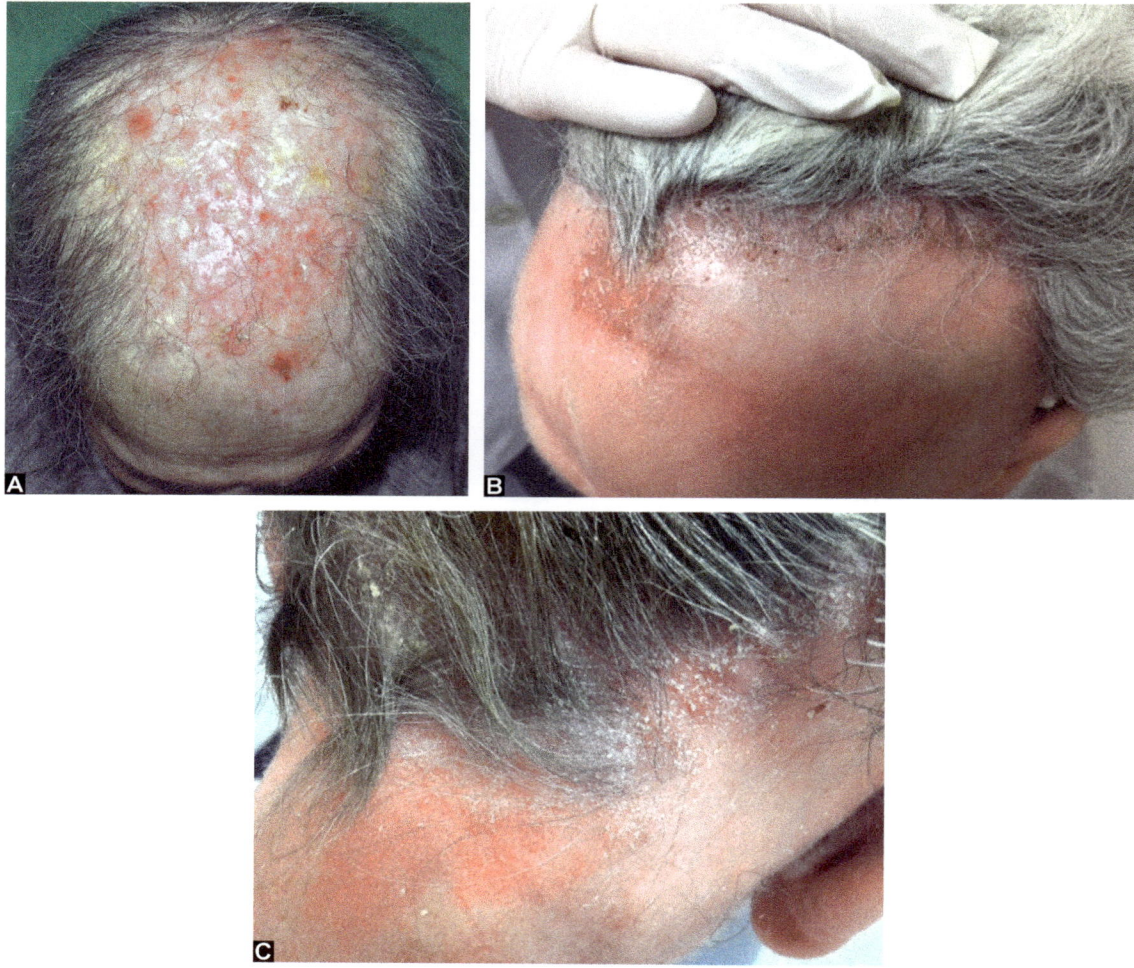

Figs. 5.13.1A to C: Erosive pustular dermatosis of the scalp. (A) Erythema, multiple sterile pustules, early scarring alopecia, and skin atrophy. (B) Band-like alopecia after skin graft for skin cancer treatment. (C) Note follicular pustules and scaling in an erythematous background.
Source: (A) Division of Dermatology, Hospital das Clínicas, University of São Paulo Medical School; (B and C) Hair Department, Division of Dermatology, Santa Casa de Misericórdia de Porto Alegre.

bacterial or fungal infections, squamous cell carcinoma, pustular psoriasis, pemphigus foliaceus, eczema, lupus erythematosus, and folliculitis decalvans.

Dermoscopy shows severe skin atrophy with erosions and crusts, and hair bulbs visible through the epidermis. Other findings include enlarged dermal vessels, follicular keratotic plugging, pili torti, milky-red areas, and white patches (Figs. 5.13.2A and B and 5.13.3).

The course of EPDS is typically chronic. Treatment options for this condition include topical high-potency corticosteroids, retinoids, calcipotriol, dapsone, and topical tacrolimus. In addition to acute treatment, long-term lesions should be monitored, because there is a risk of developing squamous cell carcinoma over EPDS scars.

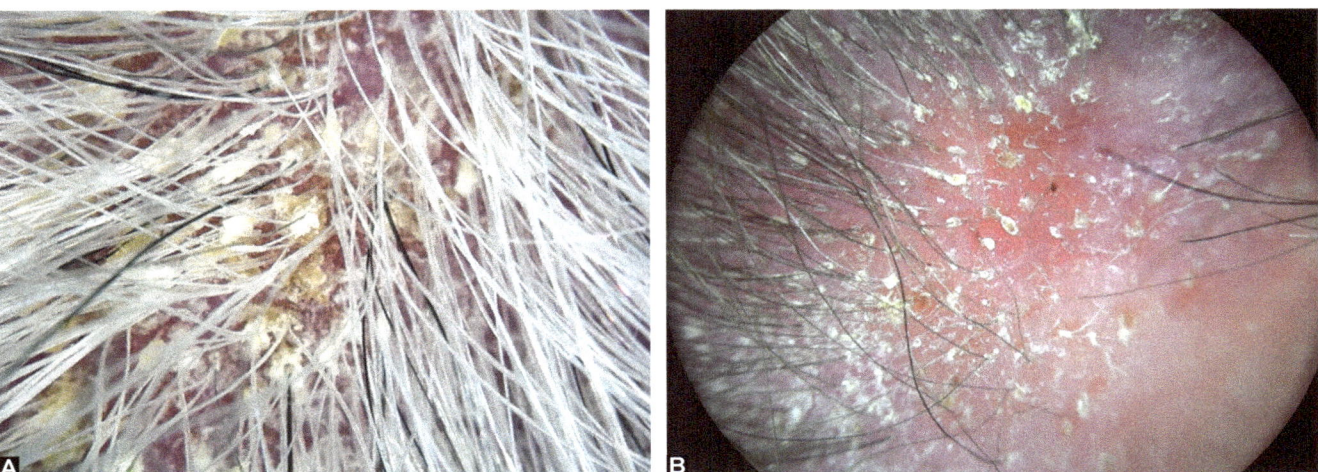

Figs. 5.13.2A and B: Erosive pustular dermatosis of the scalp. Dry dermoscopy shows erythema, scarring alopecia, and crusts.
Source: Hair Department, Division of Dermatology, Santa Casa de Misericórdia de Porto Alegre.

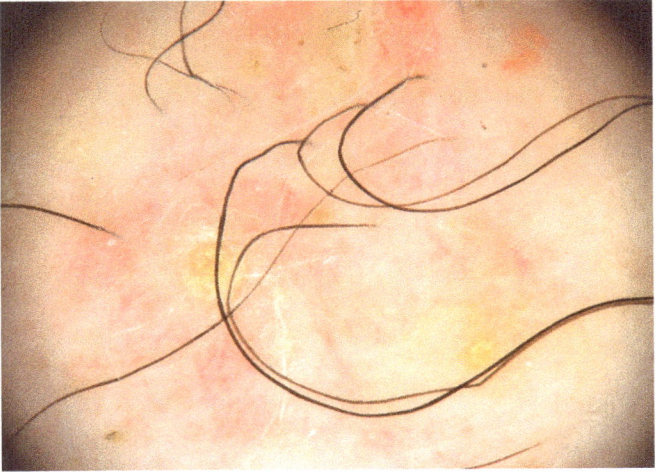

Fig. 5.13.3: Erosive pustular dermatosis of the scalp. Dermoscopy with immersion fluid shows absence of follicular openings, hair bulbs visible through epidermis, skin atrophy, pili torti, enlarged vessels, follicular keratotic plugging, and some milky-red areas.
Source: Division of Dermatology, Hospital das Clínicas, University of São Paulo Medical School.

> **Take-Home Message**
> - Erosive pustular dermatosis of the scalp is an inflammatory disease affecting elderly people with sterile pustules, erosions, and crusted lesions, resulting in scarring alopecia.
> - Dermoscopy shows absence of follicular openings, hair bulbs visible through the epidermis, follicular keratotic plugging, follicular crusts, pili torti, milky-red areas, and white patches.
> - Differential diagnoses include folliculitis decalvans, bacterial or fungus infections, pustular psoriasis, and pemphigus foliaceus.

SUGGESTED READING

1. Bolduc C, Sperling LC, Shapiro J. Primary cicatricial alopecia: Other lymphocytic primary cicatricial alopecias and neutrophilic and mixed primary cicatricial alopecias. J Am Acad Dermatol. 2016;75(6):1101-17.
2. Corradin MT, Forcione M, Giulioni E, et al. Erosive pustular dermatosis of the scalp induced by imiquimod. Case Rep Dermatol Med. 2012;2012:828749.
3. Herbst JS, Herbst AT. Erosive pustular dermatosis of the scalp after contact dermatitis from a prosthetic hair piece. JAAD Case Rep. 2017;3(2):121-3.
4. Meyer T, Lopez-Navarro N, Herrera-Acosta E, et al. Erosive pustular dermatosis of the scalp: a successful treatment with photodynamic therapy. Photodermatol Photoimmunol Photomed. 2010;26(1):44-5.
5. Starace M, Loi C, Bruni F, et al. Erosive pustular dermatosis of the scalp: Clinical, trichoscopic, and histopathologic features of 20 cases. J Am Acad Dermatol. 2017;76(6):1109-14.
6. Starace M, Patrizi A, Piraccini BM. Visualization of hair bulbs through the scalp: a trichoscopic feature of erosive pustular dermatosis of the scalp. Int J Trichology. 2016;8(2):91-3.
7. Tardio NB, Daly TJ. Erosive pustular dermatosis and associated alopecia successfully treated with topical tacrolimus. J Am Acad Dermatol. 2011;65(3)e:93-4.
8. Vaccaro M, Borgia F, Gasco L, et al. Erosive Pustular dermatoses of the scalp following topical ingenol mebutate for actinic keratoses. Dermatol Ther. 2017;30(5):e12521.

CHAPTER 6

Inflammatory Scalp Disorders

Isabella Doche, Giselle Martins, Patricia Damasco, Ricardo Romiti, Alessandra Anzai, Emilie Jane Fowler, Antonella Tosti

6.1 Seborrheic Dermatitis/Pityriasis Amiantacea

Isabella Doche

Seborrheic dermatitis is a chronic inflammatory scalp disorder affecting more frequently young male adults. Lesions are characterized by variable scaling, mild scalp erythema, and itching. Interfollicular scales are usually more pronounced than perifollicular scales, ranging from white to yellow color with a greasy surface (Figs. 6.1.1 and 6.1.2). Small follicular pustules and scalp excoriation may be noted. Dermoscopy shows white-yellowish oily scales, hair casts, increased thin arboring vessels network, occasional follicular pustules, and excoriations (Figs. 6.1.3 and 6.1.4). Atypical red vessels, comma vessels, and structureless red areas can also be found.

Pityriasis amiantacea or pseudotinea amiantacea is an exaggerated inflammatory response that affects the scalp (Fig. 6.1.5). Althoug the ethiopathogenesis remains unclear, possible causes include seborrheic dermatitis, atopic dermatitis, tinea capitis, and psoriasis. Chronic lesions may lead to secondary scarring alopecia. Dermoscopy shows thick silvery or yellowish scales, strongly adhered to hair tufts. Scarring areas may be present (Figs. 6.1.6 and 6.1.7).

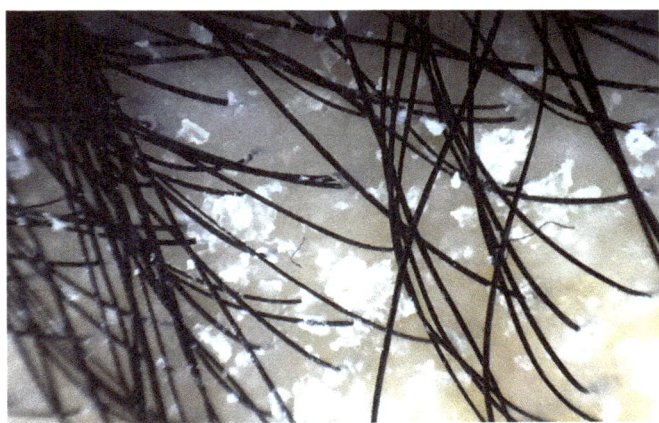

Fig. 6.1.1: Seborrheic dermatitis. Interfollicular white flaky scales.

Treatment options include antidandruff shampoos, keratolytic agents, topical steroids, oral isotretinoin, and light therapy.

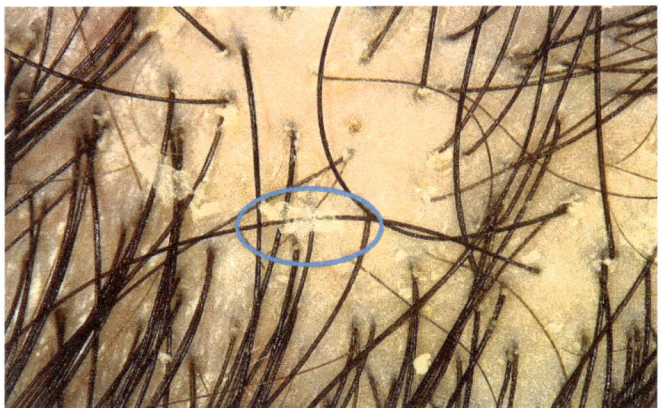

Fig. 6.1.2: Seborrheic dermatitis. Yellow greasy perifollicular and interfollicular scales. Note mild scalp erythema and hair casts (blue ring).

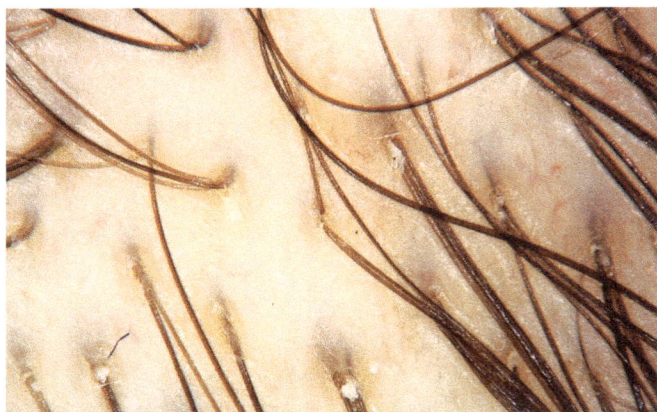

Fig. 6.1.3: Seborrheic dermatitis. Note that the peripilar scale usually does not completely encircle the hair follicle. In lichen planopilaris, peripilar scales are tubular and involve all the base of the follicles.

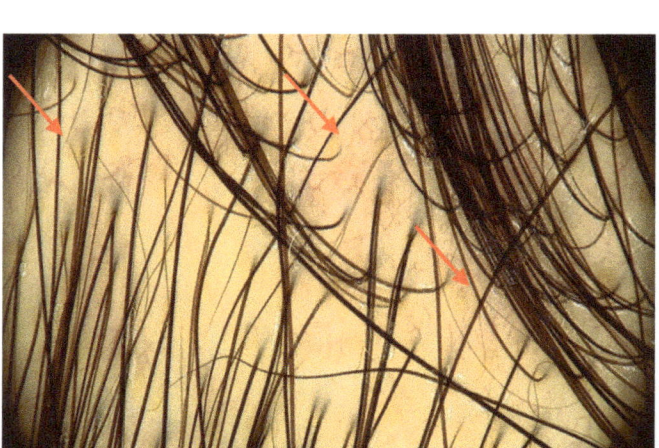

Fig. 6.1.4: Seborrheic dermatitis. Increased thin arborizing vessels network. Note yellow hues (→) surrouding some hair follicles due to increased sebum production.

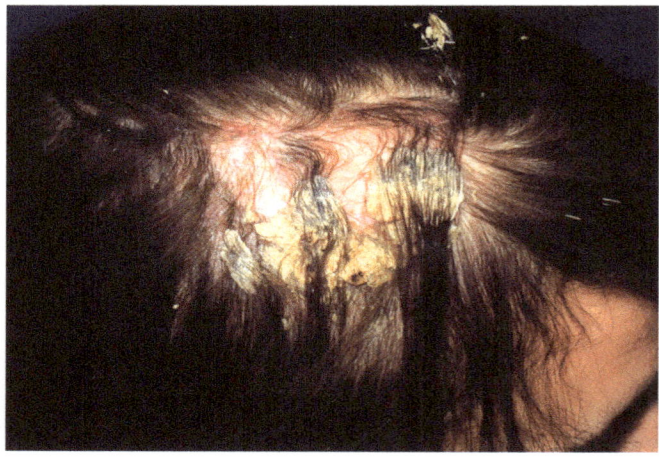

Fig. 6.1.5: Pityriasis amiantacea. Severe thick yellow crusts and partial alopecia on the scalp.

Source: Division of Dermatology, Hospital das Clínicas, University of São Paulo Medical School.

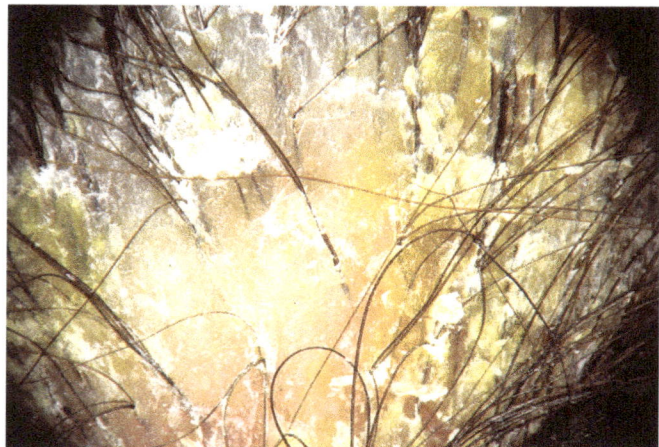

Fig. 6.1.6: Pityriasis amiantacea. On dry dermoscopy, intense interfollicular yellow crusts can be noticed.

Source: Division of Dermatology, Hospital das Clínicas, University of São Paulo Medical School.

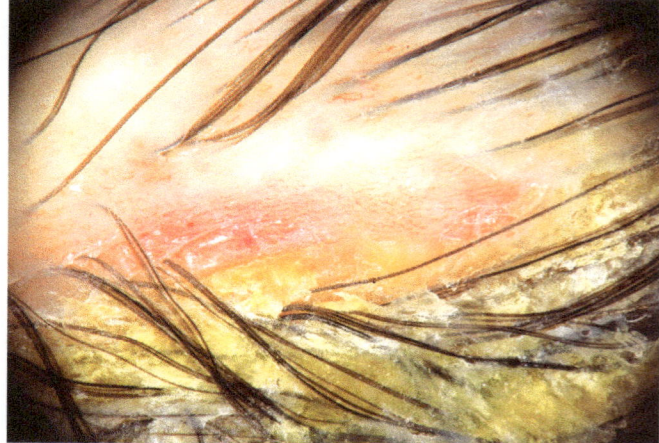

Fig. 6.1.7: Pityriasis amiantacea. Thick yellow crusts and scales, hairpin-like elongated vessels, small hair tufts, and white scarring areas. Note the absence of follicular openings in the central area.

Source: Division of Dermatology, Hospital das Clínicas, University of São Paulo Medical School.

> **Take-Home Message**
>
> Seborrheic dermatitis
> - Erythema and scaling mainly on the scalp, although other areas as glabella, and nasolabial fold can be also affected.
> - Dermoscopy shows interfollicular and perifollicular white-yellowish greasy scales, hair casts, arborizing thin vessels, and follicular pustules.
>
> Pityriasis amiantacea
> - Thick silvery or yellowish scales, strongly adhered to small hair tufts.
> - Scarring alopecia may occur.

SUGGESTED READING

1. Abdel-Hamid IA, Agha SA, Moustafa YM, et al. Pityriasis amiantacea: a clinical and etiopathological study of 85 patients. Int J Dermatol. 2003;42(4):260-4.
2. Amorim GM, Fernandes NC. Pityriasis amiantacea: a study of seven cases. An Bras Dermatol. 2016;91(5):694-6.
3. Borda LJ, Wikramanayake TC. Seborrheic dermatitis and dandruff: a comprehensive review. J Clin Investig Dermatol. 2015;3(2).
4. Errichetti E, Stinco G. Dermoscopy as a useful supportive tool for the diagnosis of pityriasis amiantacea-like tinea capitis. Dermatol Pract Concept. 2016;6(3):63-5.
5. Schwartz JR, Messenger AG, Tosti A, et al. A comprehensive pathophysiology of dandruff and seborrheic dermatitis – towards a more precise definition of scalp health. Acta Derm Venereol. 2013;93(2):131-7.
6. Verardino GC, Azulay-Abulafia L, Macedo PM, et al. Pityriasis amiantacea: clinical-dermatoscopic features and microscopy of hair tufts. An Bras Dermatol. 2012;87(1):142-5.

6.2 Psoriasis

Ricardo Romiti, Alessandra Anzai

Psoriasis is a chronic and recalcitrant inflammatory systemic disorder affecting about 2% of the population. Scalp psoriasis is present in 50–80% of the patients, as a sole manifestation of the disease or in association with body lesions. Typical lesions show well-demarcated erythematous plaques covered by silver-colored scales affecting variable areas of the scalp (Fig. 6.2.1). Patients commonly complain about hair shedding, which is noncicatricial and presents complete recovery after treatment in most cases. Psoriatic scarring alopecia is a rare complication and has been associated with constant flares of inflammation and scratching (Figs. 6.2.2A and B). Diagnosis of scalp psoriasis may require skin biopsies to rule out other inflammatory conditions, such as seborrheic dermatitis and contact dermatitis.

Dermoscopy shows thick white or white-silver scaling over a red skin (Fig. 6.2.3). When scales are removed, red dots and globular vessels can be seen in low magnifications (20X) (Fig. 6.2.4). Higher magnifications (40X or more) can show typical features of multiple twisted capillary and glomerular vessels in the entire scalp and mostly in the occipital areas (Figs. 6.2.5 and 6.2.6). Psoriatic alopecia shows scarring areas devoid of follicular openings and erythematous areas, and thick scales may be seen over the scalp (Fig. 6.2.7).

Scalp psoriasis can be treated with topical medications, such as keratolytic agents and topical steroids. Diffuse lesions may require oral medications as acitretin and methotrexate.

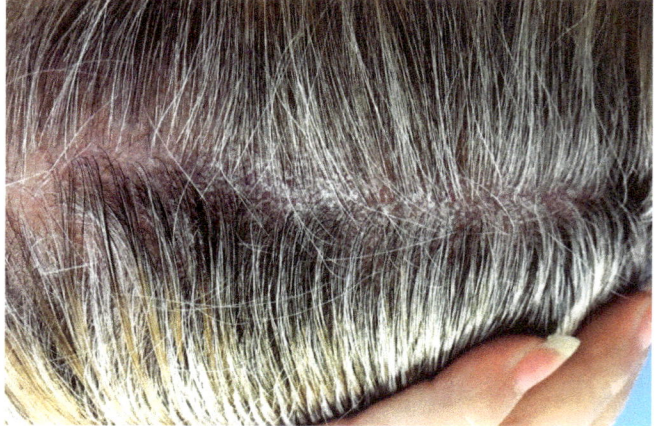

Fig. 6.2.1: Scalp psoriasis. Thick silvery-white scales over an erythematous skin.

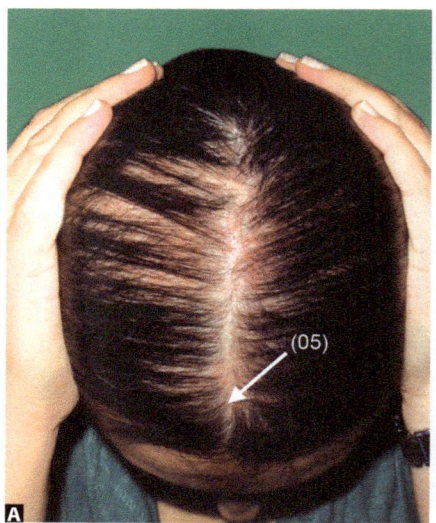
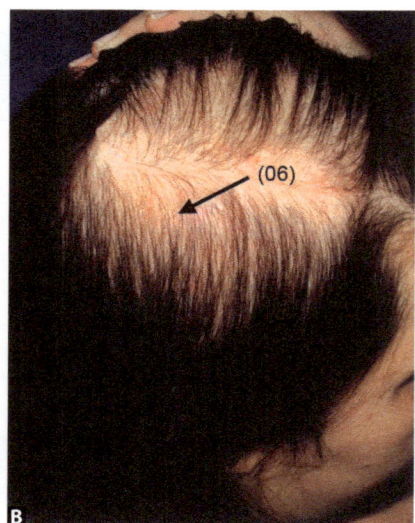

Figs. 6.2.2A and B: (A and B) Psoriatic scarring alopecia. Note decreased hair density and scarring areas with erythema and scales mostly in the frontal, vertex, and parietal areas of the scalp from a female patient.

Inflammatory Scalp Disorders

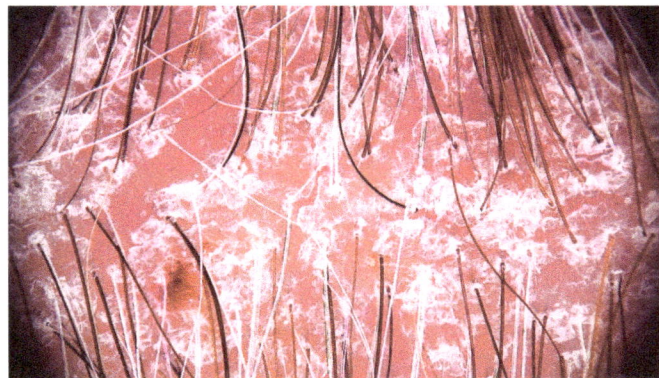

Fig. 6.2.3: Scalp psoriasis. Note interfollicular white scales over a red skin with blood extravasation.

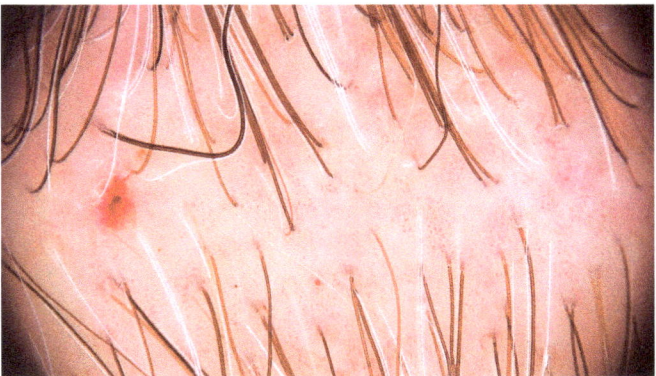

Fig. 6.2.4: Scalp psoriasis. Dermoscopy with immersion fluid shows dotted vessels (red dots) on a red background in low magnifications (20X). Note a round-shaped blood extravasation resulting from scratching.

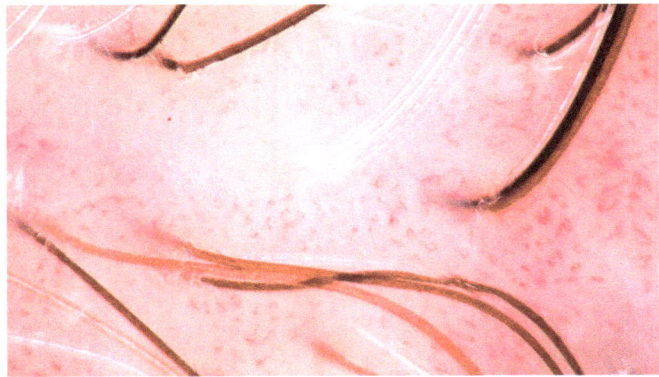

Fig. 6.2.5: Scalp psoriasis. Dermoscopy with immersion fluid shows multiple vessels as twisted loops, glomerular, comma, lace-like and hairpin-like vessels. They correspond to tortuous and dilated blood vessels of the dermal papillae (70X).

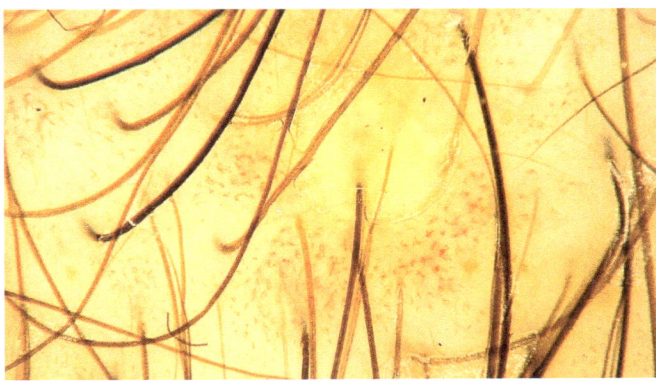

Fig. 6.2.6: Scalp psoriaisis. Clusters of multiple capillary vessels can be seen surrounding a follicular pustule.
Source: Dr. Isabella Doche

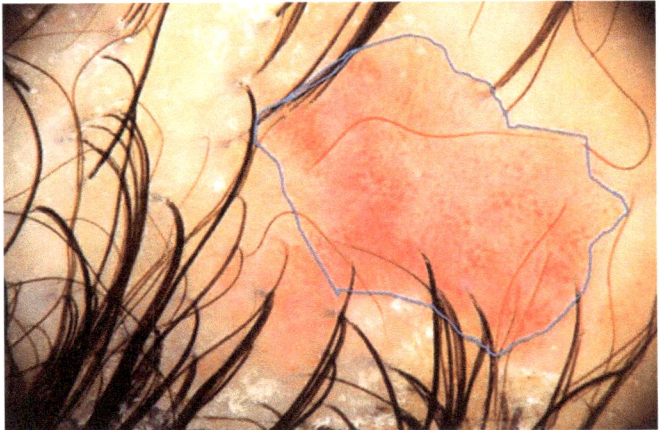

Fig. 6.2.7: Psoriatic scarring alopecia. Red dots and globules in an erythematous background area devoid of folicular openings (blue ring). Note also interfollicular thick scales (20X).

Take-Home Message

- Scalp psoriasis is present in over 50% of patients with psoriasis.
- Dermoscopy without imersion fluid shows thick silvery-white scales over an erythematous skin.
- After removing the scales, red dots and globules can be seen in low magnifications (20X).
- High magnifications (40X or above) can show typical features of twisted red loops and glomerular vessels in the entire scalp, mostly in the occipital area.
- Main differential diagnoses include seborrheic dermatitis and contact dermatitis.
- Psoriatic scarring alopecia is rare; decreased hair density, scarring areas lacking follicular openings and twisted red loops are usually present.

SUGGESTED READING

1. Almeida MC, Romiti R, Doche I, et al. Psoriatic scarring alopecia. An Bras Dermatol. 2013;88(6 Suppl. 1):29-31.
2. Kim GW, Jung HJ, Ko HC, et al. Dermoscopy can be useful in differentiating scalp psoriasis from seborrhoeic dermatitis. Br J Dermatol. 2011; 164(3):652-6.
3. Lallas A, Argenziano G, Apalla Z, et al. Dermoscopic patterns of common facial inflammatory skin diseases. J Eur Acad Dermatol Venereol. 2014;28(5):609-14.
4. Papp K, Berth-Jones J, Kragballe K, et al. Scalp psoriasis: a review of current topical treatment options. J Eur Acad Derm Venereol. 2007;21:1151-60.
5. Runne U, Kroneisen-Wiersma P. Psoriatic alopecia: acute and chronic hair loss in 47 patients with scalp psoriasis. Dermatology. 1992;185(2):82-7.
6. Shuster S. Psoriatic alopecia. Br J Dermatol. 1972;87:73-7.
7. Van de Kerkhof PC, Franssen ME. Psoriasis of the scalp. Diagnosis and management. Am J Clin Dermatol. 2001;2(3):159-65.

6.3 Contact Dermatitis

Emilie Jane Fowler, Antonella Tosti

The scalp is frequently exposed to allergens through products such as hair dyes, shampoos, and topical ointments, and to metals and rubber through objects such as brushes, hair clips, or hair rollers. However, contact dermatitis involving the scalp is relatively uncommon when compared to other areas of the body. The innate properties of the scalp such as its thick skin, numerous pilosebaceous units, and the absence of rhytids give it excellent protection against the manifestation of contact dermatitis.

When a patient does present with contact dermatitis of the scalp, they will complain of severe scalp itching, which may be accompanied by burning or hair loss, while they lack the typical eczematous lesions (Fig. 6.3.1). Associated dermatitis of the ears, eyelids, forehead, and neck may also be present. Chronic contact dermatitis on the scalp may even lead to presentations of telogen effluvium. A thorough patient history must be obtained to determine what substances their scalp is exposed to, and if they attribute their symptoms to recent use of a new product, for instance.

Dermoscopic examination, showing an increased number of arborizing vessels with or without scales, is suggestive but not diagnostic for scalp contact dermatitis (Figs. 6.3.1 to 6.3.3). In chronic, lichenified lesions, proximal trichorrhexis nodosa and prominent follicular openings can be seen on dermoscopy due to chronic scratching of the scalp (Figs. 6.3.4 and 6.3.5).

Contact dermatitis of the scalp always requires patch testing (especially of the patient's own hair products) to identify the allergen and make a definitive diagnosis. A recent study by Aleid et al. found metals such as nickel and cobalt, basalm of Peru, fragrances, carba mix, and propylene glycol among the most common allergens to cause scalp contact dermatitis.

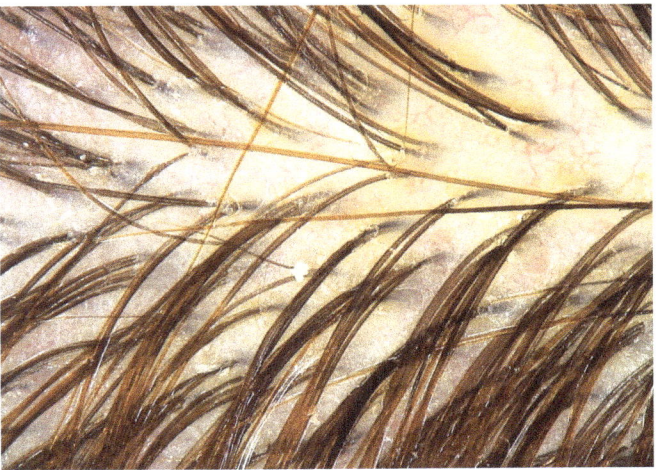

Fig. 6.3.2: Scalp contact dermatitis. Arborizing vessels and scales.

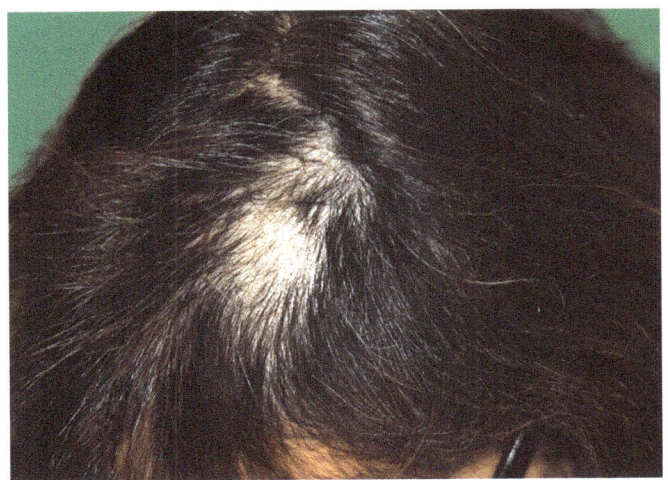

Fig. 6.3.1: Scalp contact dermatitis. Friction alopecia from scratching.

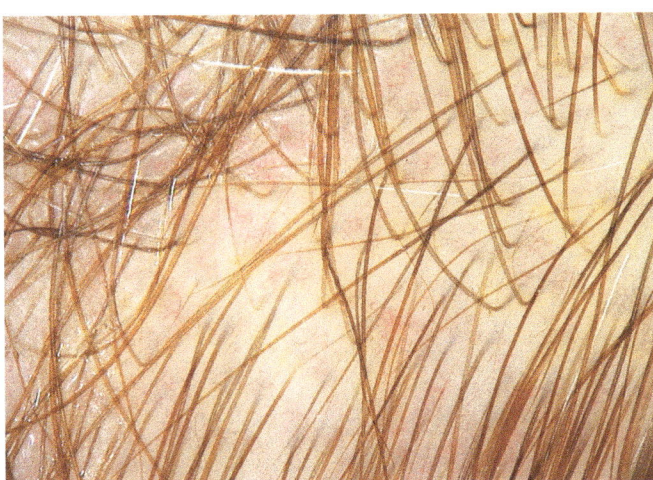

Fig. 6.3.3: Scalp contact dermatitis. Arborizing vessels.

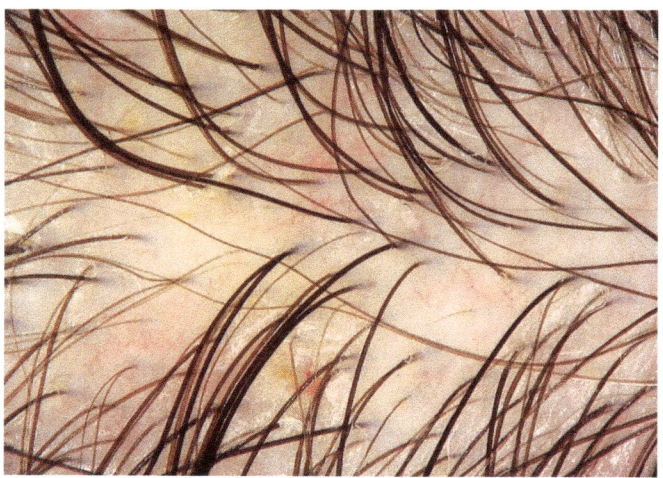

Fig. 6.3.4: Scalp contact dermatitis. Dermoscopy in androgenetic alopecia. Note arborizing vessels and hair diameter diversity.

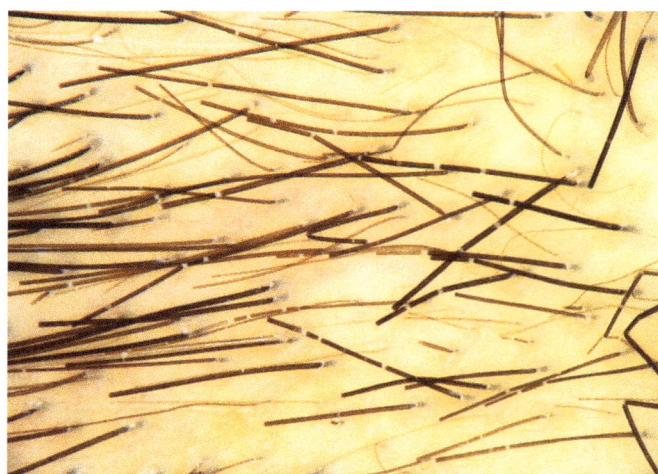

Fig. 6.3.5: Proximal trichorrhexis nodosa from scratching.

Take-Home Message

- Contact dermatitis of the scalp can cause increased hair shedding.
- Patients will present with severe scalp itching and sometimes burning.
- Dermoscopy shows arborizing vessels with or without scales.
- Proximal trichorrhexis nodosa is seen in chronic cases.

SUGGESTED READING

1. Aleid NM, Fertig R, Maddy A, et al. Common allergens identified based on patch test results in patients with suspected contact dermatitis of the scalp. Skin Appendage Disord. 2017;3(1):7-14.
2. Huynh M, Sheehan MP, Chung M, et al. Scalp. In: Lewallen R, Clark A, Feldman SR (Eds). Clinical Handbook of Contact Dermatitis: Diagnosis and Management by Body Region. Boca Raton: CRC Press; 2014. pp. 6-12.
3. Vincenzi C, Tosti A. Inflammatory scalp disorders. In: Tosti A (Ed). Dermoscopy of the Hair and Nails, 2nd edition. Boca Raton: CRC Press; 2016. pp. 120-1.
4. Tosti A, Piraccini BM, van Neste DJ. Telogen effluvium after allergic contact dermatitis of the scalp. Arch Dermatol. 2001;137(2):187-90.
5. Tosti A, Donati A, Vincenzi C, et al. Videodermoscopy does not enhance diagnosis of scalp contact dermatitis due to topical minoxidil. Int J Trichol. 2009;1(2):134-7.

6.4 Rosacea-like Dermatosis

Giselle Martins, Patricia Damasco, Isabella Doche

Rosacea is a chronic inflammatory disorder that commonly affects the central part of the face with recurrent and persistent episodes of erythema, telangiectasia, and flushing (Fig. 6.4.1). Papules, pustules, ocular lesions, and rhinophyma may occur. Extra-facial lesions are rare. Rosacea-like dermatosis is characterized by redness, itching, and burning sensations in the scalp. Patients present with follicular papules and pustules over the scalp that do not respond to potent topical steroids and antiseborrheic agents (Fig. 6.4.2). Although its exact etiology remains uncertain, excessive sun exposure and actinic damage may play a role.

Many diseases can lead to a "red scalp syndrome," such as contact dermatitis, psoriasis, seborrheic dermatitis, lichen planopilaris, lupus erythematosus, and dermatomyositis. Sometimes, facial rosacea can be also present and help the diagnosis. Histopathologic examination of the lesions can help to distinguish from other diseases.

Dermoscopy of facial lesions shows telangiectasias, polygonal vessels, and multiple follicular openings filled with keratin plugs (Figs. 6.4.3A and B). In the scalp, dermoscopy shows a nonscarring pattern of alopecia, diffuse erythema, telangiectasia in a "target pattern," follicular papules, and pustules (Figs. 6.4.4A and B). Like facial rosacea, rosacea-like dermatosis of the scalp usually improves with oral tetracyclines and protection against ultraviolet exposure.

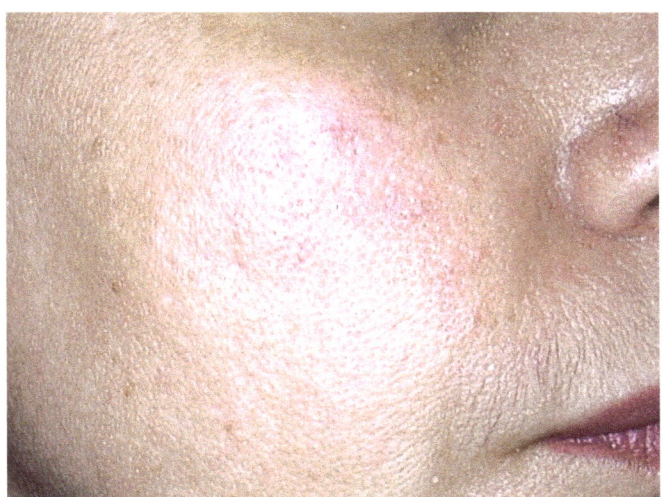

Fig. 6.4.1: Facial rosacea. Note mild erythema and telagiectasia on the midface from a female patient.

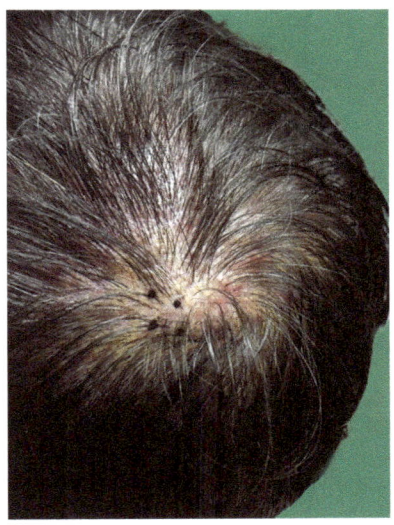

Fig. 6.4.2: Rosacea-like dermatosis of the scalp. Persistent redness and scalp itching in a 65-year-old male patient.

Source: Hair Department, Division of Dermatology, Federal University of Health Science of Porto Alegre.

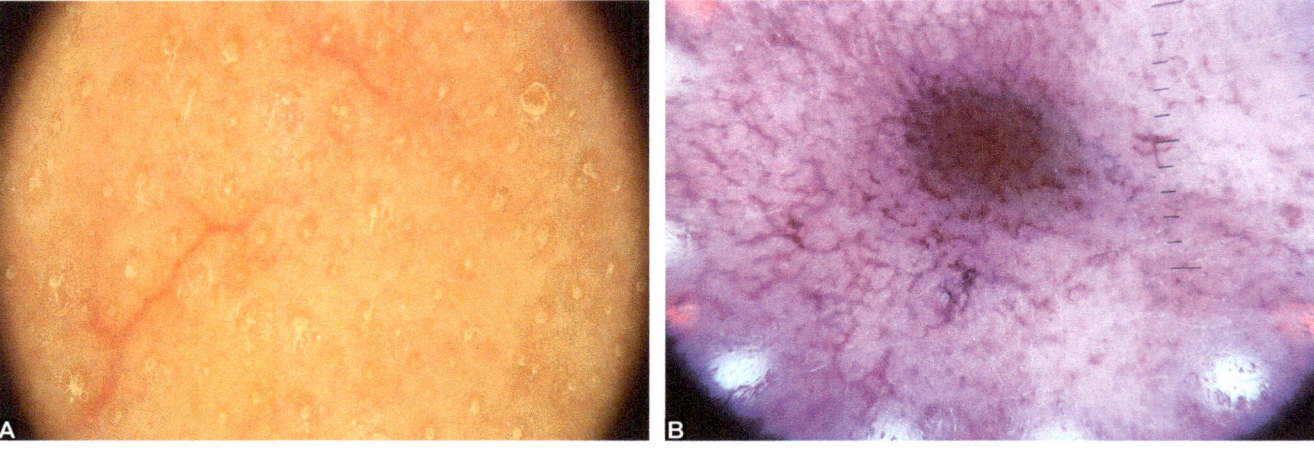

Figs. 6.4.3A and B: Facial rosacea. (A) Telangiectasic vessels and multiple follicular openings filled with keratin plugs. (B) Note the polygonal vessels.

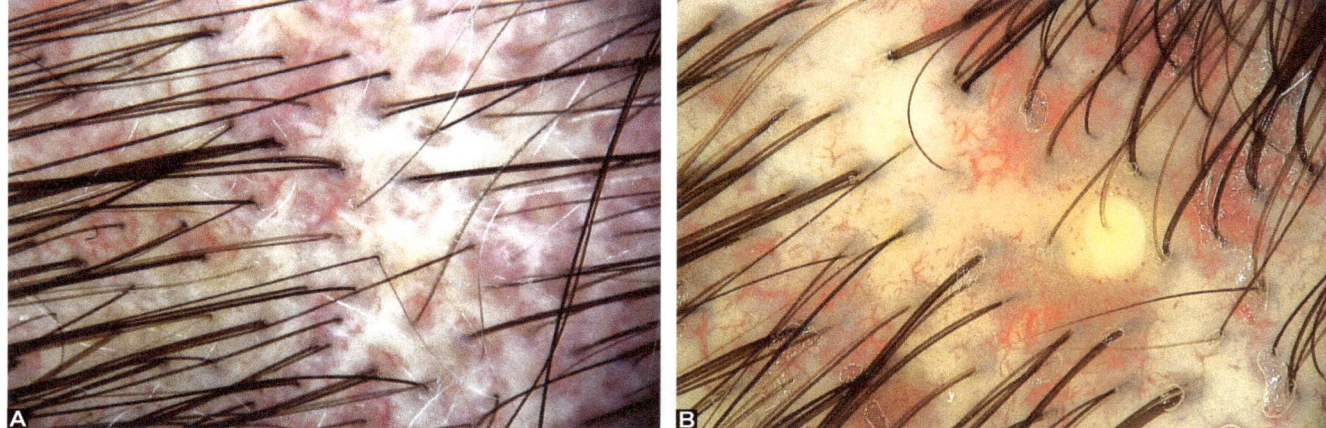

Figs. 6.4.4A and B: Rosacea-like dermatosis of the scalp. (A) Nonscarring pattern of alopecia, diffuse erythema, intense perifollicular, and interfollicular telangiectasia in a "target pattern." (B) Follicular pustules and multiple arborizing vessels.
Source: Hair Department, Division of Dermatology, Federal University of Health Science of Porto Alegre.

> **Take-Home Message**
> - Rosacea-like dermatosis of the scalp should be considered in patients with persistent scalp redness and itching.
> - Dermoscopy shows nonscarring pattern of alopecia, diffuse erythema, telangiectasia, follicular papules, and pustules.
> - Other causes of "red scalp syndrome" such as contact dermatitis, seborrheic dermatitis, psoriasis, lichen planopilaris, lupus erythematosus, and dermatomiositis must be ruled out.

SUGGESTED READING

1. Ayres S Jr. Extrafacial rosacea is rare but does exist. J Am Acad Dermatol. 1987;16:391-2.
2. Bernhard JD. Itch: Mechanisms and Management of Pruritus. New York: McGraw-Hill;1994. p. 51.
3. Lallas A, Argenziano G, Apalla Z, et al. Dermoscopic patterns of common facial inflammatory skin diseases. J Eur Acad Dermatol Venereol. 2014;28(5):609-14.
4. Lallas A, Argenziano G, Longo C, et al. Polygonal vessels of rosacea are highlighted by dermoscopy. Int J Dermatol. 2014;53(5):e325-7.
5. Lonne-Rahm SB, Fischer T, Berg M. Stinging and rosacea. Acta Derm Venereol. 1999;79(6):460-1.
6. Oberholzer PA, Nobbe S, Kolm I, et al. Red scalp disease – a rosacea-like dermatosis of the scalp? successful therapy with oral tetracycline. Dermatology. 2009;219:179-81.
7. Pereira TM, Vieira AP, Basto AS. Rosacea with extensive extrafacial lesions. Int J Dermatol. 2008;47:52-5.
8. Thestrup-Pedersen K, Hjorth N. Red scalp: a previously undescribed disease of the scalp? Ugeskr Laeger. 1987;149:2141-2.
9. Trueb RM. Is androgenetic alopecia a photoaggravated dermatosis? Dermatology. 2003;207(4)343-8.
10. Willimann B, Trüeb RM. Hair pain (trichodynia): frequency and relationship to hair loss and patient gender. Dermatology. 2002;205:374-7.
11. Wilkin J, Dahl M, Detmar M, et al. Standard classification of rosacea: report of the National Rosacea Society Expert Committee on the classification and staging of rosacea. J Am Acad Dermatol. 2002;46(4):584-7.

CHAPTER 7

Systemic Diseases

*Patricia Damasco, Giselle Martins, Isabella Doche, Maria K Hordinsky,
Ricardo Romiti, Alessandra Anzai*

7.1 Systemic Lupus Erythematosus

Patricia Damasco, Giselle Martins, Isabella Doche

Nonscarring and scarring hair loss can be observed in 20–60% of the patients with systemic lupus erythematosus (SLE). Alopecia is usually related to disease activity but can be also drug-induced. Patients with SLE may present with acute and diffuse hair shedding, nonscarring alopecia areata-like patches, and scarring discoid patches (Figs. 7.1.1A and B). Patients with telogen effluvium can show diffuse hair loss and lupus hairs may be present. They are characterized by dry, fragile, and course regrowing hairs prominently over the frontal hairline.

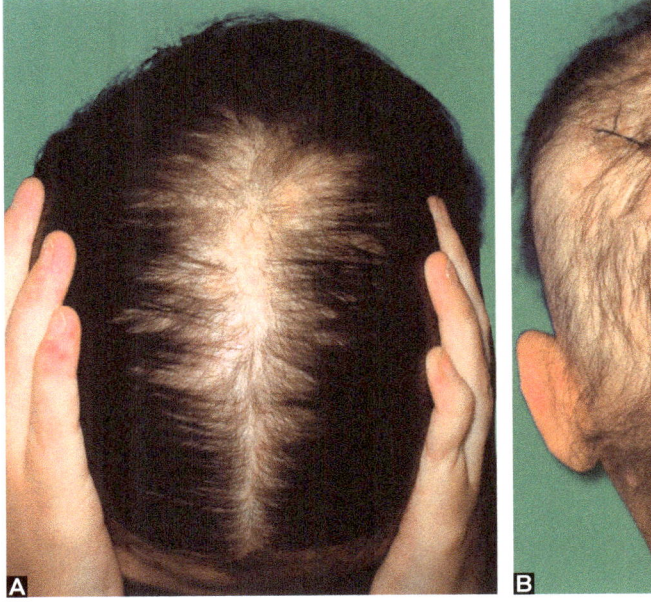 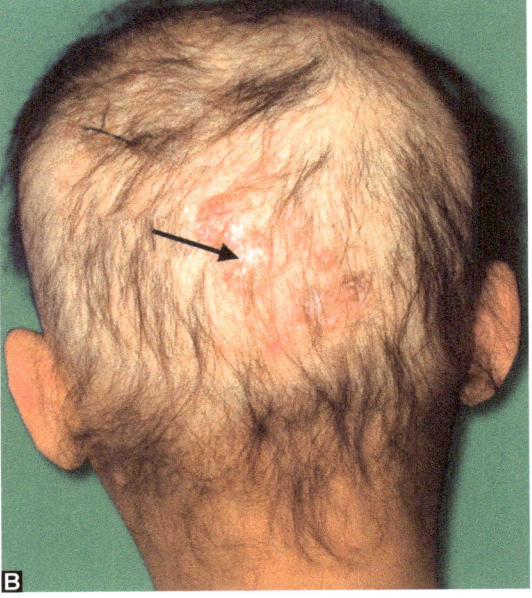

Figs. 7.1.1A and B: Systemic lupus erythematosus. (A) Nonscarring patchy alopecia. (B) Diffuse nonscarring alopecia associated with discoid lesions (black arrow) on the scalp.
Source: Division of Dermatology, Hospital das Clínicas, University of São Paulo Medical School.

Dermoscopy shows short regrowing hairs and velus hairs. Patchy nonscarring alopecic areas may resemble alopecia areata, and show the same dermoscopic typical features (Figs. 7.1.2 and 7.1.3). Sometimes the presence of associated enlarged branching vessels can help the diagnosis of lupus erythematosus (Figs. 7.1.4 and 7.1.5). Scarring discoid lesions show absence of follicular openings, scales, hyperpigmented areas, occasional keratin plugs, and enlarged giant and arborizing vessels on dermoscopy (Figs. 7.1.6A and B).

Treatment strategies depend on disease activity and extension. Topical steroid calcineurin inhibitors can be used. Oral medications as antimalarials, systemic corticosteroids, and other immunosuppressive and immunomodulatory drugs can be associated, in addition to ultraviolet protection.

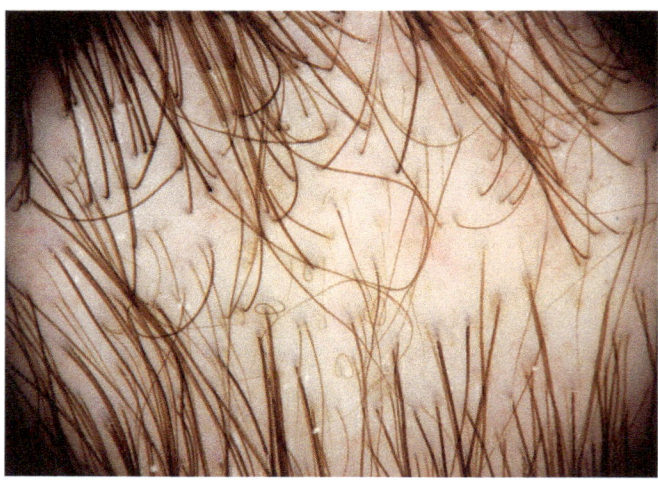

Fig. 7.1.2: Systemic lupus erythematosus. Short regrowing hairs, vellus hairs, yellow dots, and multiple circle hairs in a patient with nonscarring diffuse alopecia. Note a mild erythematous background.
Source: Division of Dermatology, Hospital das Clínicas, University of São Paulo Medical School.

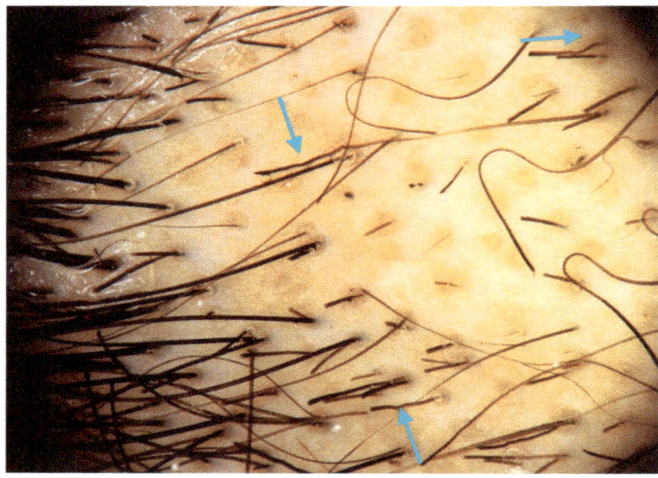

Fig. 7.1.3: Systemic lupus erythematosus. Alopecia areata-like patch showing multiple yellow dots, broken hairs, black dots, and pili torti (blue arrows). No vascular pattern can be seen in this case.
Source: Division of Dermatology, Hospital das Clínicas, University of São Paulo Medical School.

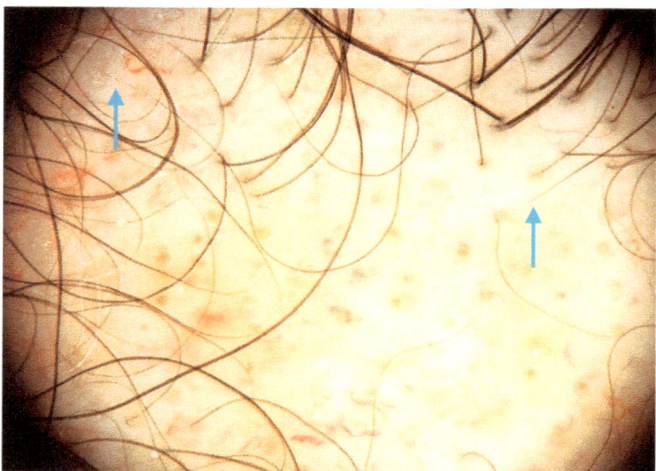

Fig. 7.1.4: Systemic lupus erythematosus. Nonscarring alopecic patch with yellow dots, thinned hairs, and caudability hairs (blue arrows). Note some enlarged arborizing vessels.
Source: Division of Dermatology, Hospital das Clínicas, University of São Paulo Medical School.

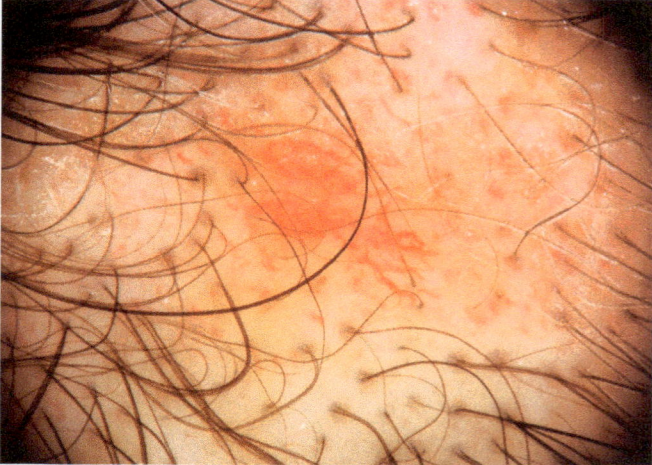

Fig. 7.1.5: Systemic lupus erythematosus. Polymorphous enlarged and giant capillary vessels within a nonscarring alopecic patch.
Source: Division of Dermatology, Hospital das Clínicas, University of São Paulo Medical School.

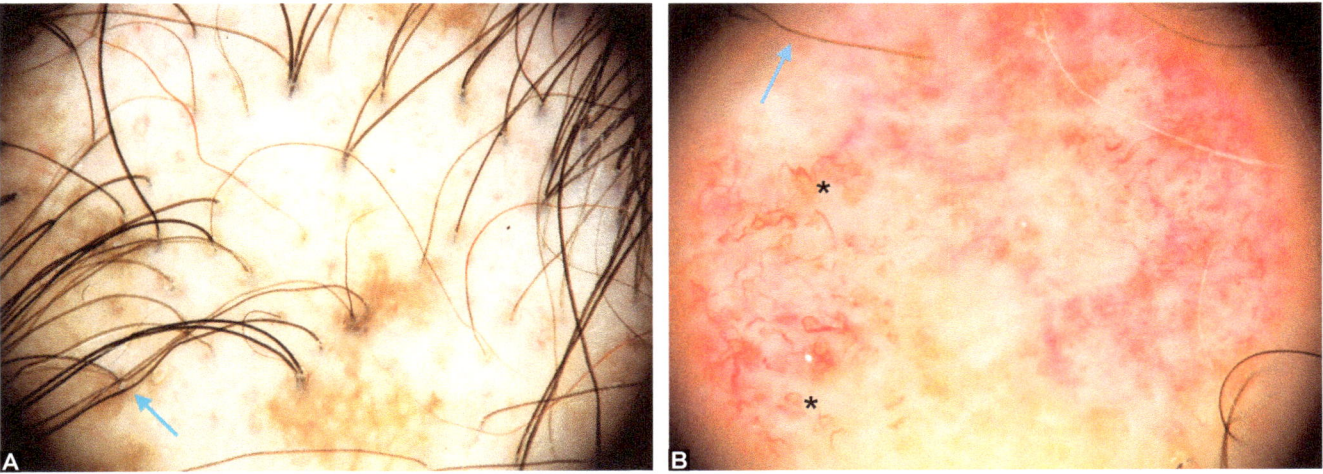

Figs. 7.1.6A and B: Systemic lupus erythematosus. (A) Dyschromia and peripilar scales in a scarring discoid alopecic patch. (B) Enlarged vessels surrounding a scarring patch of alopecia devoid of follicular openings. Note the presence of thin arborizing vessels surrounding some yellow spiders ("red spiders" in a yellow dot) (*) and pili torti (blue arrows).
Source: Division of Dermatology, Hospital das Clínicas, University of São Paulo Medical School.

Take-Home Message

- Systemic lupus erythematous mostly presents as a nonscarring diffuse or patchy alopecia.
- Nonscarring alopecia presents as alopecia areata-like patches and/or acute telogen effluvium.
- Scarring alopecia may occur and show features of discoid lesions.
- Dermoscopy usually shows features of nonscarring alopecia. However, some features of scarring process may be associated.

SUGGESTED READING

1. Cardinali C, Caproni M, Bernacchi E, et al. The spectrum of cutaneous manifestations in lupus erythematous – the italian experience. Lupus. 2000;9(6):417-23.
2. Gong Y, Ye Y, Zhao Y, et al. Severe diffuse non-scarring hair loss in systemic lupus erythematosus – clinical and histopathological analysis of four cases. J Eur Acad Dermatol Venereol. 2013;27(5):651-4.
3. Moghadam-Kia S, Franks AG Jr. Autoimmune disease and hair loss. Dermatol Clin. 2013;31(1):75-91.
4. Rigopoulos D, Stamatios G, Ioannides D. Primary scarring alopecias. Curr Probl Dermatol. 2015;47:76-86.
5. Ross EK, Shapiro J. Primary cicatricial alopecia. In: Blume-Peytavi U, Tosti A, Whiting D, et al. (Eds). Hair Growth and Disorders. Leipzig:Springer;2008. pp. 293-4.
6. Trueb RM. Hair and nail involvement in lupus erythematosus. Clin Dermatol. 2004; 22(2):139-47.
7. Yell JA, Mbuagbaw J, Burge SM. Cutaneous manifestations of systemic lupus erythematous. Br J Dermatol. 1996;135(3):355-62.
8. Yun SJ, Lee JW, Yoon HJ, et al. Cross-sectional study of hair loss patterns in 122 Korean systemic lupus erythematous patients: a frequent finding of non-scarring patch alopecia. J Dermatol. 2007;34(7):451-5.

7.2 Dermatomyositis

Isabella Doche, Maria K Hordinsky

Dermatomyositis is a rare autoimmune inflammatory disorder characterized by muscle weakness and skin rash. Although it can occur in both genders with all ages, women are usually more affected. Symptoms may involve many organs and can be insidious or sudden. The most specific skin signs are Gottron papules over the knuckles and a periorbital heliotropic rash. Complications can include visceral involvement and cancer.

Scalp involvement is a common manifestation of dermatomyositis. Patients usually present a nonscarring alopecia with diffuse hair thinning and variable scalp erythema (Fig. 7.2.1A). Severe scalp itching is a prominent symptom and sometimes may be misdiagnosed as other scalp dermatitis, such as seborrheic dermatitis and contact dermatitis. Scarring alopecia is rare; scalp atrophy and scales may occur (Fig. 7.2.1B).

Dermoscopy of nonscarring alopecia shows hair thinning, irregularly giant capillary vessels, and thick arborizing vessels (Figs. 7.2.2 and 7.2.3). Scarring lesions shows the absence of follicular openings and erythema. Scalp scaling and pili torti may be present (Figs. 7.2.4A and B). Vascular changes in nail fold capillaroscopy can help the diagnosis and assess disease activity (Fig. 7.2.5).

Diagnosis is by clinical findings and abnormalities on muscle tests, which may include muscle enzymes, magnetic resonance imaging, electromyography, and muscle biopsy. Treatment options include corticosteroids, usually combined with immunosuppressants or intravenous immune globulin besides avoiding drugs that could induce skin rashes.

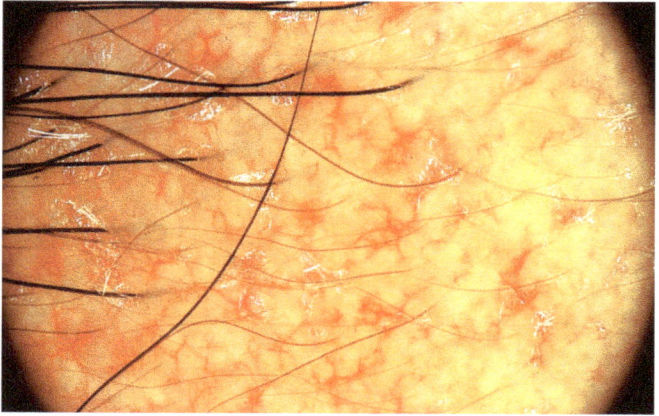

Fig. 7.2.2: Dermatomyositis. Nonscarring alopecia shows hair thinning and marked scalp telangiectasia with irregularly enlarged interfollicular vessels.

Source: Dr Giselle Martins.

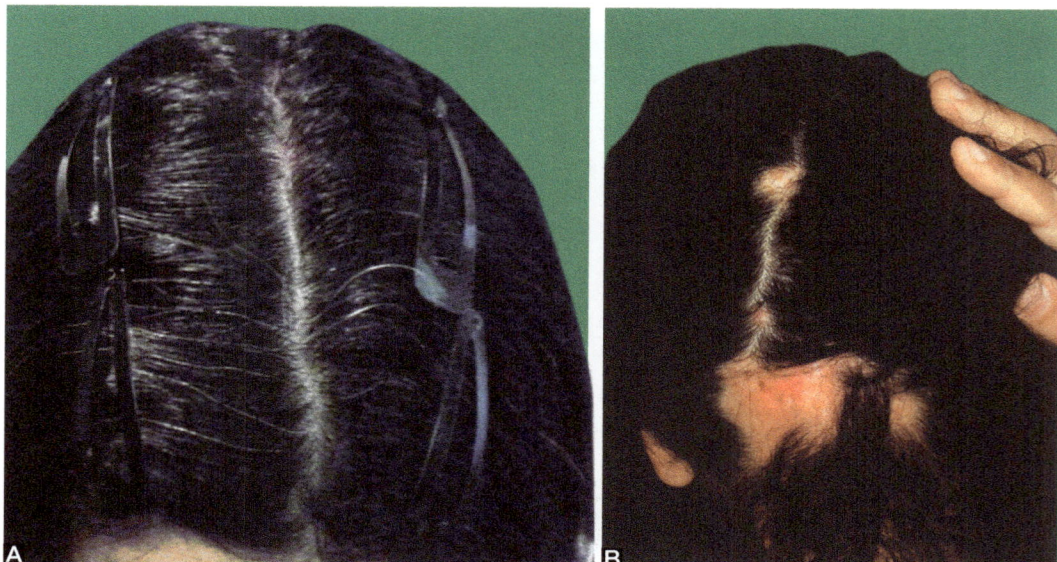

Figs. 7.2.1A and B: Dermatomyositis. (A) Nonscarring alopecia with mild scalp erythema and scaling on the vertex area of the scalp. (B) Scarring patches of alopecia in the posterior scalp from a female patient.

Source: (A) Dr Giselle Martins. (B) Division of Dermatology, Hospital das Clínicas, University of São Paulo Medical School.

Systemic Diseases

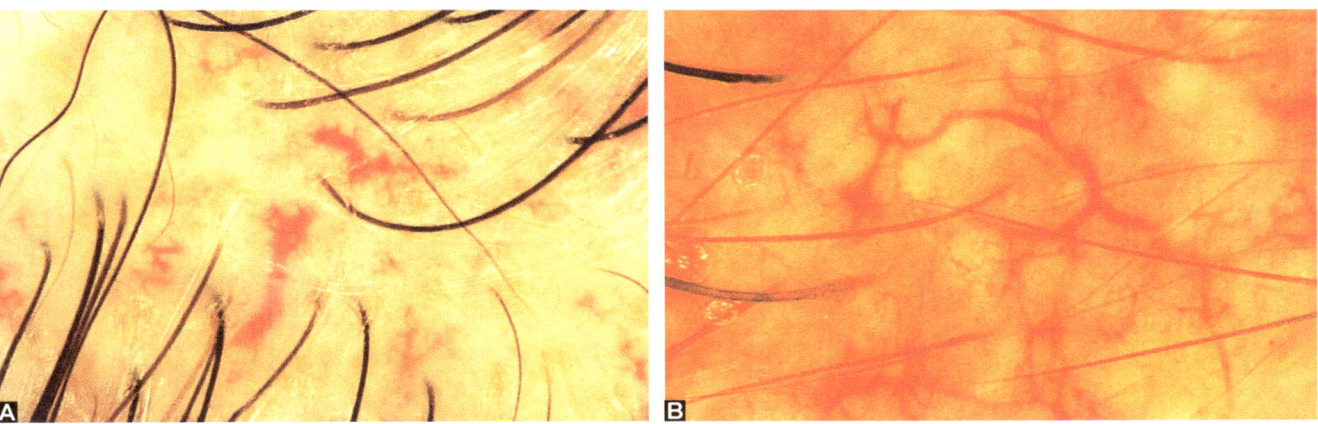

Figs. 7.2.3A and B: (A and B) Dermatomyositis. Note giant and tortuous interfollicular capillaries.
Source: Dr Giselle Martins

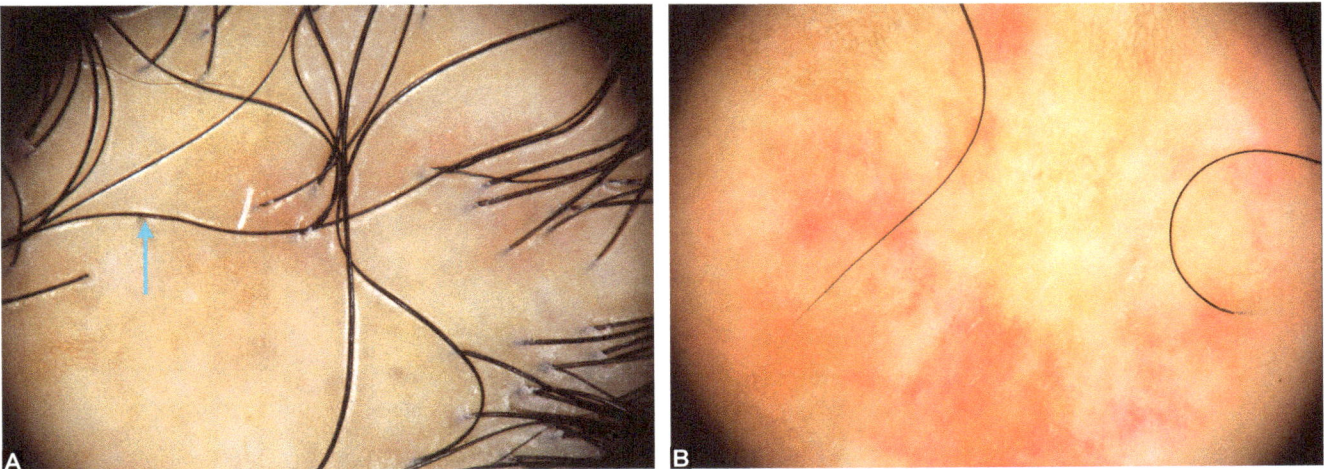

Figs. 7.2.4A and B: Dermatomyositis. (A) Dry dermoscopy shows a mild peripilar scale and one pili torti (blue arrow). (B) Dermoscopy with imersion fluid shows a scarring white patch lacking follicular openings, absence of honeycomb pattern, and an erythematous background.
Source: Division of Dermatology, Hospital das Clínicas, University of São Paulo Medical School.

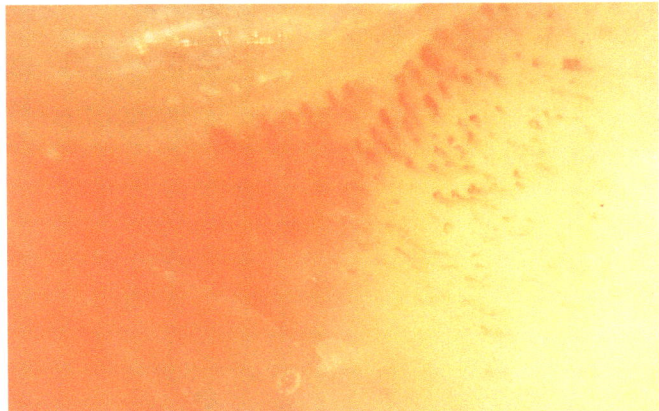

Fig. 7.2.5: Dermatomyositis. Capillaroscopy shows capillary enlargement and avascular areas on the proximal nail fold.
Source: Dr Giselle Martins.

> **Take-Home Message**
> - Scalp alopecia occurs in most cases of dermatomyositis.
> - Nonscarring alopecia with hair thinning, scale, and erythema is the most frequent clinical feature.
> - Severe scalp itching may be misdiagnosed as other scalp dermatoses.
> - Scarring alopecia is rare.
> - Dermoscopy of nonscarring lesions shows hair thinning and thick polymorphous giant vessels.
> - Nail fold capillaroscopy may help the diagnosis and assess disease activity.

SUGGESTED READING

1. Callen JP. Dermatomyositis. Lancet. 2000;355(9197):53-7.
2. Jasso-Olivares JC, Tosti A, Miteva M, et al. Clinical and Dermoscopic Features of the Scalp in 31 Patients with Dermatomyositis. Skin Appendage Disord. 2017;3(3):119-24.
3. Kasteler JS, Callen JP. Scalp involvement in dermatomyositis. Often overlooked or misdiagnosed. JAMA. 1994;272(24):1939-41.
4. Manfredi A, Sebastiani M, Cassone G, et al. Clin Rheumatol. 2015;34(2):279-84.
5. Mugii N, Hasegawa M, Matsushita T, et al. Association between nail-fold capillary findings and disease activity in dermatomyositis. Rheumatology. 2011;50(6):1091-8.
6. Oremović L, Lugović L, Vucić M, et al. Cicatricial alopecia as a manifestation of different dermatoses. Acta Dermatovenereol Croat. 2006;14(4):246-52.
7. Parodi A, Cozzani E. Hair loss in autoimmune systemic diseases. G Ital Dermatol Venereol. 2014;149(1):79-81.
8. Tilstra J, Prevost N, Khera P, English JC III. Scalp dermatomyositis revisited. Arch Dermatol. 2009;145(9):1062-3.

7.3 Scleroderma

Ricardo Romiti, Alessandra Anzai

Scleroderma is a rare connective tissue disease characterized by cutaneous sclerosis and variable systemic involvement. Two types of scleroderma are known—systemic sclerosis (cutaneous sclerosis and visceral involvement, especially the esophagus, lung, and vascular system) and localized scleroderma or morphea.

Localized scleroderma or morphea is a chronic and benign connective tissue disease of unknown etiology, which lesions are restricted to the skin and/or underlying tissues. There are several types of morphea with variable clinical manifestations and connective tissue involvement. All types are characterized by increasing amounts of collagen fibers and skin thickening, resulting in an indurative lesion with pigmented edges. Localized scleroderma can be linear, involving the head and face areas, such as linear scleroderma "en coup de sabre" and progressive facial hemiatrophy. Other types of morphea include plaque, deep, bullous, and generalized lesions.

Linear scleroderma is characterized by one or more linear streaks of cutaneous induration that may involve dermis, subcutaneous tissue, muscle, and underlying bone. Linear scleroderma is often observed in children and adolescents, and is the most frequent form of scleroderma in childhood.

"En coup de sabre" morphea is the variant that most frequently affects the scalp. Variable degrees of deformity and cicatricial alopecia of linear distribution following Blaschko´s lines can be found. The plaque is usually unilateral, atrophic, and slightly depressed, and the skin is smooth, shiny, hard, and sometimes pigmented (Fig. 7.3.1). Frontal depressed lesions may extend to the malar and nasal regions, and even to the upper lip resulting in bone depression and severe impact in the quality of life. Association with various systemic disorders has been reported.

Dermoscopy of early-onset scleroderma en coup de sabre lesions shows broken hairs, black dots, and vellus hairs (Fig. 7.3.2). In long-standing lesions, whitish fibrotic beams, the absence of follicular openings, elongated vessels, and pigment network-like structures can be seen

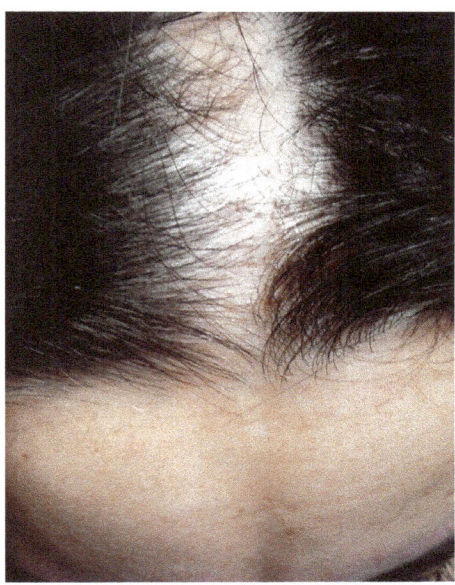

Fig. 7.3.1: Localized scleroderma. Scleroderma "en coup de sabre" affecting the paramedian forehead and frontal scalp region. Note the depressed and slightely pigmented skin.

(Fig. 7.3.3). In active systemic scleroderma, patients may have diffuse hair loss and dermoscopy of the scalp does not reveal any abnormalities. Pili torti and typical elongated vessels may be found in chronic cases (Fig. 7.3.4).

Nail fold capillaroscopy is useful both as a diagnostic tool and as a predictor of disease progression. Active scleroderma shows capillary enlargement with hemorrhagic lesions. Chronic lesions may show bushy vessels and avascular areas with loss of capillaries in the proximal nail fold (Fig. 7.3.5). Magnifications of 30–50X can help to identify the severity of capillary changes and disease activity.

Main differential diagnoses include dermatomyositis and systemic lupus erythematosus. Treatment options are vasodilators, antiinflammatory, immunosuppressive, and antifibrotic drugs.

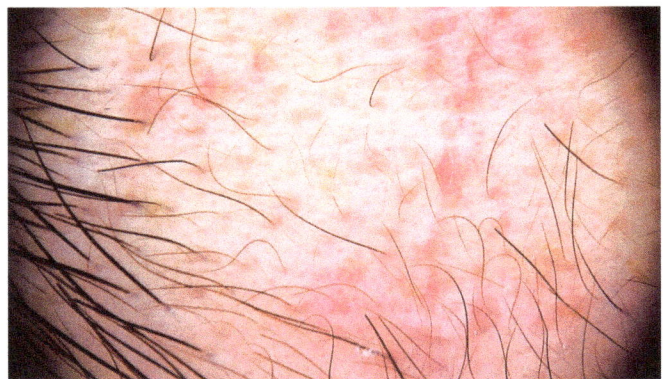

Fig. 7.3.2: Localized scleroderma. Early stages show a nonscarring process with vellus hairs, broken hairs, black dots, and some yellow dots. Note some linear vessels.

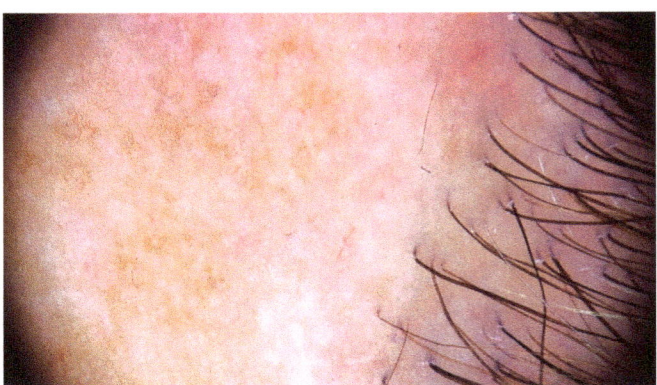

Fig. 7.3.3: Localized scleroderma. Long-standing lesions show whitish fibrotic beams, absence of follicular openings, elongated vessels, within an irregular pigmented network.

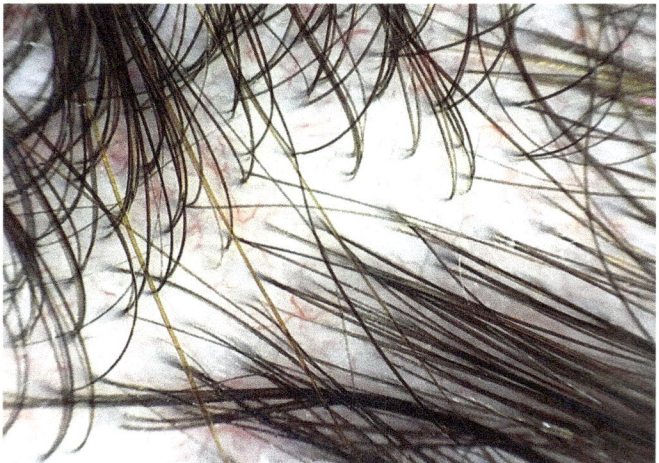

Fig. 7.3.4: Systemic scleroderma. Typical elongated vessels can be seen in this patient with longstanding disease. Early onset cases usually do not reveal any tricoscopic abnormalities.
Source: Dr Isabella Doche.

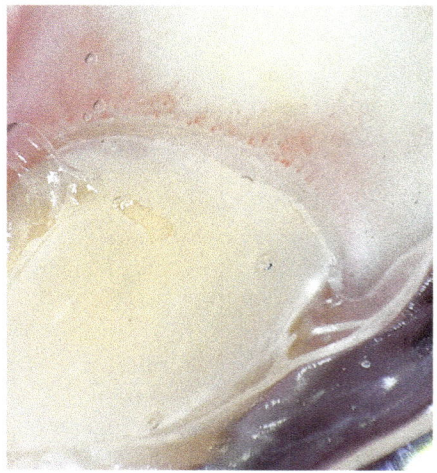

Fig. 7.3.5: Systemic scleroderma. Areas with mild capillary loss and enlarged and bushy (ramified) capillaries in the proximal nail fold in a patient with longstanding disease.
Source: Dr Isabella Doche.

Take-Home Message

- Scleroderma is classified into systemic and localized scleroderma.
- In localized scleroderma (morphea), dermoscopy findings include whitish fibrotic beams, crossed by linear branching vessels, and pigment network-like structures.
- In systemic scleroderma, peripheral microvascular morphology is generally assessed using nail fold capillaroscopy, which also allows the detection of disease activity.

SUGGESTED READING

1. Campione E, Paternó EJ, Diluvio L, et al. Localized morphea treated with imiquimod 5% and dermoscopic assessment of effectiveness. J Dermatol Treat. 2009;20(1):10–3.
2. Careta MF, Leite Cda C, Cresta F, et al. Prospective study to evaluate the clinical and radiological outcome of patients with scleroderma of the face. Autoimmun Rev. 2013;12(11):1064-9.
3. Cassidy JT, Petty RE. The systemic scleroderma and related disorders. In: Cassidy JT, Petty RE, (Eds). Textbook of Pediatric Rheumatology. Philadelphia. 2001. pp. 505-34.
4. Fett N, Werth VP. Update on morphea: part I. Epidemiology, clinical presentation, and pathogenesis. J Am Acad Dermatol. 2011;64(2):217-28.
5. Nelson A. Localized sclerodermas. In: Cassidy JT, Petty RE (Eds). Textbook of pediatric rheumatology. Philadelphia: W.B. Saunders; 2001. pp. 535-44.
6. Shim WH, Jwa SW, Song M, et al. Diagnostic usefulness of dermatoscopy in differentiating lichen sclerous et atrophicus from morphea. J Am Acad Dermatol. 2012;66(4):690-1.

7. Tiodorovic-Zivkovic D, Argenziano G, Popovic D, et al. Clinical and dermoscopic findings of a patient with co-existing lichen planus, lichen sclerosus and morphea. Eur J Dermatol. 2012;22(1):143-4.
8. Tollefson MM, Witman PM. En coup de sabre morphea and Parry-Romberg syndrome: a retrospective review of 54 patients. J Am Acad Dermatol. 2007;56:257-63.
9. Uziel Y, Miller ML, Laxer RM. Scleroderma in children. Pediatr Clin North Am. 1995;42:1171-203.
10. Weibel L, Harper JI. Linear morphea follows Blaschko's lines. Br J Dermatol. 2008;159(1):175-81.

7.4 Sarcoidosis

Isabella Doche

Scalp sarcoidosis is a very rare disease mostly affecting African descent patients. Initial lesions start with itching folliculitis-like lesions that progress to patches of scarring alopecia, with erythematous, hyperpigmented, and violaceous areas (Fig. 7.4.1).

Dermoscopy shows white scarring patches, telangiectasias, hyperpigmented violaceous areas, few pili torti, mild peripilar scale, with a pale-to-orange discoloration (Figs. 7.4.2 to 7.4.4).

About 50% of the patients will require systemic treatment, while the remaining will present spontaneous resolution of the disease. Systemic treatments include long-term regimens in order to prevent relapses. Systemic corticosteroids are the first line treatment in sarcoidosis. The main differential diagnosis of chronic lesions is discoid lupus erythematosus.

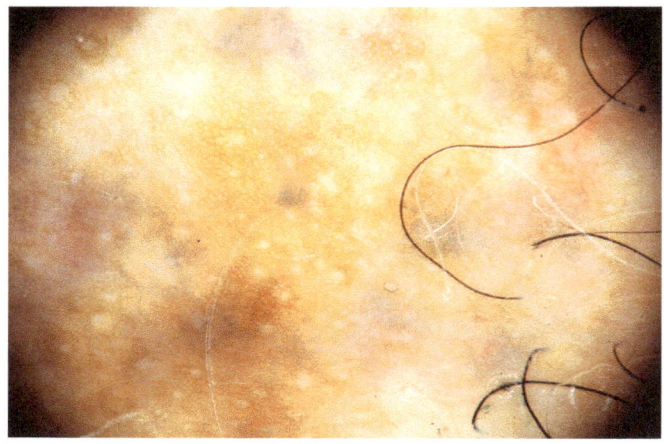

Fig. 7.4.2: Sarcoidosis. White scarring dots/patches and violaceous and erythematous lesions.
Source: Division of Dermatology, Hospital das Clínicas, University of São Paulo Medical School.

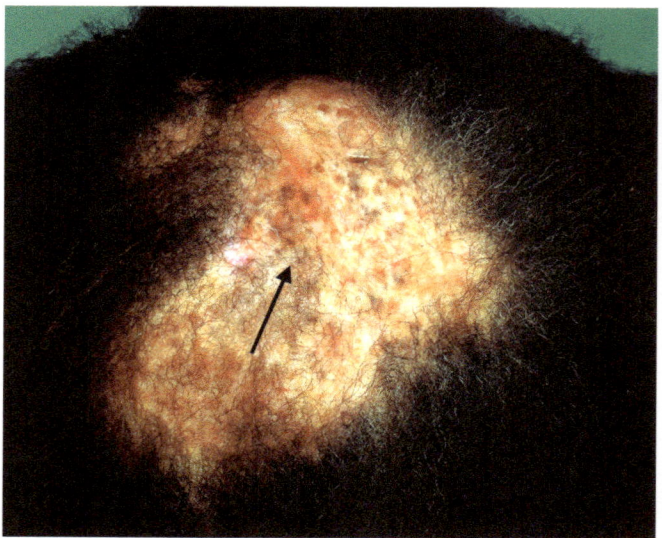

Fig. 7.4.1: Sarcoidosis. Longstanding scarring patch of alopecia with atrophic, erythematous, and hyperpigmented lesions (black arrow) on the scalp from an African descent patient.
Source: Division of Dermatology, Hospital das Clínicas, University of São Paulo Medical School.

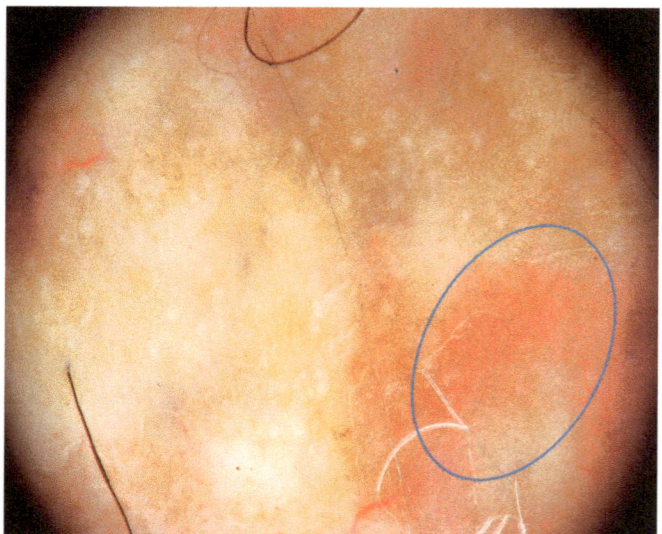

Fig. 7.4.3: Sarcoidosis. Pale-to-orange discoloration areas (blue ring).
Source: Division of Dermatology, Hospital das Clínicas, University of São Paulo Medical School.

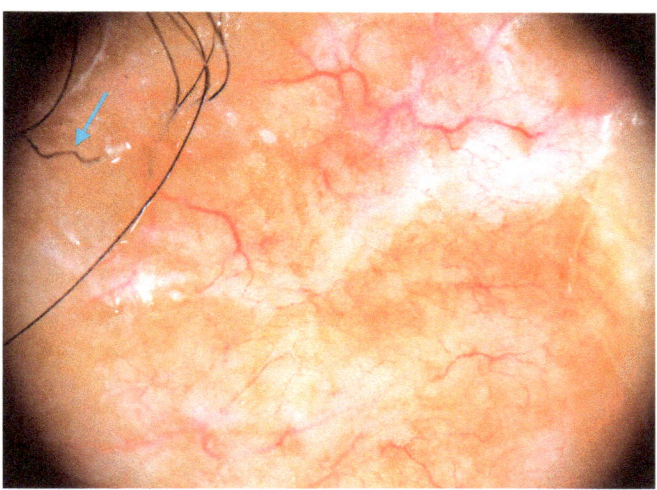

Fig. 7.4.4: Sarcoidosis. Prominent telangiectasias. Note one pili torti on the border (→).

Source: Division of Dermatology, Hospital das Clínicas, University of São Paulo Medical School.

Take-Home Message
- Sarcoidosis can affect different systems of the body including the scalp.
- Scalp presentation is very rare and mostly occurs in African descent patients.
- Early lesions can start with an itching folliculitis that progresses to scarring alopecia.
- Dermoscopy shows white scarring areas, absence of follicular openings, hyperpigmented violaceous lesions, telangiectasia, mild peripilar scale, and few pili torti.

SUGGESTED READING

1. Argraves M, Sloan SB, Dadras SS. Cutaneous sarcoidosis masquerading as psoriatic plaques. Dermatol Online J. 2015;21(4):13030/qt0pq3r2qv.
2. Bhushan P, Thatte SS, Singh A. Ket messages from a rare case of anular sarcoidosis of scalp. Indian Dermatol Online J. 2016;7(3):192-4.
3. Cheraghi N, Robinson A, O'Donnell P, et al. Scalp sarcoidosis: a sign of systemic sarcoidosis. Dermatol Online J. 2014; 20(3).
4. Dan L, Relic J. Sarcoidosis presenting as non-scarring non-scalp alopecia. Australas J Dermatol. 2016;57(3):e112-3.
5. Ghosh A, Sengupta S, Coondoo A, et al. Single lesion of sarcoidosis presenting as cicatricial alopecia: a rare report from India. Int J Trichology. 2014;6(2):63-6.
6. Henderson CL, Lafleur L, Sontheimer RD. Sarcoidal alopecia as a mimic of discoid lupus erythematosus. J Am Acad Dermatol. 2008;59(1):143-5.
7. House NS, Welsh JP, English JC III. Sarcoidosis-induced alopecia. Dermatol Online J. 2012;18(8):4.
8. Katta R, Nelson B, Chen D, et al. Sarcoidosis of the scalp: a case series of the literature. J Am Acad Dermatol. 2000;42(4):690-2.
9. La Placa M, Vincenzi C, Misciali C, et al. Scalp sarcoidosis with systemic involvement. J Am Acad Dermatol. 2008;59(5 Suppl):S126-7.
10. Rochat TS, Janssens JP, Soccal PM, et al. Update on the treatment of sarcoidosis. Rev Med Suisse. 2016;12(539): 1966-71.
11. Torres F, Tosti A, Misciali C, et al. Trichoscopy as a clue to the diagnosis of scalp sarcoidosis. Int J Dermatol. 2011;50(3): 358-61.
12. Yamamoto T, Yokozeki H. Scalp sarcoidosis mimicking organoid nevus. Eur J Dermatol. 2015;25(1):78-9.

7.5 Amyloidosis

Giselle Martins, Patricia Damasco, Isabella Doche

Systemic amyloidosis rarely causes alopecia. However, in most reports, it preceded the diagnosis of systemic amyloidosis by up to 6 years. Clinically, patients present with a patchy or diffuse nonscarring progressive thinning of the scalp hairs (Fig. 7.5.1).

Dermoscopy shows a nonscarring pattern, with dystrophic hairs, black dots, and broken hairs. These features are not specific. A typical feature is the presence of a salmon-colored halo (0.3–1 mm in diameter) surrounding the follicular ostia (Fig. 7.5.2). These halos can be seen around empty follicles or follicles with terminal and vellus hairs and correspond to perifollicular deposition of amyloid substance in the pathology. Depending on the type of amyloidosis, steroids, immunossupressive drugs, chemotherapy or stem-cell transplant may be necessary.

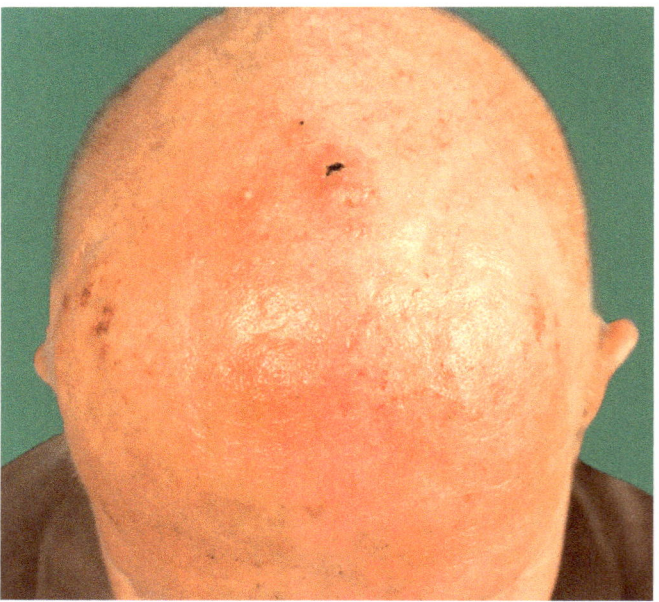

Fig. 7.5.1: Systemic amyloidosis. Diffuse and nonscarring pattern alopecia.
Source: Dr Mariya Miteva.

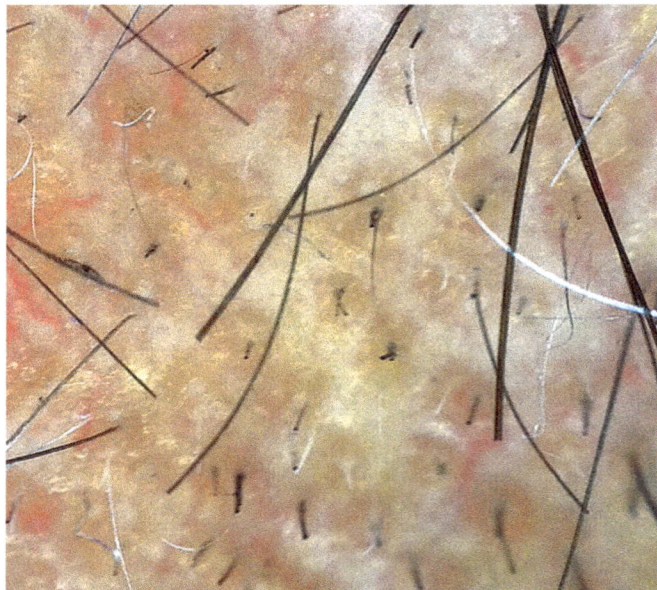

Fig. 7.5.2: Systemic amyloidosis. Note multiple broken hairs and a salmon-colored halo surrounding the follicular ostia.
Source: Dr Mariya Miteva.

Take-Home Message
- Systemic amyloidosis can cause a patchy or diffuse nonscarring alopecia.
- Dermoscopy shows broken hairs, black dots, and a salmon-colored halo surrounding the follicular ostia.

SUGGESTED READING

1. Barja J, Piñeyro F, Almagro M, et al. Systemic amyloidosis with an exceptional cutaneous presentation. Dermatol Online J. 2013;19(1):11.
2. Bedlow AJ, Sampson SA, Holden CA. Primary systemic amyloidosis of the hair and nails. Clin Exp Dermatol. 1998;23(6):298-9.
3. Hunt SJ, Caserio RJ, Abell E. Primary systemic amyloidosis causing diffuse alopecia by telogen arrest. Arch Dermatol. 1991;127(7):1067-8.
4. Lutz ME, Pittelkow MR. Progressive generalized alopecia due to systemic amyloidosis. J Am Acad Dermatol. 2002;46(3):434-6.
5. Miteva M, Wei E, Milikowski C. Alopecia in systemic amyloidosis: trichoscopic-pathologic correlation. Int J Trichology. 2015;7(4):176-8.
6. Renker T, Haneke E, Röcken C, et al. Systemic light-chain amyloidosis revealed by progressive nail involvement, diffuse alopecia and sicca syndrome: Report of an unusual case with a review of the literature. Dermatology. 2014;228(2):97-102.
7. Rudnicka L, Olszewska M, Rakowska A (eds). Atlas of Trichoscopy. London: Springer Verlag;2012. p. 507.
8. Wheeler GE, Barrows GH. Alopecia universalis. A manifestation of occult amyloidosis and multiple myeloma. Arch Dermatol. 1981;117:815-6.

CHAPTER 8

Infections and Infestations

Daniel Asz-Sigall, Maria Abril Martínez-Velasco, Norma Elizabeth Vásquez-Herrera, Roberto Arenas, Antonella Tosti, Maria de Fátima Maklouf Amorim Ruiz, Valeria Petri, Isabella Doche

8.1 Localized Infectious Diseases

Daniel Asz-Sigall, Maria Abril Martínez-Velasco, Norma Elizabeth Vásquez-Herrera, Roberto Arenas, Antonella Tosti

INTRODUCTION

Infections and infestations of the scalp and hair shafts are common diseases in Latin American patients. Dermoscopy can be a useful tool to confirm the diagnosis and treatment follow-up.

PEDICULOSIS

Pediculosis is a pruritic infestation of the scalp (*Pediculus capitis*) and/or pubis (*Phthirus pubis*). It is one of the main differential diagnoses of nodular lesions along the hair shaft (Fig. 8.1.1). Dermoscopy is useful to confirm the diagnosis by observing the lice (Fig. 8.1.2A) and nits, provide treatment follow-up, and assess if the parasites are dead or viable (Fig. 8.1.3). Pharmacological treatment includes permethrin 1% lotion or shampoo and oral ivermectin. Multiple novel treatments have shown limited evidence of efficacy. Nits must be removed.

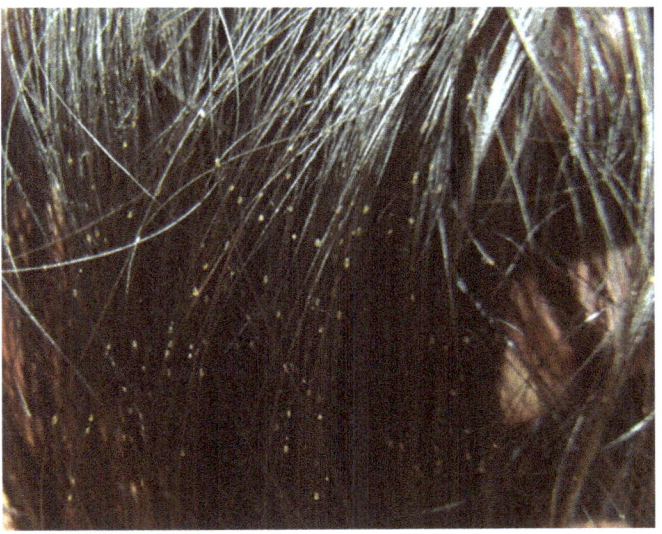

Fig. 8.1.1: Pediculosis. Dermoscopy with low magnifications shows nodular lesions along the hair shaft.

134 Fundamentals of Hair and Scalp Dermoscopy

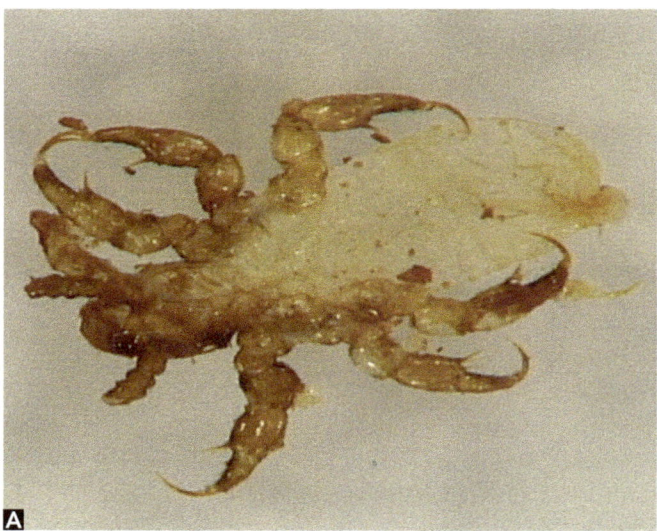
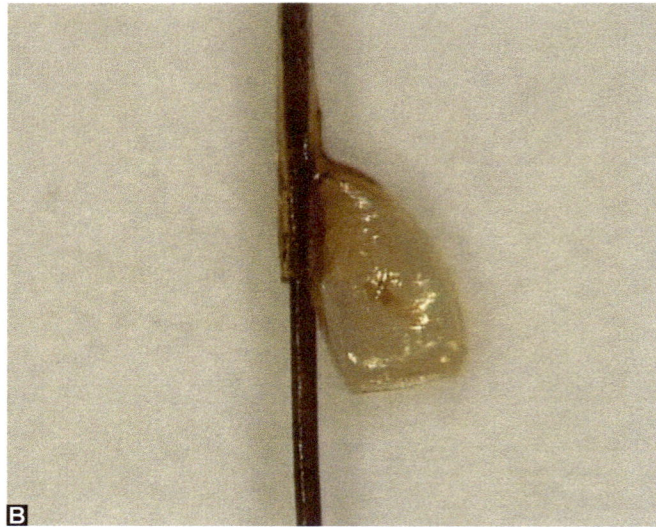

Figs. 8.1.2A and B: Pediculosis. Lice (A) and nits (B) on high magnification.

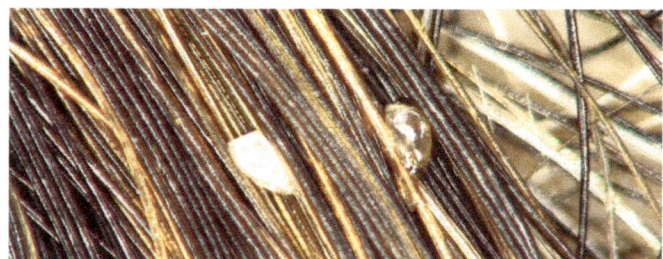

Fig. 8.1.3: Pediculosis. High magnifications are useful for treatment follow-up: Empty (white) and full (black) nits (70x). Differently from true casts and pseudocasts, note that nits attach to the hair shaft but do not encircle it.

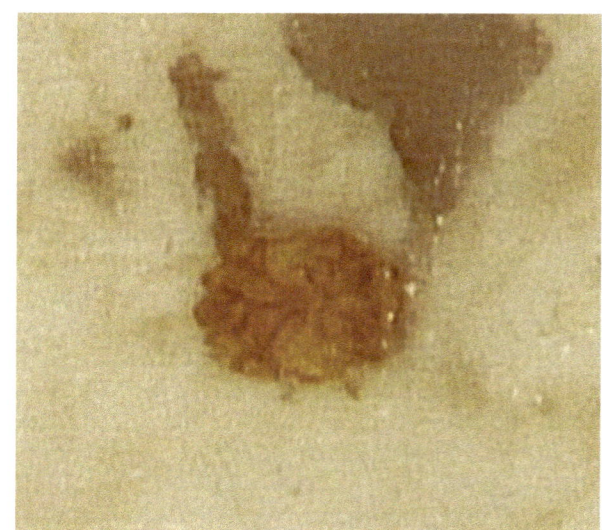

Fig. 8.1.4: Scabies mite.

Take-Home Message
- Pruritic nodular lesions mostly in the back area of the scalp.
- Look for lices and nits.
- Dermoscopy useful for diagnosis and treatment follow-up.

SCABIES

Infestation caused by *Sarcoptes scabiei var hominis*. The classical form affects families with nocturnal pruritus and nonscalp affection (Hebra lines). Crusted scabies (Norwegian form) can affect all the body and are mainly present in immunosuppressed patients. By dermoscopy, we can find the mites (Fig. 8.1.4), crusts, and tunnels with the triangle sign which corresponds to the mite head (Fig. 8.1.5). Treatment includes topical permethrin and oral ivermectin. Sulfur preparation is preferred for infants younger than 2 months. Itching may persist for up to a month, even following successful treatment.

Infections and Infestations

Fig. 8.1.5: Scabies. Tunnel with the triangle sign (mite head) seen in high magnification.

> **Take-Home Message**
> - Nocturnal itch in families.
> - Look for mites and tunnels with the triangle sign (mite head).

TINEA CAPITIS

Noninflammatory infection of the scalp caused by dermatophytes. There are two main forms: Microsporic (well-defined big patches, Fig. 8.1.6) and Trichophytic (irregular small patches, Fig. 8.1.7). Scales are present in both forms. Dermoscopy shows comma hairs, corkscrew hairs, morsecode hairs, zigzag hairs, scales, peripilar casts, black dots, and broken hairs (Figs. 8.1.8 and 8.1.9) Diagnosis can be confirmed by KOH (potassium hydroxide) test or culture. Oral griseofulvin and terbinafine are the treatment of choice in all forms of tinea capitis. However, oral itraconazole, and fluconazole can also be used with good results.

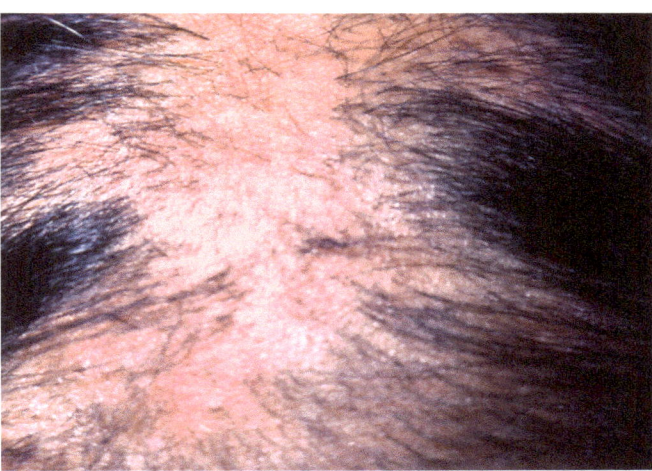

Fig. 8.1.7: Trichophytic tinea capitis. Irregular patches with scales.

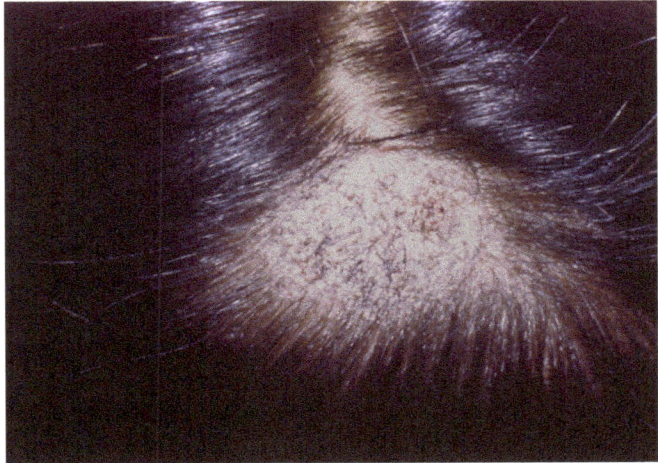

Fig. 8.1.6: Microsporic tinea capitis. Well-defined patches with scales.

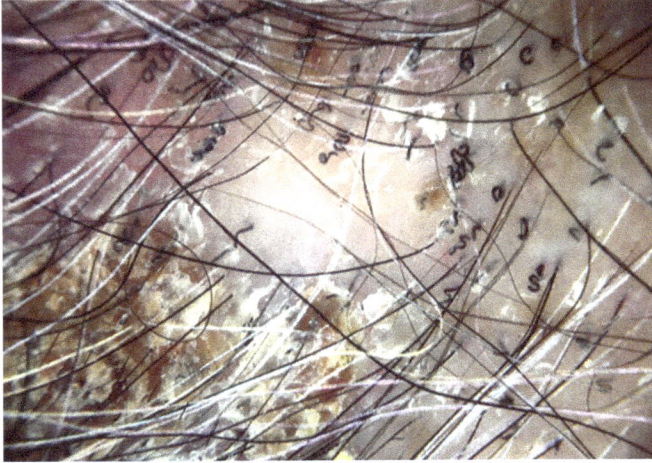

Fig. 8.1.8: Tinea capitis. Comma and corkscrew hairs.

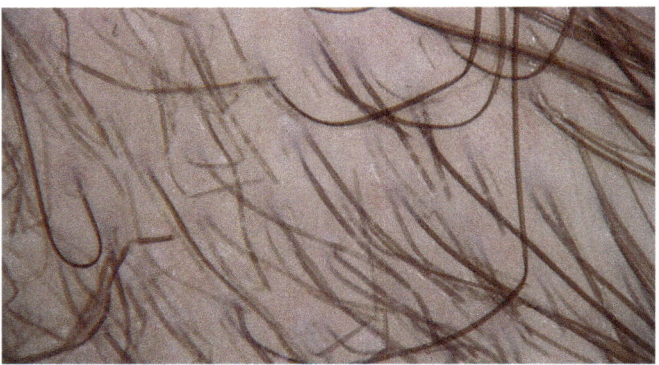

Fig. 8.1.9: Tinea capitis. Horizontal white bands ('Morse code' hairs) and broken hairs.

Source: Dr Patricia Damasco

Take-Home Message
- Pseudoalopecia patches with scales.
- Dermoscopy shows comma and corkscrew hairs.
- Diagnosis confirmed by KOH test or culture.

KERION CELSI

Inflammatory tinea capitis caused mainly by *Microsporum canis* or *Trichophyton mentagrophytes*. It is characterized by an inflammatory cicatricial patch with pustules, ulcers and crusts (Fig. 8.1.10). Dermoscopy shows cicatricial alopecia, pustules, and crusts. Diagnosis can be confirmed by KOH test or culture. Oral steroids are often recommended along with oral antifungals in the treatment of kerion celsi.

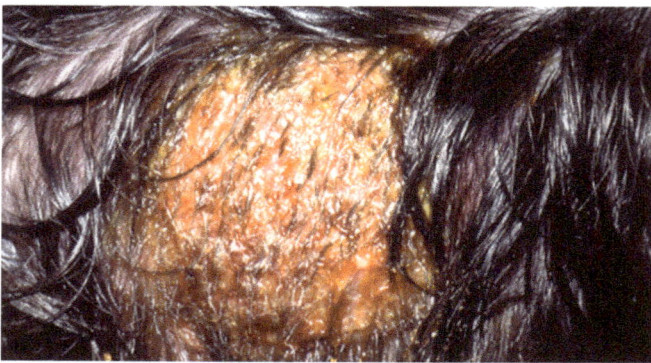

Fig. 8.1.10: Kerion celsi. Inflammatory and cicatricial scalp patch with pustules and crusts.

Take-Home Message
- Cicatricial patch with pustules and crusts.
- Diagnosis confirmed by KOH test or culture.

PIEDRAS

Asymptomatic nodular fungal infection of the hair shafts. There are two forms: White (*Trichosporon* spp., mainly *T. asahii*) and black (*Piedraia hortae*). Dermoscopy shows the ectothrix parasitation (concretion of hyphae) surrounding the hair (Figs. 8.1.11A and B). Diagnosis can be confirmed by KOH test or culture. Shaving or cutting the hair is the treatment of choice as topical and oral antifungals may not completely eradicate the infection.

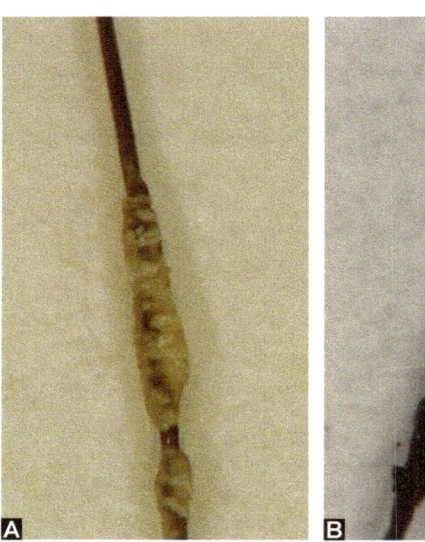 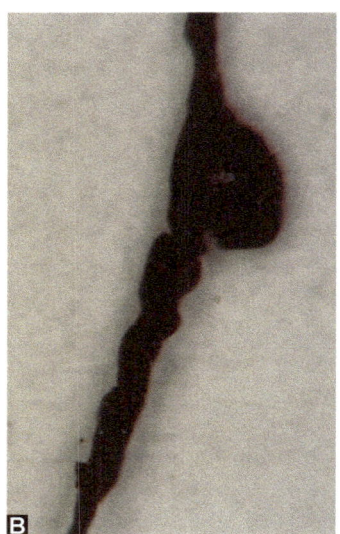

Figs. 8.1.11A and B: (A and B) White and black piedras seen in high magnification.

Take-Home Message
- Asymptomatic nodular lesions of hair shafts.
- Diagnosis confirmed by KOH test or culture.

TRICHOMYCOSIS

Pseudomycosis caused by *Corynebacterium tenuis*. Soft yellow concretions along the hair shafts of axillary and pubic hairs. Dermoscopy shows an opaque material surrounding the involved hair, without invasion of the hair cortex (Fig. 8.1.12). Diagnosis can be confirmed by KOH test or culture. The fastest method to treat the infection is shaving the affected hairs. Benzoyl peroxide formulations and antiperspirant agents can help to prevent recurrence. Topical antibiotics such as erythromycin or clindamycin are also effective.

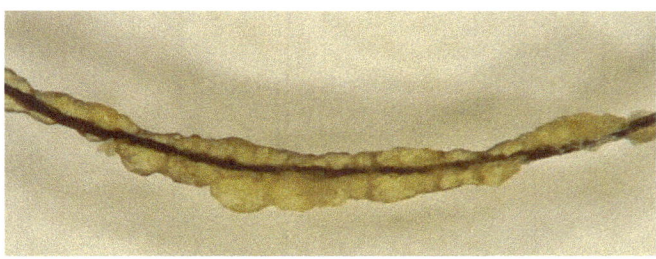

Fig. 8.1.12: Trichomycosis. Opaque material surrounding the involved hair seen on high magnification.

Take-Home Message

- Axillary or pubic asymptomatic soft yellow concretions surrounding hair shafts.
- Diagnosis can be confirmed by KOH test or culture.

MYIASIS

Myiasis is an infestation of the skin by the larval stage of botflies mainly *Dermatobia hominis* (Fig. 8.1.13). It clinically presents as furunculoid lesions that drain a serosanguineous fluid from a central pore. Dermoscopy shows a central opening surrounded by dilated blood vessels containing a yellowish structure with black barb-like spines extruding intermittently at the periphery. The occlusion of the respiratory orifice by dermatoscope stimulates the emergence of the caudal end of the larva, improving visualization. Therapy in the use of oclussive agents producing localized hypoxia to force the emergence of the larva, and removing the maggots.

Take-Home Message

- Furunculoid lesions usually on the scalp.
- Dermoscopy shows a central opening surrounded by dilated blood vessels containing a yellowish structure with black barb-like spines.

SUGGESTED READING

1. Abraham LS, Azulay-Abulafia L, Aguiar DP, et al. Dermoscopy features for the diagnosis of furuncular myiasis. An Bras Dermatol. 2011;86(1):160-2.
2. Almazán-Fernández FM, Fernández-Crehuet Serrano P. Trichomycosis axillaris dermoscopy. Dermatol Online J. 2017;23(6):13030/qt5hp5x1kz.
3. Bonifaz A, Ramírez-Ricarte I, Rodríguez-Leviz A, et al. Trichomycosis (trichobacteriosis) capitis in an infant: microbiological, dermoscopic and ultrastructural features. Rev Chil Pediatr. 2017;88(2):258-62.
4. Campos-Muñoz L, Fueyo-Casado A, Carranza-Romero C, et al. Peripilar hair casts. J Am Acad Dermatol. 2017;76(2Suppl 1):S3-S4.
5. Doche I, Vincenzi C, Tosti A. Casts and pseudocasts. J Am Acad Dermatol. 2016;75(4):e147-48.
6. Elghblawi E. Idiosyncratic findings in trichoscopy of tinea capitis: comma, zigzag hairs, corkscrew, and morse code-like hair. Int J Trichology. 2016;8(4):180-83.
7. Graveriau C, Peyron F. Cutaneous myiasis. Travel Med Infect Dis. 2017;16:70-1.
8. Hay RJ. Tinea capitis: current status. Mycopathologia. 2017;182(1-2):87-93.
9. Lacarrubba F, Verzì AE, Dinotta F, et al. Dermatoscopy in inflammatory and infectious skin disorders. G Ital Dermatol Venereol. 2015;150(5):521-31.
10. Micali G, Lacarrubba F, Verzì AE, et al. Scabies: advances in noninvasive diagnosis. PLOS Negl Trop Dis. 2016;10(6):e0004691.
11. Navarrete-Dechent C, Fich F, Gonzalez S. Trichomycosis (trichobacteriosis) capitis misdiagnosed as poliosis: the utility of dermoscopy and why it should always be done. J Eur Acad Dermatol Venereol. 2017;31(6):e275-76.
12. Sandoval-Tress C, Arenas-Guzmán R, Guzmán-Sánchez DA. Hair shaft yellow nodules in a pediatric female patient. Skin Appendage Disord. 2015;1(2):62-4.
13. Zhuang K, Ran X, Dai Y, et al. An unusual case of white piedra due to Trichosporon inkin mimicking trichobacteriosis. Mycopathologia. 2016;181(11-12):909-14.

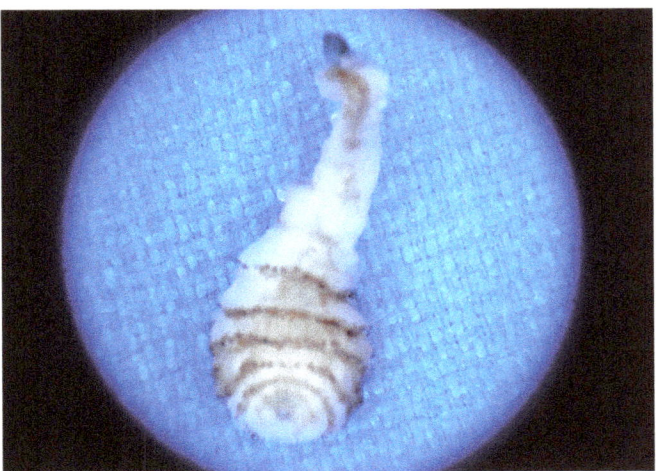

Fig. 8.1.13: Myiasis. *Dermatobia homonis* larva.

8.2 Systemic Infectious Diseases

Maria de Fátima Maklouf Amorim Ruiz, Valeria Petri, Isabella Doche

Hair loss can be a common clinical finding in patients with chronic systemic diseases. Diffuse hair shedding is expected in association with fever, nutrition deficiencies, and multiple drug therapy. However, the possible cause of hair loss may also include the infection itself, recurrent secondary infections, immunological and endocrine dysregulation. Variable types of scarring and nonscarring alopecias have been reported in association with hepatitis C, human immunodeficiency virus (HIV) and syphilis infections.

In HIV patients, the majority of hair disorders usually occurs with helper T cell numbers of less than $150/mm^3$. According to a project developed by Ruiz, patients with HIV infection have decreased numbers of telogen and anagen hairs, and decreased hair shaft diameter comparing to healthy subjects. Papulosquamous problems, as seborrheic dermatitis and psoriasis are the most frequent hair disorders. Trichorrhexis nodosa, trichomegaly, fragile hairs, anagen and telogen effluvium, and autoimune alopecias may also occur during the course of the infection and multiple drug treatment, especially anti-HIV regimens and pegylated interferon and ribavirin combination therapy for hepatitis C.

Syphilitic alopecia can occur as a rare manifestation of secondary syphilis (incidence of 2.9–11.2%). Basically, there are two types of secondary syphilitic alopecia: symptomatic and nonsymptomatic. The first in very uncommon and can be found in association with papulosquamous skin lesions. The second, also known as essential syphilitic alopecia, is characterized by alopecia in the absence of syphilitic typical lesions (Figs. 8.2.1A and B). Syphilitic alopecia can be divided into three types: classic patchy 'moth-eaten' alopecia, diffuse alopecia and a combination of both types. Although patchy moth-eaten alopecia is the most frequent type, diffuse alopecia can be the sole manifestation of the disease in some cases (Fig. 8.2.1C). Penicillin is the drug of choice to treat syphilis. Doxycycline is the best alternative to treat early and late latent cases.

Dermoscopy of hair loss in chronic infections is not specific. Eczematous lesions may show a more intense interfollicular erythema and scaling (Fig. 8.2.2). Syphilitic alopecia shows decreased hair density, empty follicles, yellow dots, and broken hairs. Zigzag hairs may also be present (Figs. 8.2.3A and B). Diffuse forms may resemble telogen effluvium and alopecia areata both on clinical and dermoscopic examinations. Dermoscopy features in syphilic alopecia usually disappear within 3 months of treatment.

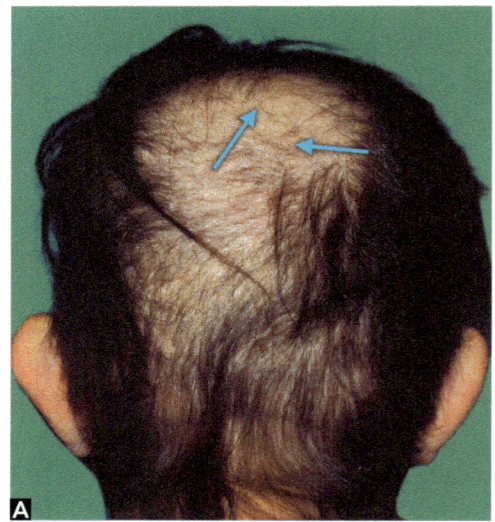

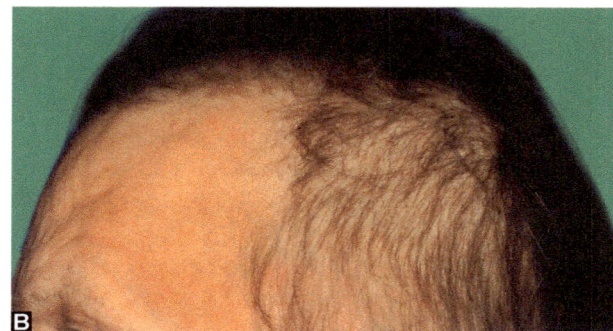

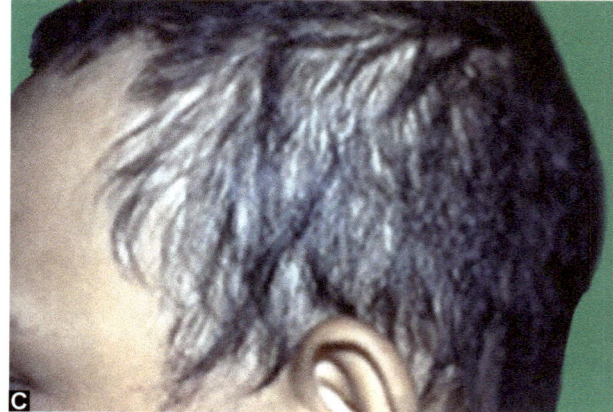

Figs. 8.2.1A to C: Syphilitic alopecia in a patient with associated hepatitis C infection. (A) Diffuse alopecia, mostly on the vertex area of the scalp. (B) Eyebrow and parietal scalp alopecia. (C) Syphilitic alopecia—moth-eaten pattern. Irregular patches of nonscarring alopecia over the scalp.

Source: (A, B) Division of Dermatology, Hospital das Clínicas, University of São Paulo Medical School.

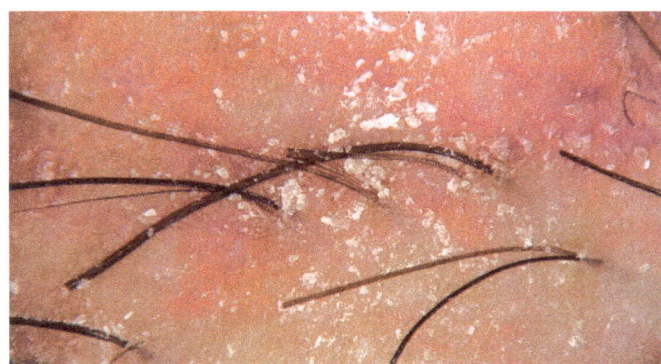

Fig. 8.2.2: Seborrheic dermatitis in a patient with HIV infection. Note intense interfollicular erythema and scaling.
Source: Dr Patricia Damasco

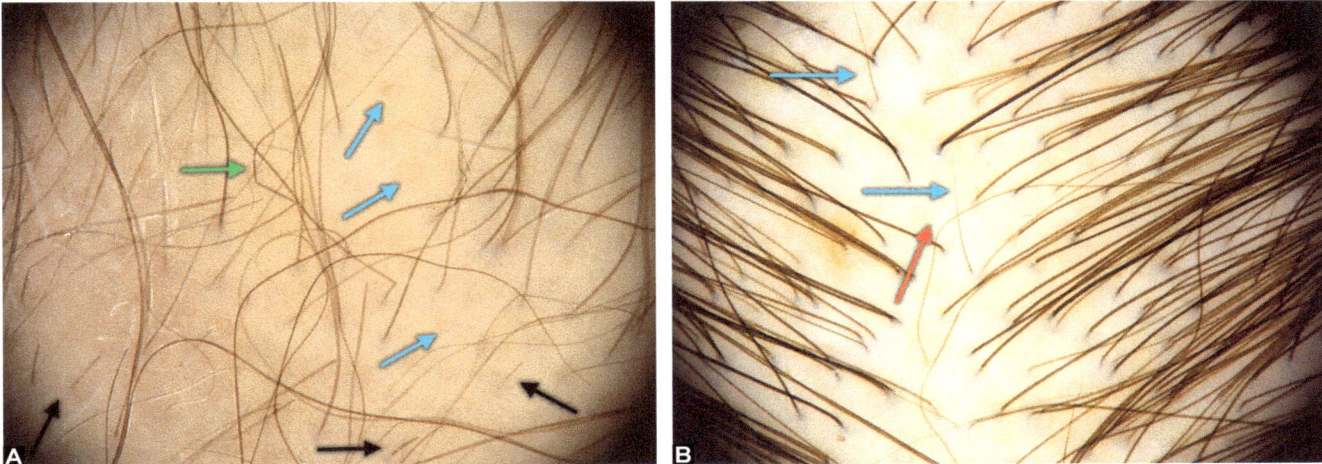

Figs. 8.2.3A and B: Syphilitic alopecia. (A) Decreased hair density, broken hairs with different lenghts (black arrows), yellow dots (blue arrows) and zigzag hairs (green arrow) before treatment. (B) Note short regrowing hairs (blue arrows) and one yellow dot (red arrow) after treatment.
Source: Division of Dermatology, Hospital das Clínicas, University of São Paulo Medical School; (A) *Credits to original source: Karger AG, Basel.*

Take-Home Message

- Nonscarring and scarring alopecia may occur in association with chronic systemic infections.
- Seborrheic dermatitis, psoriasis, and tellogen effluvium are the most frequent hair disorders.
- Syphilitic alopecia may mimic alopecia areata and telogen effluvium both on clinical and dermoscopic examinations.
- Dermoscopy is not specific.

SUGGESTED READING

1. Doche I, Hordinsky MK, Valente NYS, et al. Syphilitic alopecia: case reports and trichoscopic findings. Skin Appendage Disord. 2017;3(4):222-24.
2. Gamal N, Brodosi L, Misciali C, et al. Alopecia universalis after discontinuation of pegylated interferon and ribavirin combination therapy for hepatitis C: a case report. Ann Hepatol. 2014;13(2):293-6.
3. Guzmán-Sánchez D, Asz-Sigall D. Alopecias due to drugs and other skin and systemic disorders. Curr Probl Dermatol. 2015;47:97-106.
4. Jan V, Roudier-Pujol C. Hair loss associated with human immunodeficiency virus. Ann Dermatol Venereol. 2000; 127(Suppl 1):1S34-6.
5. Kim HS, Shin HS. Alopecia areata associated with abacavir therapy. Infect Chemother. 2014;46(2):103-5.
6. Lin RL, Garibyan l, Kimball AB, et al. Systemic causes of hair loss. Ann Med. 2016;48(6):393-402.
7. Navarrete-Dechent C, Ortega R, Fich F, et al. Dermatologic manifestations associated with HIV/AIDS. Rev Chil Infect. 2015;32(Suppl 1):S57-71.
8. Piraccini BM, Broccoli A, Starace M, et al. Hair and scalp manifestations in secondary syphilis: epidemiology, clinical features and trichoscopy. Dermatology. 2015;231(2):171-6.

9. Ruiz MFMA. Histomorfometria dos foliculos pilosos em indivíduos com infecção pelo vírus da imunodeficiência humana (HIV1). Dissertação, Universidade Federal de São Paulo, São Paulo;2003.
10. Sadick NS. Clinical and laboratory evaluation of AIDS trichopathy. Int J Dermatol. 1993;32(1):33-8.
11. Schön MP, Reifenberger J, Gantke B, et al. Progressive cicatricial psoriatic alopecia in AIDS. Hautarzt. 2000;51(12):935-8.
12. Smith KJ, Skelton HG, DeRusso D, et al. Clinical and histopathologic features of hair loss in patients with HIV-1 infection. J Am Acad Dermatol. 1996;34(1):63-8.
13. Türker K, Tas B, Altinay S, et al. Widespread dystrophic-anagen alopecia and drug eruption due to usage of PEG-IFN α-2a /ribavirin combination therapy. Hair Ther Transplant. 2014;4(3):1-5.
14. Vafaie J, Weinberg JM, Smith B, et al. Alopecia in association with sexually transmitted disease: a review. Cutis. 2005;76(6):361-6.
15. Verma P, Dayal S, Jain VK, et al. Aloepcia universalis as a side effect of pegylated interferon α-ribavirin combination therapy for hepatitis C: a rare case report. J Chemother. 2017;29(6):380-82.
16. Ye Y, Zhang X, Zhao Y, et al. The clinical and trichoscopic features of syphilitic alopecia. J Dermatol Case Rep. 2014;8(3):78-80.

CHAPTER 9

Alopecia During Childhood

Giselle Martins, Patricia Damasco, Isabella Doche

9.1 Aplasia Cutis Congenita

Giselle Martins, Patricia Damasco, Isabella Doche

Aplasia cutis congenita is a rare congenital disease characterized by localized absence of skin mostly affecting the scalp. Patients present with an oval-shape shiny and hairless area. Erosions and underlying bone and brain defects may be present (Figs. 9.1.1A and B).

Dermoscopy shows an atrophic skin with an absence of follicular openings (Fig. 9.1.2). Mild erythematous background, telangiectasia around the lesion and few pili torti may be present (Figs. 9.1.3A and B). Hair roots can be seen through the skin at the periphery of the patch, forming a 'hair collar sign' or 'starburst hair follicles' (Fig. 9.1.4). The main differential diagnoses are sebaceous nevus and congenital triangular alopecia, both present in childhood.

Treatment is scarce and depends on the size, depth, location of the cutaneous defects, and associated lesions. Local agents can be used to prevent secondary infection. Surgical repair can be an option for small lesions.

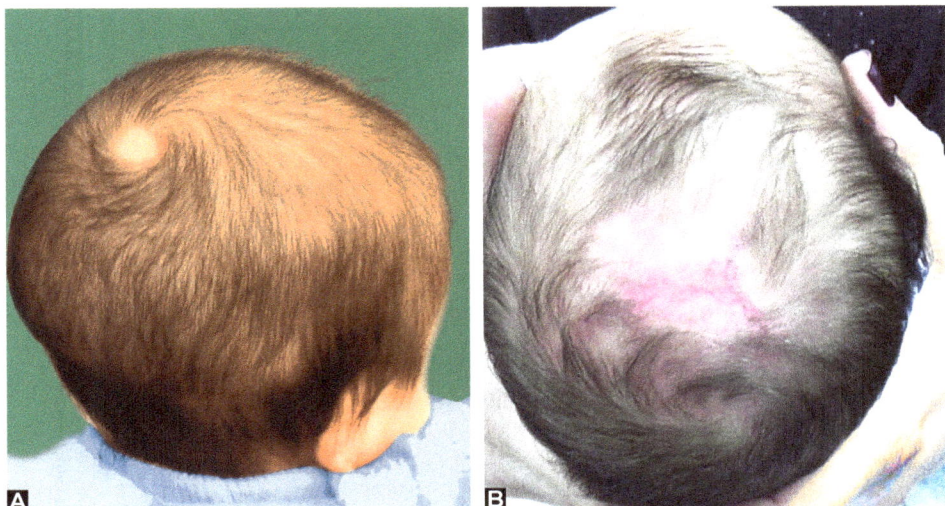

Figs. 9.1.1A and B: Aplasia cutis congenita. (A) Focal round-shape atrophic skin patch devoid of hairs. (B) Erosions and deep ulceration may occur.
Source: Hair Department, Division of Dermatology, Santa Casa de Misericórdia de Porto Alegre.

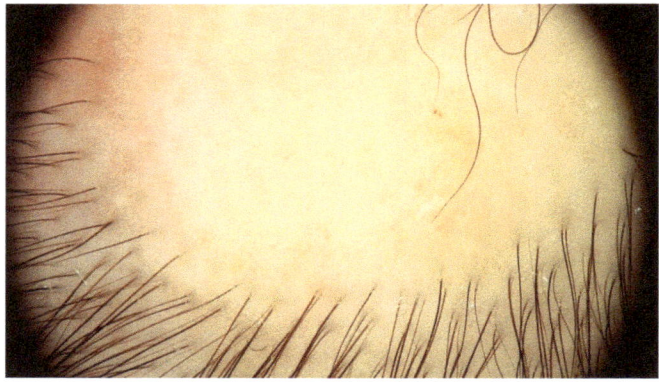

Fig. 9.1.2: Aplasia cutis congenita. Atrophic patch with loss of follicular openings.
Source: Hair Department, Division of Dermatology, Santa Casa de Misericórdia de Porto Alegre.

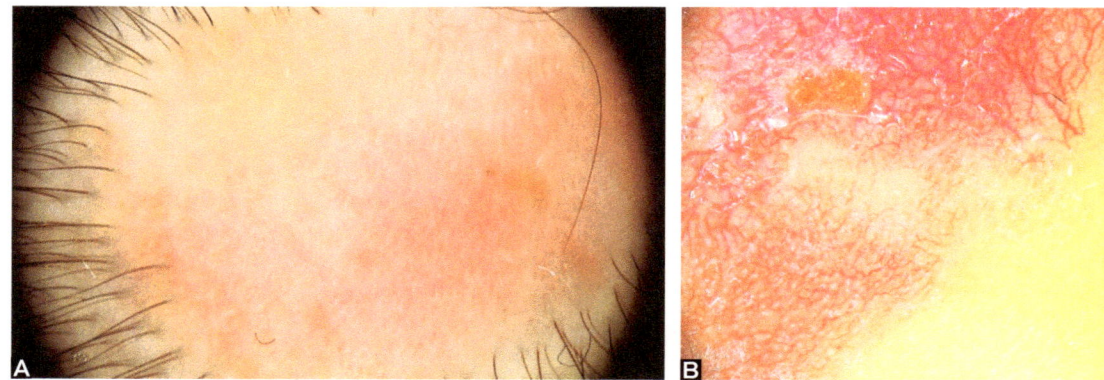

Figs. 9.1.3A and B: Aplasia cutis congenita. Mild erythema (A) and marked telangiectasia can be seen surrounding the atrophic area (B).
Source: Hair Department, Division of Dermatology, Santa Casa de Misericórdia de Porto Alegre.

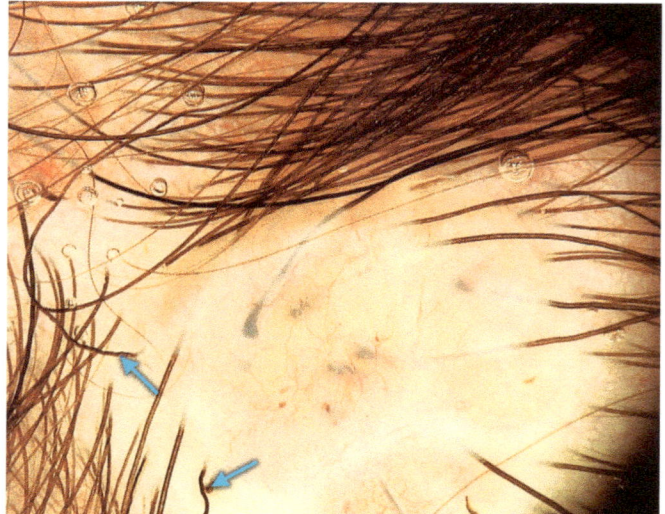

Fig. 9.1.4: Aplasia cutis congenita. Elongated and pigmented hair roots can be seen through the margins of the translucent skin, forming a "hair collar sign" or "starburst-hair follicles." Note some pili torti on the periphery of the lesion (blue arrows).
Source: Dr Ana Maria Pinheiro.

> **Take-Home Message**
> - Rare congenital skin atrophy mostly affecting the scalp.
> - Oval-shape hairless patch with a shiny appearance.
> - Dermoscopy shows absence of follicular openings; hair roots can be visible through the skin forming a 'hair-collar sign' or 'starburst hair follicles'.
> - Should be distinguished from sebaceous nevus and congenital triangular alopecia.

SUGGESTED READING

1. Colon-Fontanez F, Fallon Friedlander S, Newbury R, et al. Bullous aplasia cutis congenita. J Am Acad Dermatol. 2003;48(5 Suppl):S95-8.
2. Damiani L, Aguiar FM, da Silva MV, et al. Dermoscopic findings of scalp aplasia cutis congenita. Skin Appendage Disord. 2017;2(3-4):177–79.
3. Lozano-Masdemont B. A Case of membranous aplasia cutis congenita and dermoscopic features. Int J Trichology. 2017;9(1):33-4.
4. Neri I, Savoia F, Giacomini F, et al. Usefulness of dermatoscopy for the early diagnosis of sebaceous naevus

and differentiation from aplasia cutis congenital. Clin Exp Dermatol. 2009; 34(5):e50-2.
5. Pinheiro AMC, Mauad EBS, Fernandes LFA, et al. Aplasia cutis congenita: trichoscopy findings. Int J Trichology. 2016;8(4):184-85.
6. Rakowska A, Maj M, Zadurska M, et al. Trichoscopy of focal alopecia in children - new trichoscopic findings: hair bulbs arranged radially along hair-bearing margins in aplasia cutis congenita. Skin Appendage Disord. 2016; 2(1-2):1-6.
7. Verzì AE, Lacarrubba F, Micali G. Starburst hair follicles: a dermoscopic clue for aplasia cutis congenita. J Am Acad Dermatol. 2016; 75(4):e141-42.

9.2 Congenital Triangular Alopecia

Giselle Martins, Patricia Damasco, Isabella Doche

Congenital triangular alopecia (CTA) is a noninflammatory and nonscarring form of alopecia that usually affects the frontotemporal scalp. Although most cases are present at birth, some children may develop lesions during the first 6 years of life that remain stable thereafter.

Etiology remains unknown. Most cases are sporadic, but reports of familial cases suggest a genetic inheritance. Patients present with a well-demarcated triangular or oval-shaped alopecic area over the frontotemporal line of the scalp (Figs. 9.2.1A and B). Atypical presentations may resemble alopecia areata, trichotillomania, traction alopecia and aplasia cutis congenita (Fig. 9.2.1C).

Dermoscopy shows an alopecic patch with decreased hair density, empty follicles and vellus hairs surrounded by terminal hairs. No broken hairs, no black dots, or dystrophic hairs are present (Figs. 9.2.2A to C).

There is no effective treatment for CTA. Topical minoxidil and hair transplantation can be tried with variable results.

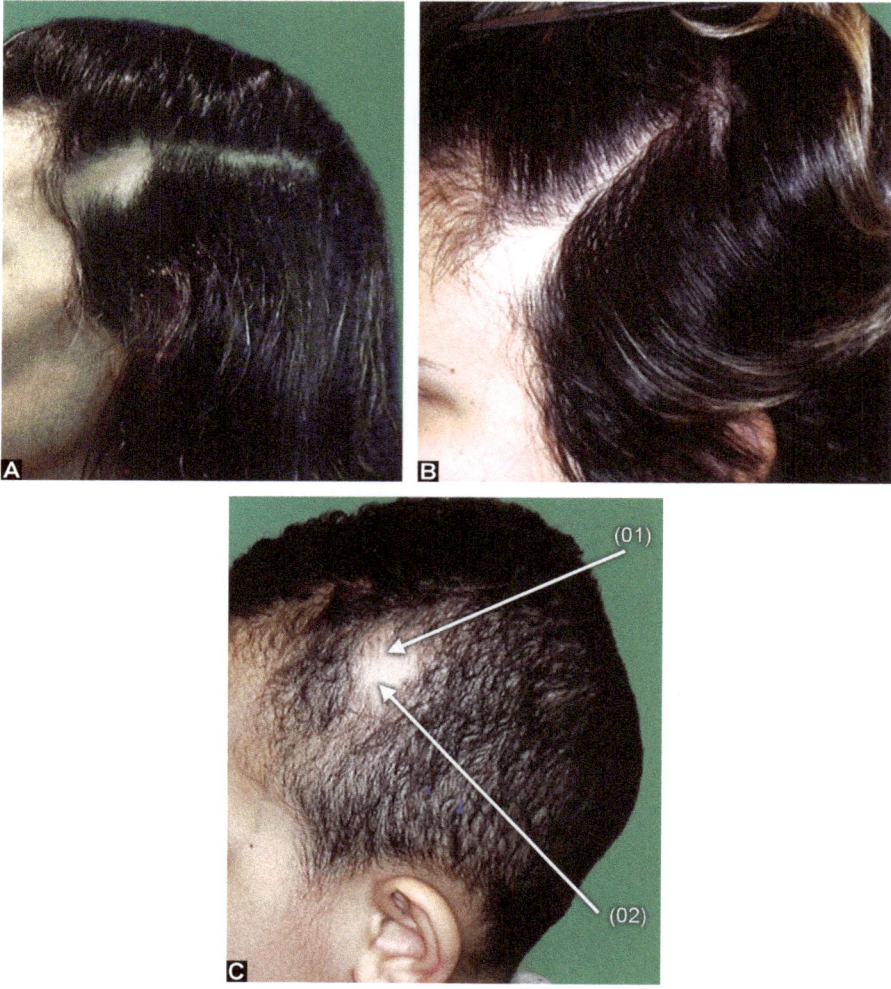

Figs. 9.2.1A to C: Congenital triangular alopecia. (A and B) Clinical presentation shows a nonscarring, oval-shaped area of alopecia in the frontotemporal line of the scalp. (C) Atypical presentations may mimic other nonscarring alopecias.

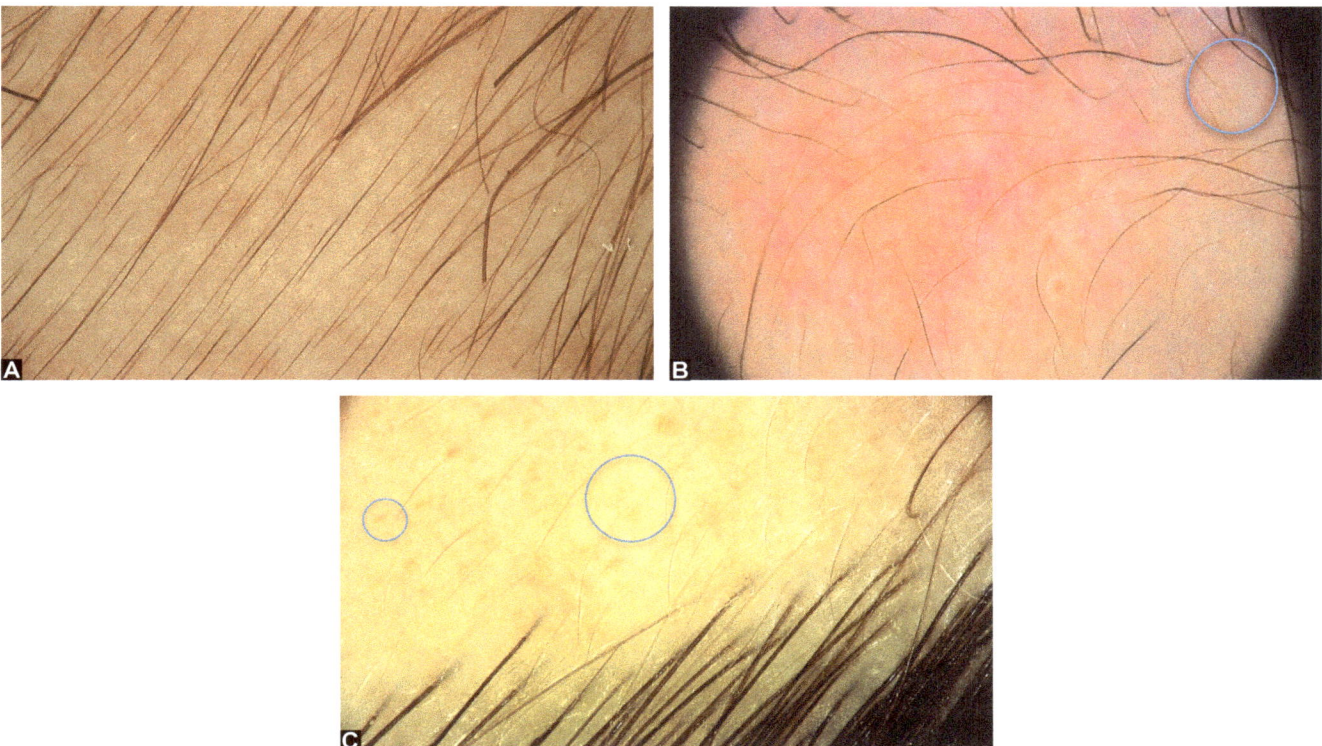

Figs. 9.2.2A to C: Congenital triangular alopecia. (A) Alopecic area with decreased hair density and multiple vellus hairs surrounded by terminal hairs. (B and C) Note the empty follicle (blue circles). No broken hairs and black dots can be seen.

Take-Home Message

- Present at the birth or during the first 6 years of life.
- Nonscarring and noninflammatory alopecic patch over the frontotemporal line of the scalp.
- Dermoscopy shows decreased hair density, multiple vellus hairs surrounded by terminal hairs and empty follicles.
- Atypical presentations should be distinguished from alopecia areata, trichotillomania, traction alopecia, and congenital aplasia cutis.

SUGGESTED READING

1. Assouly P, Happle R. A hairy paradox: congenital triangular alopecia with a central hair tuft. Dermatology. 2010;221(2):107-9.
2. Bang CY, Byun JW, Kang MJ, et al. Successful treatment of temporal triangular alopecia with topical minoxidil. Ann Dermatol. 2013;25(3):387-8.
3. Campos JG, Oliveira CM, Romero SA, et al. Use of dermoscopy in the diagnosis of temporal triangular alopecia. An Bras Dermatol. 2015;90(1):123-5.
4. Chung J, Sim JH, Gye J, et al. Successful hair transplantation for treatment of acquired temporal triangular alopecia. Dermatol Surg. 2012;38(8):1404-6.
5. Fernández-Crehuet P, Vaño-Galván S, Martorell-Calatayud A, et al. Clinical and trichoscopic cheractersfies of temporal triangular alopecia: a multicenter study. J Am Acad Dermatol. 2016;75(3):634-7.
6. Inui S, Nakajima T, Itami S. Temporal triangular alopecia: trichoscopic diagnosis. J Dermatol. 2012;39(6):572-4.
7. Iorizzo M, Pazzaglia M, Starace M, et al. Videodermoscopy: a useful tool for diagnosing congenital triangular alopecia. Pediatr Dermatol. 2008;25(6):652-4.
8. Pereira JM. Congenital triangular alopecia occurring in sisters. An Bras Dermatol. 2001;76:695-700.
9. Shim WH, Jwa SW, Song M, et al. Dermoscopic approach to a small round to oval hairless patch on the scalp. Ann Dermatol. 2014;26(2):214-20.
10. Yin Li VC, Yesudian PD. Congenital triangular alopecia. Int J Trichology. 2015;7(2):48-53.
11. Yamazaki M, Irisawa R, Tsuboi R. Temporal triangular alopecia and a review of 52 past cases. J Dermatol. 2010;37(4):360-2.

9.3 Loose Anagen Syndrome

Giselle Martins, Patricia Damasco, Isabella Doche

Loose anagen syndrome (LAS) is a disorder of abnormal anagen hair anchorage, leading to anagen easily extraction from the scalp. It is a self-limiting and benign condition, mainly reported in young girls between 2 old and 6 years. There are three phenotypes of LAS: Type A (decreased hair density with sparse and patchy hair loss), type B (mainly unruly and curly hairs), and type C [normal-appearing hair with excessive shedding of LA hairs (LAHs)]. These phenotypes appear to be age-dependent with types A and B occurring mostly in children, and type C affecting children around the age of 8 years and adults.

In most cases, LAS is sporadic. However, it can be an autosomal dominant disorder associated with many other defects such as coloboma, Noonan syndrome, hypohidrotic ectodermal dysplasia, (EEC) ectrodactyly–ectodermal dysplasia–clefting syndrome, trichorhinophalangeal syndrome, nail-patella syndrome, neurofibromatosis, and woolly hair. The differential diagnoses include alopecia areata, trichotillomania, congenital hair shafts disorders, and telogen effluvium.

Clinical presentation is diverse. Physical examination reveals sparse growth of thin, fine hair, and diffuse or patchy alopecia. Gentle traction results in hair that is painlessly removed; however, the hair is not fragile. The occipital area of the head is the most affected because of the trauma against the pillow. However, the presence of loose anagen hairs at the pull test is not specific for LAS since it may also occur in healthy individuals. Diagnosis of LAS therefore relies on the number and percentage of LAHs at the pull test and on the trichogram.

The trichogram reveals a predominance of loose anagen hairs (≥50–70%). A few or no telogen hairs are present. Loose anagen hairs have absent inner and outer root sheaths, ruffling of the cuticle on the proximal hair shaft (floppy sock appearance), and deformed-pigmented anagen bulbs that may appear long and tapered, twisted, or positioned at an acute angle to the long axis of the hair shaft (Fig. 9.3.1).

Dermoscopy shows solitary rectangular black granular structures, yellow dots, and a major predominance of follicular units with single hairs. However, those are no specific for LAS (Figs. 9.3.2A and B). The main differential diagnosis is alopecia areata which shows dense black structures (black dots).

LAS typically is considered a benign condition that resolves with age, although it is possible to have persistent symptoms after puberty. Treatment options include biotin supplementation and topical minoxidil with variable results.

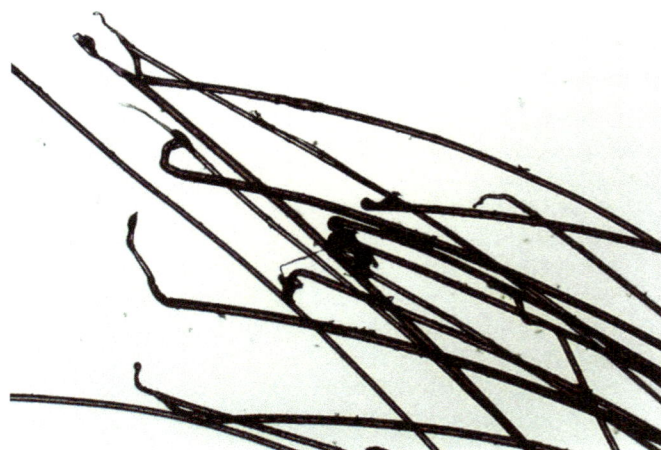

Fig. 9.3.1: Loose anagen syndrome. Note deformed pigmented anagen bulbs and the ruffling of the cutticle on the proximal hair shafts.

Source: Dr Neusa Valente

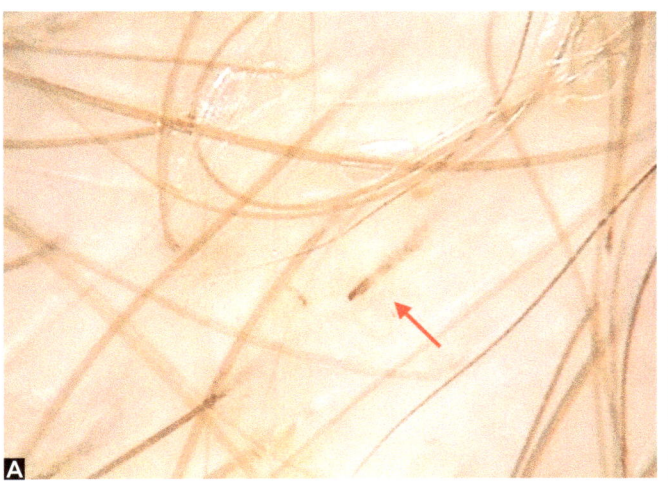 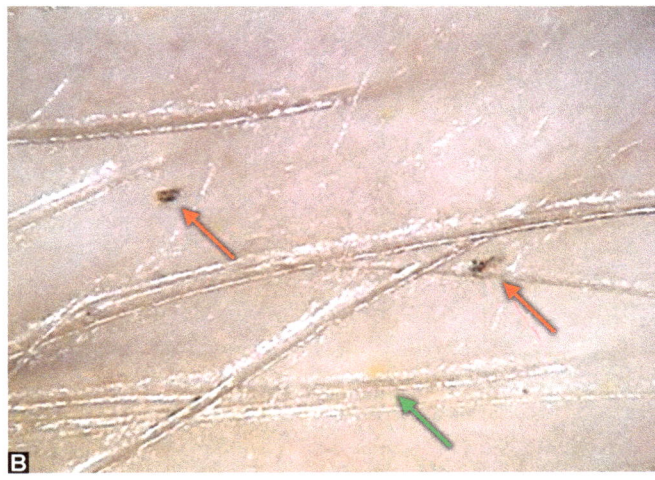

Figs. 9.3.2A and B: Loose anagen syndrome. Dermoscopy shows black rectangular features with granular structure (A and B; red arrows) and solitary yellow dots. (B; green arrow) (x70). It is important to differentiate these rectangular structures from black dots in alopecia areata.

Source: Rakowska A, et al. Trichoscopy findings in loose anagen hair syndrome: rectangular granular structures and solitary yellow dots. J Dermatol Case Rep. 2015;9(1):1-5.

Take-Home Message

- Loose anagen syndrome is a benign, self-limiting condition in which the anagen hairs are easily and painlessly extracted from the scalp.
- Hair does not grow long and patchy or diffuse alopecia may be present.
- Pull test can be either positive or negative.
- Trichogram shows around 50–70% of anagen hairs with ruffled cuticle (floppy sock appearance).
- Dermoscopy shows rectangular black granular structures, yellow dots, predominance of follicular units with one hair.
- The main differential diagnosis is alopecia areata.

SUGGESTED READING

1. Alves R, Grimalt R. Hair loss in children. Curr Probl Dermatol. 2015;47:55-66.
2. Avhad G, Ghuge P, Jerajani H. Loose anagen hair syndrome. Indian Dermatol Online J. 2014;5(4):548-9.
3. Chandran NS, Oranje AP. Minoxidil 5% solution for topical treatment of loose anagen hair syndrome. Pediatr Dermatol. 2014;31(3):389-90.
4. Dhurat RP, Deshpande DJ. Loose anagen hair syndrome. Int J Trichology. 2010;2(2):96-100.
5. Price VH. What looks like alopecia areata is not always alopecia areata. J Investig Dermatol Symp Proc. 2013;16(1):S63-4.
6. Rakowska A, Zadurska M, Czuwara J, et al. Trichoscopy findings in loose anagen hair syndrome: rectangular granular structures and solitary yellow dots. J Dermatol Case Rep. 2015;9(1):1-5.
7. Srinivas SM. Loose anagen hair syndrome. Int J Trichology. 2015;7(3):138-9.
8. Swink SM, Castelo-Soccio L. Loose anagen syndrome: a retrospective chart review of 37 cases. Pediatr Dermatol. 2016;33(5):507-10.

9.4 Short Anagen Syndrome

Giselle Martins, Patricia Damasco, Isabella Doche

Short anagen syndrome (SAS) is a congenital disease clinically characterized by very short hairs (less than 6 cm) and recurrent hair shedding. Patients complain that the hair never grows and they never had a haircut. Telogen effluvium is also a common complaint because of the shortened anagen phase. Although most cases occur in Caucasian blond-haired girls, there are a few reports in African-American, Asian, and Hispanic women in the literature (Fig. 9.4.1).

The disease can be sporadic or congenital. Some reports of familial cases may suggest an autosomal dominant inheritance. SAS is usually a benign condition, but some cases can be associated with trichodental syndrome, congenital hypotrichosis, linear scleroderma, and occluded lacrimal duct.

The most important differential diagnosis is loose anagen syndrome which also presents with short hair, but the hair is shed during the anagen phase. Other differential diagnoses include telogen effluvium, Noonan syndrome, and peeling skin syndrome (Fig. 9.4.2).

Dermoscopy is not specific for SAS. Some short regrowing hairs can be seen (Fig. 9.4.3).

Hair length tends to improve spontaneously after puberty in most cases. Treatment options for SAS are limited, however, improvement with minoxidil and cyclosporine has been reported.

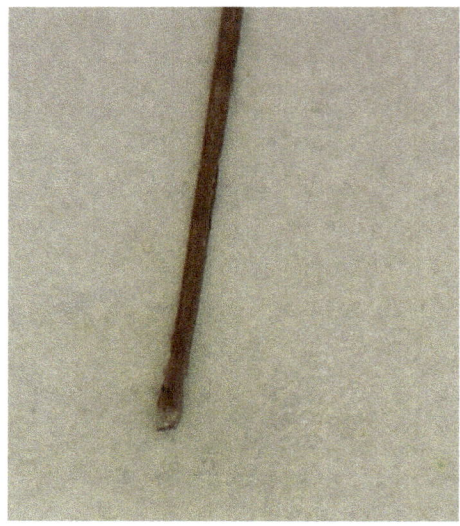

Fig. 9.4.2: Pull test is usually positive with multiple telogen hairs. Note the pointed tip.

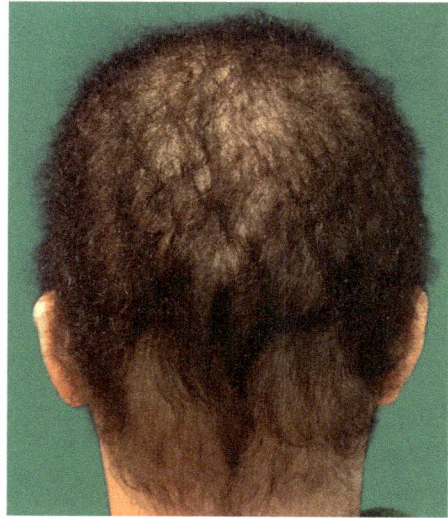

Fig. 9.4.1: Short anagen syndrome. Note short hairs (less than 6 cm) that had never been cut in a female teenager.

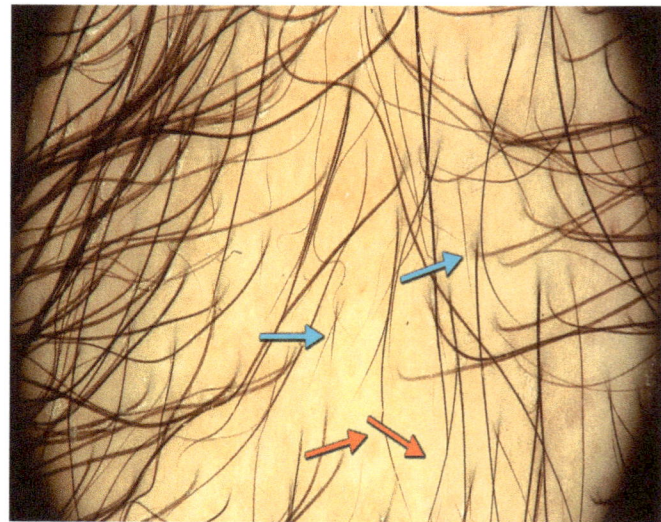

Fig. 9.4.3: Short anagen syndrome. Dermoscopy is not specific. Note multiple short regrowing hairs (blue arrows) and some empty follicles (red arrows).

> **Take-Home Message**
> - Short anagen syndrome is characterized by very short hairs and recurrent shedding of telogen hairs.
> - The main complaint is that the hair does not grow long and had never been cut.
> - Dermoscopy is not specific. Some short regrowing hairs and empty follicle can be present.

SUGGESTED READING

1. Avashia N, Woolery-Lloyd H, Tosti A, et al. Short anagen syndrome in an African American Woman. J Am Acad Dermatol. 2010;63(6):1092-3.
2. Cheng YP, Chen YS, Lin SJ, et al. Minoxidil improved hair density in an Asian girl with short anagen syndrome: a case report and review of literature. Int J Dermatol. 2016;55(11):1268-71.
3. Doche I, Donati A, Valente NS, et al. Short anagen syndrome in a girl with curly dark hair and consanguineous parents. J Am Acad Dermatol. 2012;67(6):e279-80.
4. Giacomini F, Starace M, Tosti A. Short anagen syndrome. Pediatr Dermatol. 2011;28(2):133-4.
5. Herskovitz I, de Sousa IC, Simon J, et al. Short anagen hair syndrome. Int J Trichology. 2013;5(1):45-6.
6. Jung HD, Kim JE, Kang H. Short anagen syndrome successfully controlled with topical minoxidil and systemic cyclosporine A combination treatment. J Dermatol. 2011;38(11):1108-10.
7. Martin JM, Montesinos E, Sanchez S, et al. Clinical, microscopic and ultrastructural findings in a case of short anagen syndrome. Pediatr Dermatol. 2017;34(4):e221-2.

CHAPTER 10

Genetic Skin Diseases

*Marina Lino Vieira, Maria Cecilia da Matta Rivitti Machado,
Zilda Najjar Prado de Oliveira, Isabella Doche*

10.1 Ichthyosis

Marina Lino Vieira, Maria Cecilia da Matta Rivitti Machado, Zilda Najjar Prado de Oliveira, Isabella Doche

Ichthyosis comprises a group of heterogeneous rare disorders characterized by dry, thickened, and scaly skin. Ichthyosis may be either inherited or acquired. Inherited ichthyosis appears in the first years of life or at birth. Acquired ichthyosis usually occurs as a result of internal causes, such as hormonal, inflammatory, or malignant disorders.

Clinical signs and symptoms depend on the particular form. Patients usually present with dry scaly skin, redness, blistering, or excessive skin peeling associated with overheating, and pain. Scalp scales and dry scalp can be extremely uncomfortable for individuals with ichthyosis (Figs. 10.1.1A to C). Hair breakage can occur in scalp areas exposed to friction. Alopecia may be severe in some cases with associated eyebrow and eyelash abnormalities.

Main types of ichthyosis are:

- *Ichthyosis vulgaris*: Common, mild skin scaling and dryness

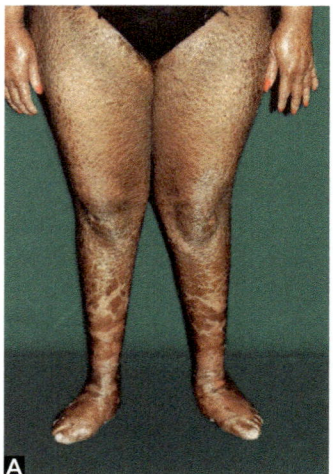
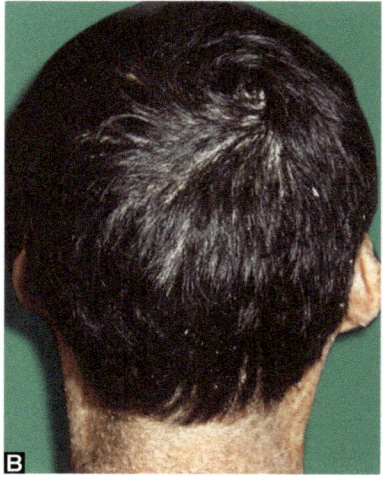
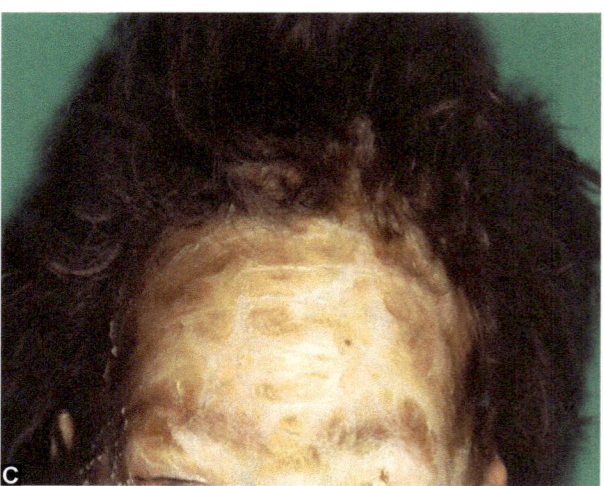

Figs. 10.1.1A to C: Ichthyosis. Lamellar ichthyosis with dark and thick scales on the (A) Limbs and (B) Neck. Note thick scales over the scalp. (C) Severe scaling on the face and scalp of this child with Harlequin ichthyosis.
Source: Division of Dermatology, Hospital das Clínicas, University of São Paulo.

Genetic Skin Diseases

- *Retinopatic ichthyosis*: Thick and dark scales, skin fragility with blisters after trauma
- *Lamellar ichthyosis*: Large and thick scales
- *Congenital ichthyosiform erythroderma*: Red skin and fine scales.

There are no specific features in dermoscopy. Dry dermoscopy can show variable interfollicular and perifollicular thick scales, hair casts, and scalp erythema (Figs. 10.1.2 to 10.1.4). Dermoscopy with immersion fluid can show some broken hairs due to scratching and areas of secondary cicatricial alopecia may be present.

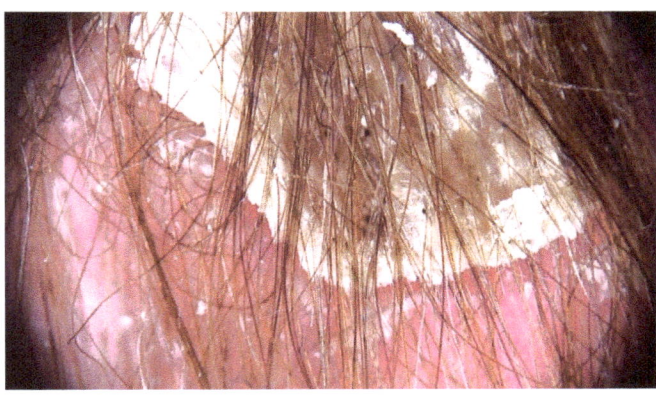

Fig. 10.1.4: Ichthyosis. Dry dermoscopy shows diffuse erythema, severe yellow scaling and broken hairs in a child with Harlequin ichthyosis.

Source: Division of Dermatology, Hospital das Clínicas, University of São Paulo.

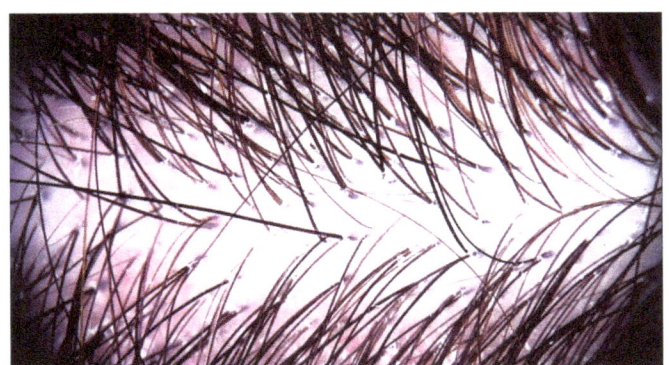

Fig. 10.1.2: Ichthyosis. Dry dermoscopy shows mild peripilar scale, hairs casts, and a mild erythematous scalp in a patient with congenital ichthyosiform erythroderma.

Source: Division of Dermatology, Hospital das Clínicas, University of São Paulo.

There is no cure for ichthyosis and the therapeutic options aim to manage dryness and scaling. Treatment includes moisturizers, keratolytic agents and, oral retinoids. Scales should be removed with caution in order to prevent secondary cicatricial alopecia.

Take-Home Message

- Ichthyoses are characterized by dry and scaly skin, redness and blisters.
- The scalp is usually affected with scaly and pruritic lesions.
- Secondary cicatricial alopecia and decreased hair density can occur after chronic scale removal.
- Dermoscopy does not show any specific features.

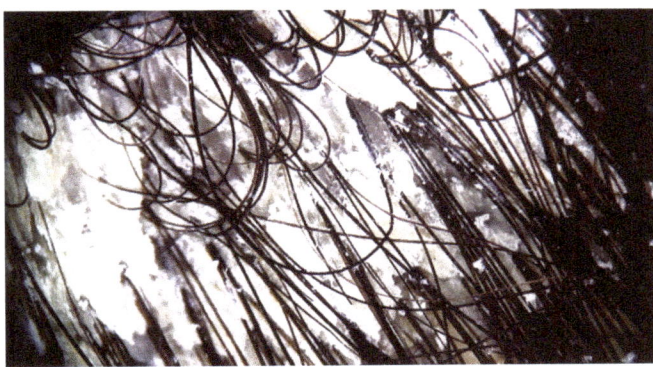

Fig. 10.1.3: Ichthyosis. Dry dermoscopy shows severe and diffuse white-yellowish scales over the scalp in a patient with lamellar ichthyosis.

Source: Division of Dermatology, Hospital das Clínicas, University of São Paulo.

SUGGESTED READING

1. DiGiovanna JJ, Robinson-Bostom L. Ichthyosis: etiology, diagnosis, and management. Am J Clin Dermatol. 2003;4(2):81-95.
2. Ma JE, Hand JL. What's new with common genetic skin disorders? Minerva Pediatr. 2017;69(4):288-97.
3. Oji V, Tadini G, Akiyama M, et al. Revised nomenclature and classification of inherited ichthyoses: results of the First Ichthyosis Consensus Conference in Sorèze 2009. J Am Acad Dermatol. 2010;63(4):607-41.
4. Rakowska A, Slowinska M, Kowalska-Oledzka E, et al. Trichoscopy in genetic hair shaft abnormalities. J Dermatol Case Rep. 2008;2(2):14-20.

10.2 Ectodermal Dysplasia

Marina Lino Vieira, Maria Cecilia da Matta Rivitti Machado, Zilda Najjar Prado de Oliveira, Isabella Doche

Ectodermal dysplasia (ED) is a group of hereditary diseases comprising around 200 genetic disorders caused by more than 50 different genes. It is characterized by abnormalities of two or more ectoderm-derived structures such as hair, teeth, nails, sweat glands, and salivary glands.

Clinically, patients may not sweat (anhidrotic type) or may have decreased sweating (hypohidrotic type) because of a lack of sweat glands. In the hypo/anhidrotic form, that encompasses 70% of ED cases, patients are not able to control temperature, which is often misdiagnosed as recurrent episodes of fever. Hyperpigmented skin around the eyes, nose and mouth areas; absent or abnormal teeth (cone-shaped), scalp and body hair abnormalities are also present. Scalp hairs grow slowly and are usually sparse, thin, fragile, and dry. Eyebrow and eyelash partial alopecia can occur and body hairs may be absent (Figs. 10.2.1 and 10.2.2). In some cases, scalp hairs can become fuller after adolescence, and male patients may develop beard hairs.

Dermoscopy shows follicular units with single hair shafts. Diverse hair shaft pigmentation with gray, white and dark brown colors, pili torti, pili canaliculi (hair shafts with longitudinal grooves), trichothiodystrophy, monilethrix-like hairs, trichorrhexis nodosa, and rarely, scarring areas may also be present (Fig. 10.2.3).

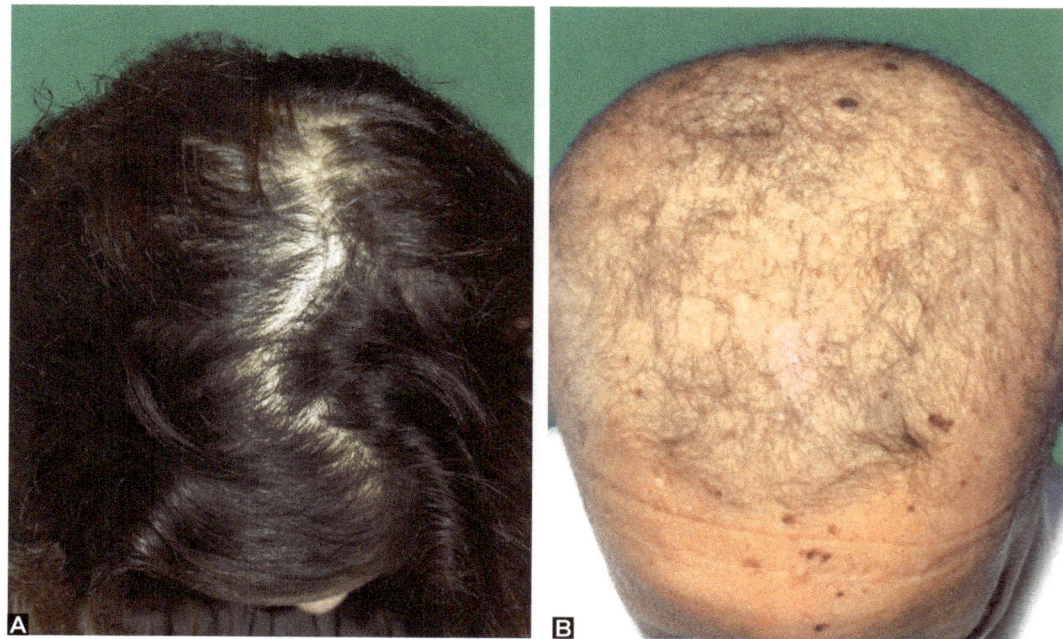

Figs. 10.2.1A and B: Ectodermal dysplasia. Note variable scalp hypotrichosis.
Source: Division of Dermatology, Hospital das Clínicas, University of São Paulo.

Genetic Skin Diseases

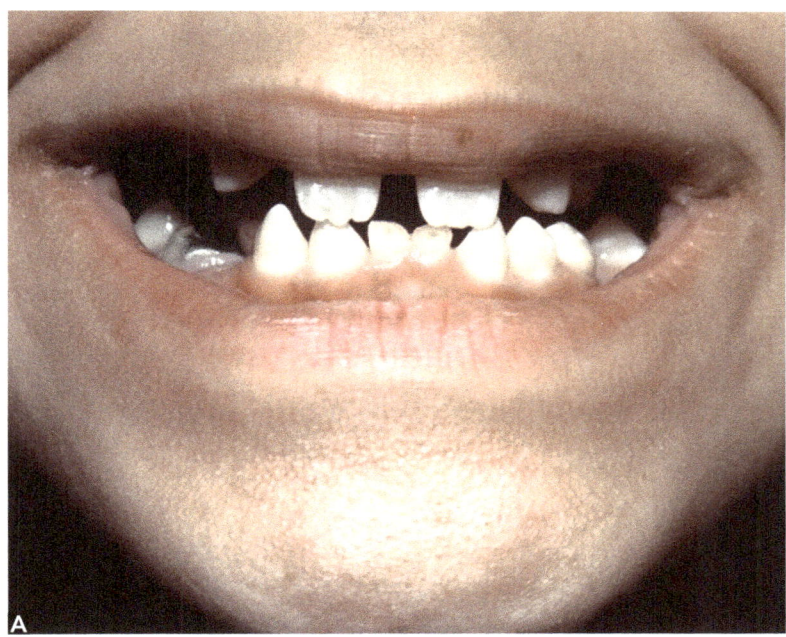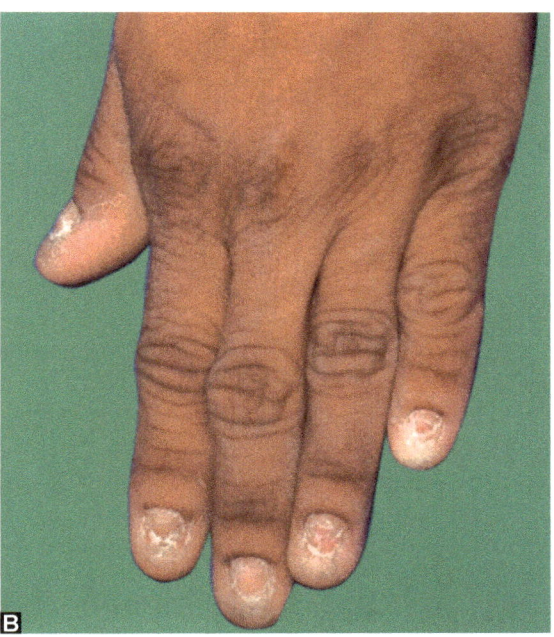

Figs. 10.2.2A and B: Ectodermal dysplasia. (A) Dental abnormalities. Note typical peg-shaped teeth and some missing teeth. (B) Nail dystrophy.
Source: Division of Dermatology, Hospital das Clínicas, University of São Paulo.

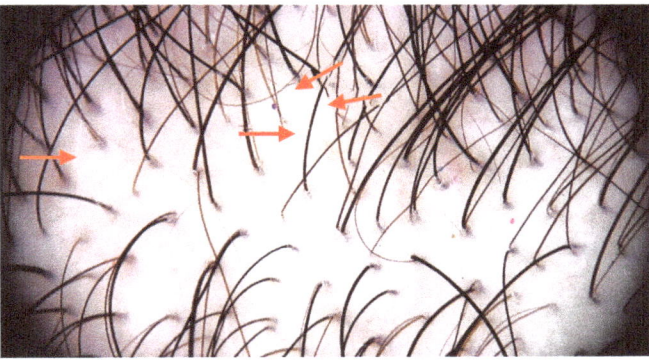

Fig. 10.2.3: Ectodermal dysplasia. Dry dermoscopy shows multiple follicular units with one single hair, thin hairs, and some white hair shafts (red arrows) in a 16-year-old patient.
Source: Division of Dermatology, Hospital das Clínicas, University of São Paulo.

There is no specific treatment for ED patients. Symptoms should be managed according to the affected organ.

Take-Home Message

- Ectodermal dysplasia is characterized by sparse, thin, fragile, eccrine and dry scalp hairs usually associated with teeth, nail, and eccrine gland abnormalities.
- Dermoscopy shows follicular units with single hairs and few hypopigmented shafts may be present.
- Pili torti, pili canaliculi, trichothiodystrophy, trichorrhexis nodosa and cicatricial alopecia may occur.

SUGGESTED READING

1. Carvalho MV, Sousa JRS, Melo FPC, et al. Hypohidrotic and hidrotic ectodermal dysplasia: a report of two cases. Dermatol Online J. 2013;19(7):18985.
2. García-Martín P, Hernández-Martín A, Torrelo A. Ectodermal dysplasias: a clinical and molecular review. Actas Dermosifiliogr. 2013;104(6):451-70.
3. Itin PH. Etiology and pathogenesis of ectodermal dysplasias. Am J Med Genet A. 2014;164A(10):2472-7.
4. Rakowska A, Górska R, Rudnicka L, et al. Trichoscopic hair evaluation in patients with ectodermal dysplasia. J Pediatr. 2015;167(1):193-5.

10.3 Congenital Epidermolysis Bullosa

Zilda Najjar Prado de Oliveira, Maria Cecilia da Matta Rivitti Machado, Marina Lino Vieira, Isabella Doche

Congenital epidermolysis bullosa (EB) is a group of hereditary diseases characterized by a marked fragility of the skin and mucous membranes. It is a result of a defect in anchoring between the epidermis and dermis leading to blisters and ulcers in response to minor trauma. The severity of the disease ranges from mild to lethal. Congenital EB is divided according to the level of cleavage into four large groups, (simplex, junctional, dystrophic and mixed or Kindler syndrome) and in at least 20 different clinical phenotypes.

Blistering of the scalp often occur in junctional and dystrophic EB, usually resulting in scarring alopecia (Figs. 10.3.1A to D). Not only severe cases of EB present alterations in the scalp; other types of alopecia may also occur, such as telogen effluvium due to anemia or sepsis, typical androgenetic alopecia pattern, and traction alopecia (especially in woman), and the complete absence of hairs in acantholytic EB simplex. Dermoscopy of alopecic areas secondary to blisters shows features of cicatricial alopecia, such as white areas with absence of follicular openings (Figs. 10.3.2A and B). Milky-red areas can also be present. Milia can be present in some skin lesions (Fig. 10.3.3).

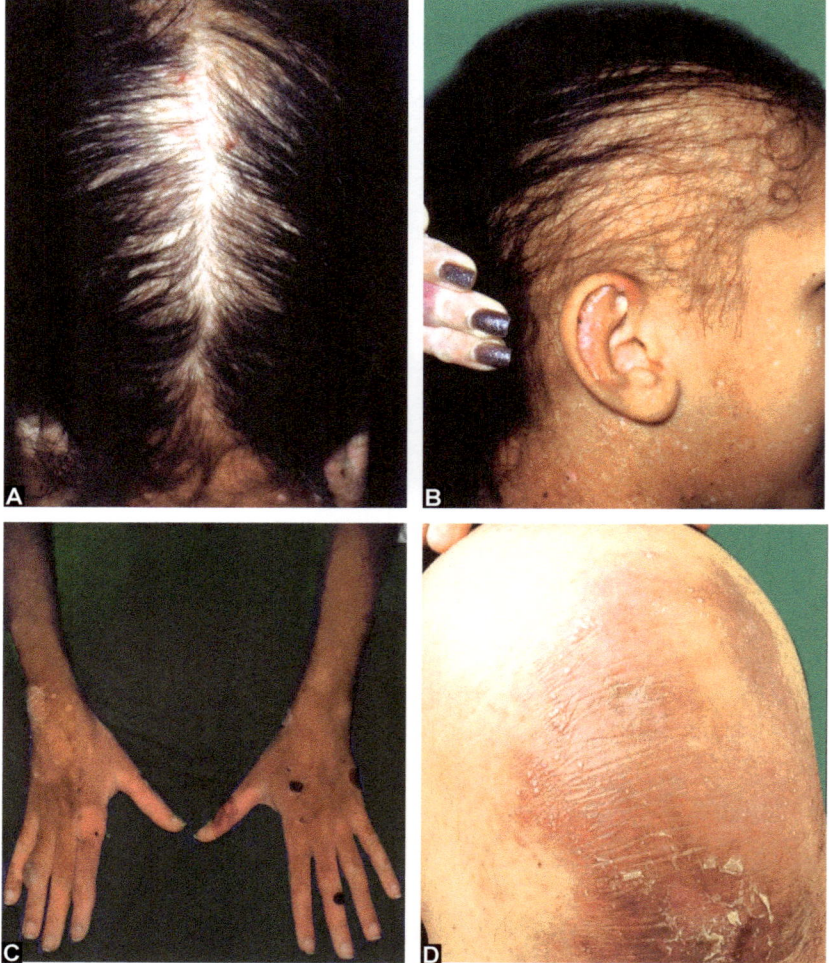

Figs. 10.3.1A to D: Dystrophic epidermolysis bullosa. (A) Scalp cicatricial alopecia. (B) Diffuse alopecia. (C) Blisters and erosions on the arms and hands. (D) Milia lesions in the knee.
Source: Division of Dermatology, Hospital das Clínicas, University of São Paulo.

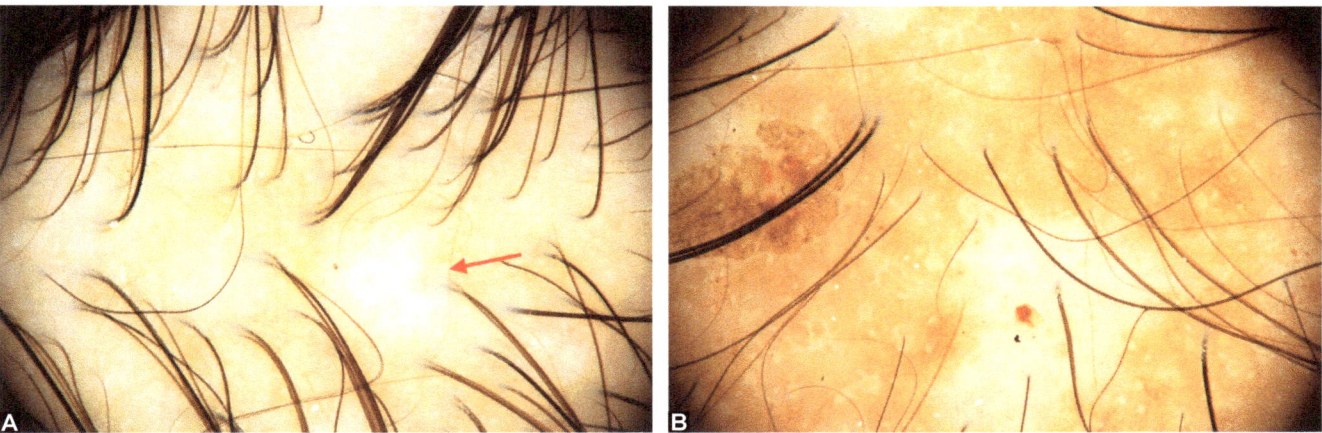

Figs. 10.3.2A and B: Dystrophic epidermolysis bullosa. (A) Decreased hair density, thin hairs, and follicular units with only one hair. Note white scarring areas lacking follicular openings. (B) Note also the honeycomb pigmentation between the sparse follicular units in a dark-skinned child.

Source: Division of Dermatology, Hospital das Clínicas, University of São Paulo.

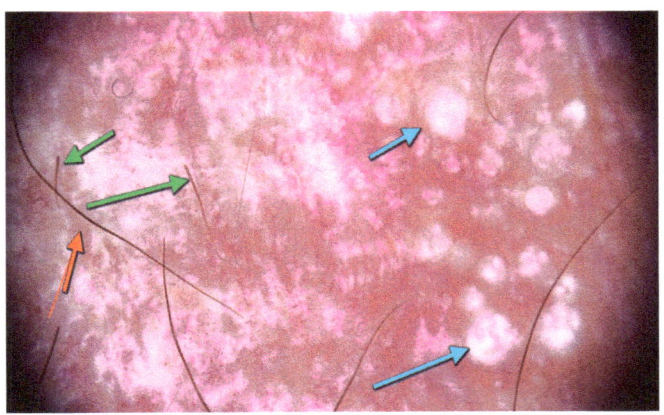

Fig. 10.3.3: Dystrophic epidermolysis bullosa. Scarring area, milia (small white cysts, blue arrows), pili torti (red arrow), and broken hairs (green arrows).

Source: Division of Dermatology, Hospital das Clínicas, University of São Paulo.

> **Take-Home Message**
> - Congenital EB is characterized by a defect in anchoring epidermis to dermis, leading to blisters and skin fragility in response to minor trauma.
> - Four groups: simplex, junctional, dystrophic and mixed with variable phenotypes.
> - Secondary cicatricial alopecia is common, except in EB simplex.
> - Other types of alopecia may occur, such as telogen effluvium, androgenetic alopecia pattern and traction alopecia.
> - Dermoscopy of alopecic areas secondary to blisters shows absence of follicular openings.

SUGGESTED READING

1. Boeira VL, Souza ES, Rocha BO, et al. Inherited epidermolysis bullosa: clinical and therapeutic aspects. An Bras Dermatol. 2013;88(2):185-98.
2. Fine JD, Eady RA, Bauer EA, et al. The classification of inherited epidermolysis bullosa (EB): report of the third international consensus meeting on diagnosis and classification of EB. J Am Acad Dermatol. 2008;58(6):931-50.
3. Rakowska A, Slowinska M, Kowalska-Oledzka EW, et al. Trichoscopy of cicatricial alopecia. J Drugs Dermatol. 2012;11(6):753-8.
4. Siañez-González C, Pezoa-Jares R, Salas-Alanis JC. Congenital epidermolysis bullosa: a review. Actas Dermosifiliogr. 2009;100(10):842-56.
5. Tosti A, Duque-Estrada B, Murrell DF. Alopecia in epidermolysis bullosa. Dermatol Clin. 2010;28(1):165-9.

There is still no specific treatment for congenital EB. The therapy is essentially supportive and based on the combination of general care, infection control, surgical procedures when needed, mainly for correction of pseudosyndactyly, and nutritional support.

CHAPTER 11

Autoimmune Bullous Disorders

Marta Kurzeja

PEMPHIGUS VULGARIS AND FOLIACEUS

Pemphigus is a severe autoimmune disease characterized by intraepidermal blisters affecting the skin and/or mucous membranes. Two main subtypes of pemphigus may be distinguished: pemphigus vulgaris (PV) and pemphigus foliaceus (PF). In PV, the blisters and erosions are observed on the skin and mucosa, whereas in PF lesions are present only in the skin (Figs. 11.1 to 11.3). Scalp involvement in pemphigus ranges from 5% to 50% of the cases, probably as a result of high concentration of pemphigus autoantigens in hair follicles. In many cases, scalp erosions are the first manifestation of the disease. There are some reports describing long-lasting and therapy-resistant scalp lesions in the course of the pemphigus.

The type of alopecia in patients with pemphigus remains controversial. Some authors indicate that anagen effluvium is a frequent finding in nonlesional and lesional scalp areas. However, tufted hair folliculitis in persistent PV and scarring alopecia have also been described so far.

Dermoscopy can be a useful diagnostic tool in the autoimmune skin disorders, especially when the lesions are limited to the scalp. One of the most characteristic dermoscopic features of pemphigus is blood extravasations visible as red, sharply, demarcated hemorrhagic areas (Figs. 11.4A to D). In recent studies in 76.9% of patients with PV and in 70.6% of patients with PF. Also, various types of scaling (yellow and white diffuse scaling—Figs. 11.5A to D;

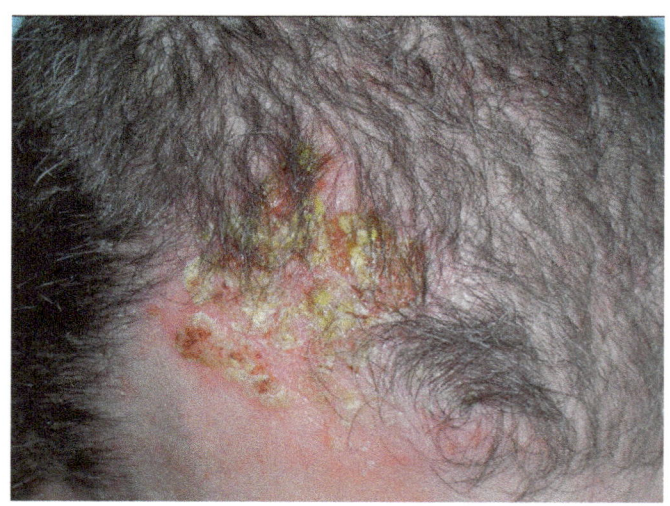

Fig. 11.1: Scalp lesions in pemphigus vulgaris. Crusted erosions on an erythematosus background and hair loss in a 44-year-old patient with pemphigus vulgaris.

scaling forming polygonal structures—Figs. 11.6A and B) may be visible. This feature is more common occurring in PF than in PV. Perifollicular tubular scaling (Figs. 11.7A and B) and hair casts can also be present, due to acantholysis within the outer root sheath. Large yellow dots with a whitish halo ("fried egg sign") may be observed in both types of pemphigus (Figs. 11.8A to D).

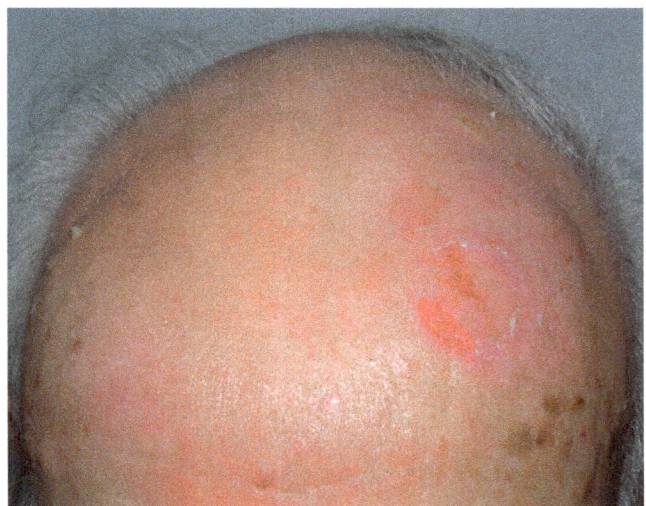

Fig. 11.2: Scalp lesions in pemphigus vulgaris. Sharply demarcated erosions and whitish scale on erythematosus background in a 72-year-old patient with long-lasting pemphigus vulgaris.

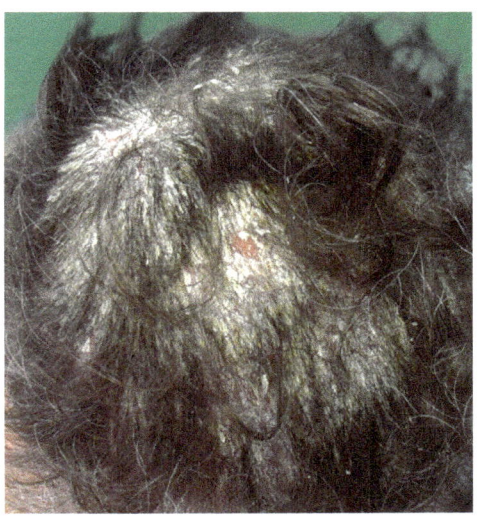

Fig. 11.3: Scalp lesions in pemphigus foliaceus. Sharply demarcated small erosion and diffuse, whitish scale on erythematosus background in a 65-year-old patient.

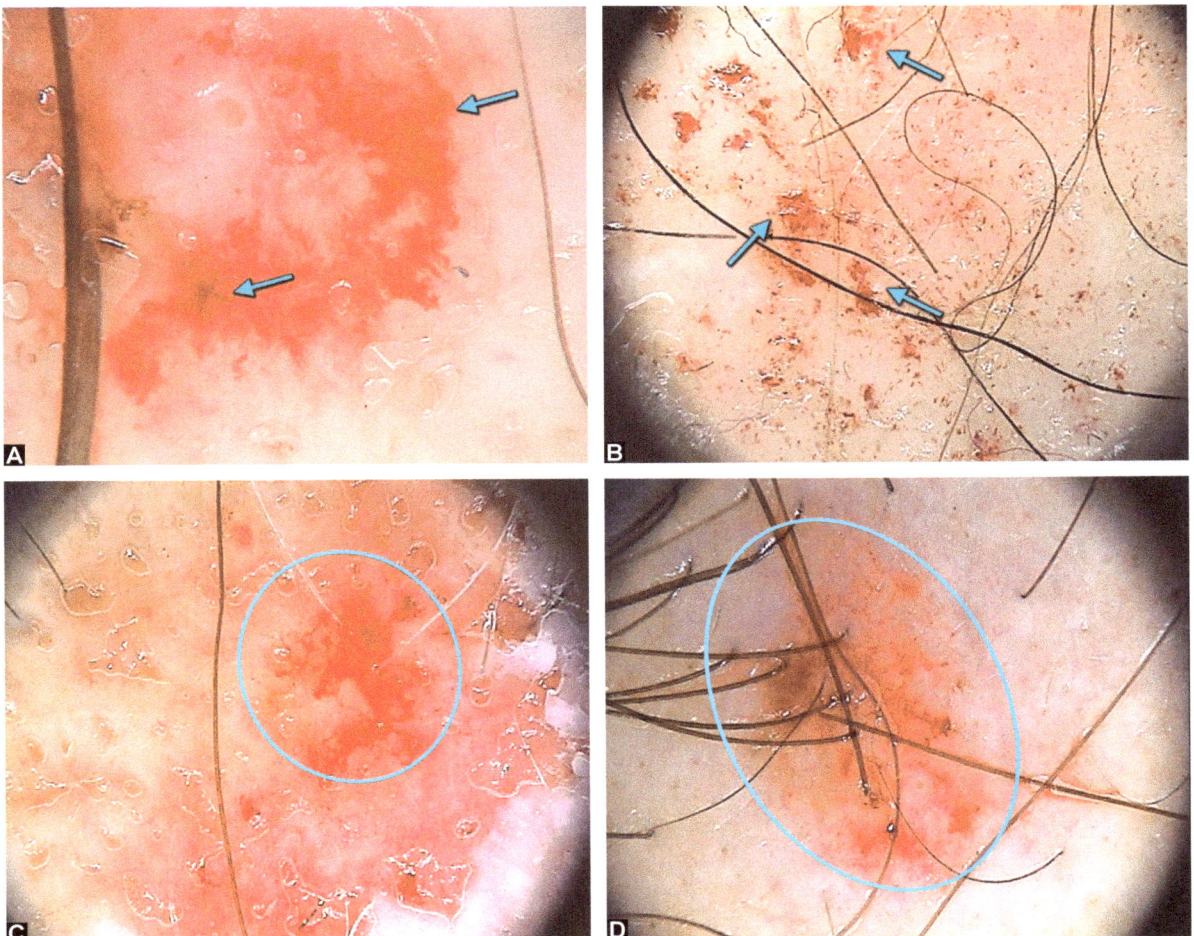

Figs. 11.4A to D: Blood extravasation in pemphigus vulgaris and foliaceus. Red, sharply demarcated, polygonal hemorrhagic areas (A and B—blue arrows, and C and D—blue circles). This feature usually develops within pemphigus vulgaris and foliaceus of recent onset. (A: x70; B to D: x20).

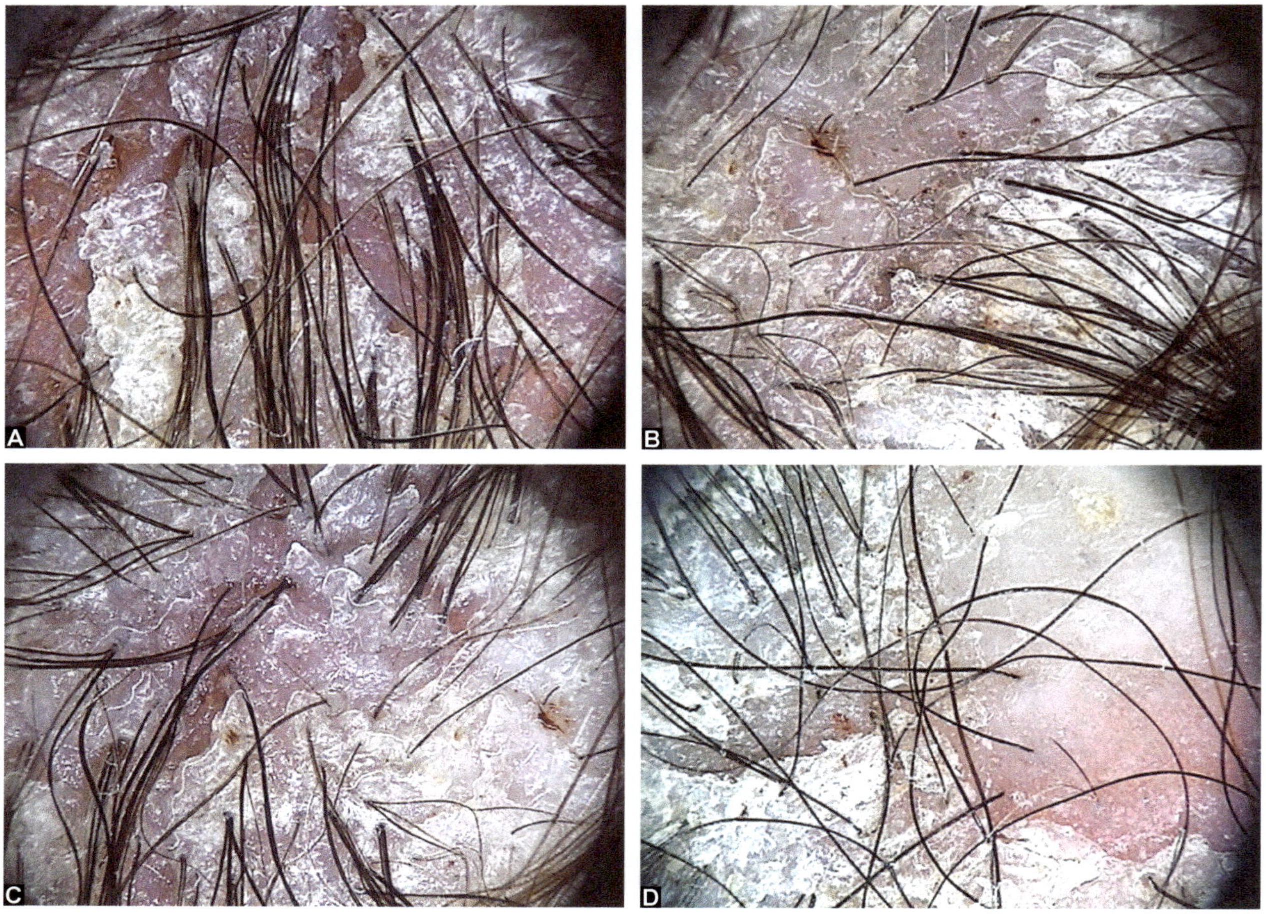

Figs. 11.5A to D: Diffuse white and yellow scaling on an erythematosus background in the scalp from a patient with pemphigus foliaceus (A to C) and pemphigus vulgaris (D) (x20).

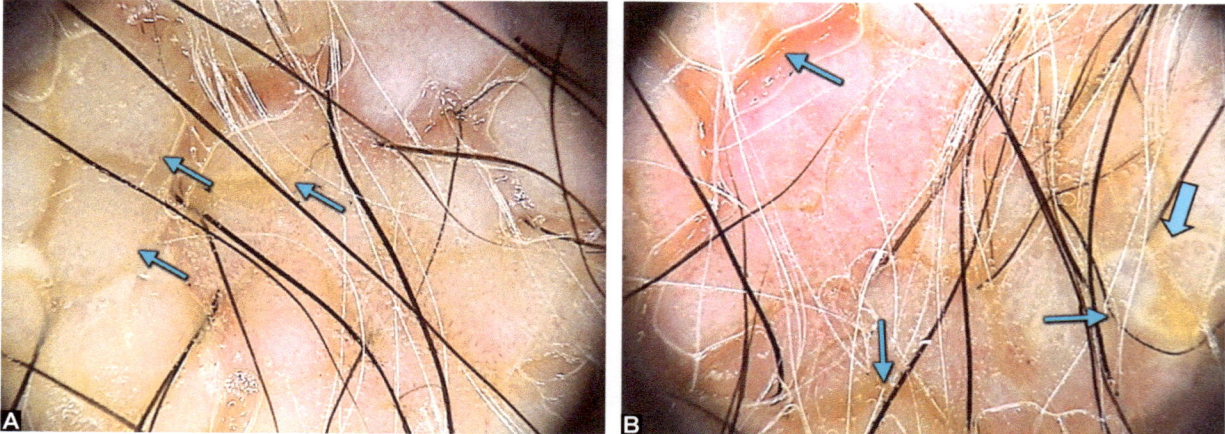

Figs. 11.6A and B: Scaling forming polygonal structures (blue arrows) in a patient with pemphigus vulgaris. Large yellowish thick polygonal scales with sharp edges correspond to partly detached elements of the epidermis (x20).

Autoimmune Bullous Disorders

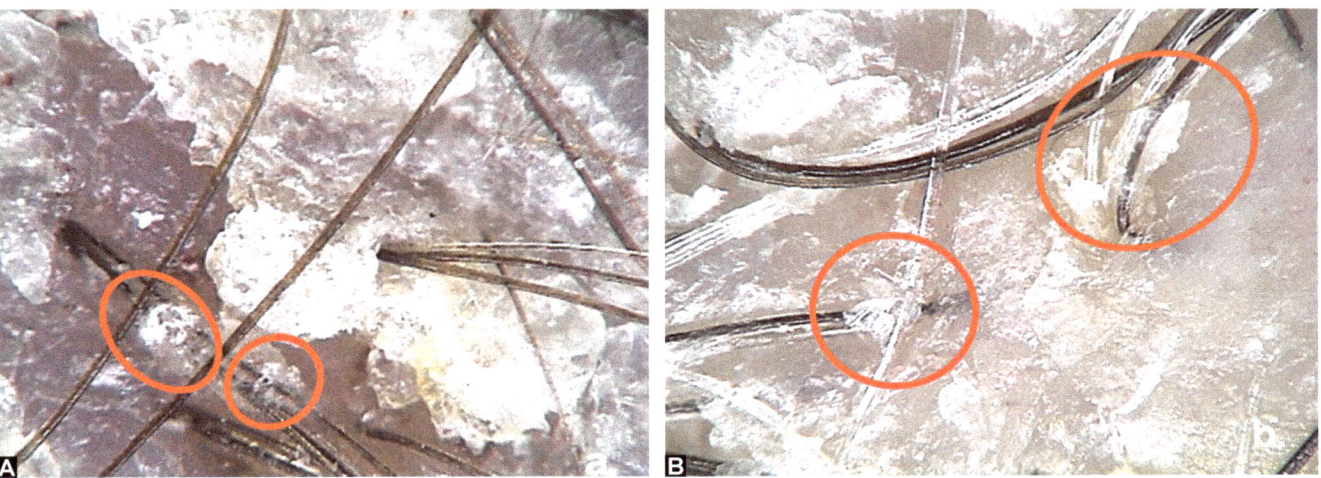

Figs. 11.7A and B: Perifollicular tubular whitish scaling (red oval) in a patient with pemphigus vulgaris (x70).

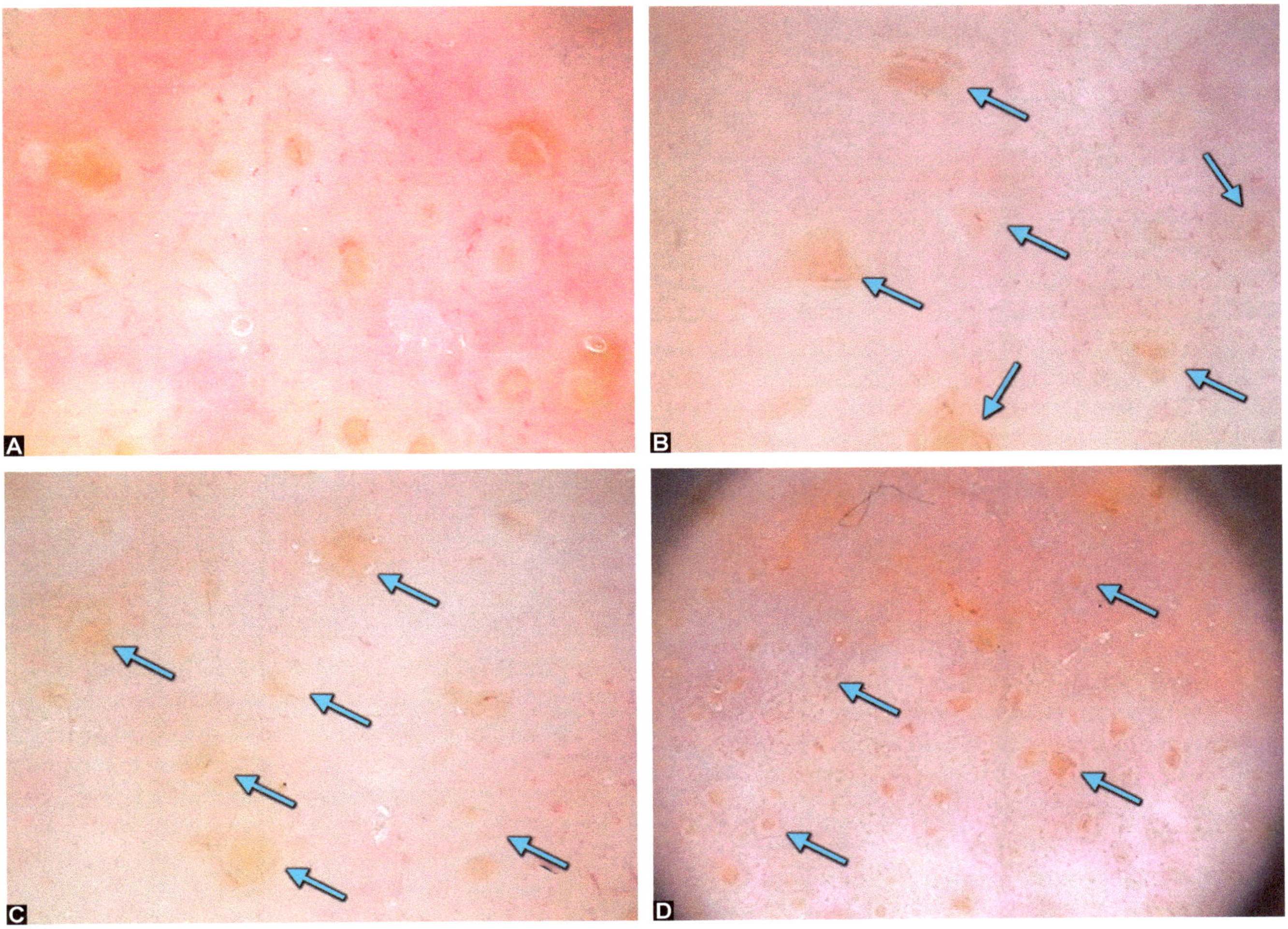

Figs. 11.8A to D: Large yellow dots with a whitish halo—"fried egg sign" (blue arrows) in a patient with pemphigus vulgaris. These yellow dots appear to correspond to follicular openings covered by residues of detached epidermis. Dotted vessels with a whitish halo (red circle; A). This sign is a hallmark of pemphigus vulgaris. White lamellar structures (black bracket; A) correspond to a partly detached epidermis overlying the erosion (A to C: x70; D: x70).

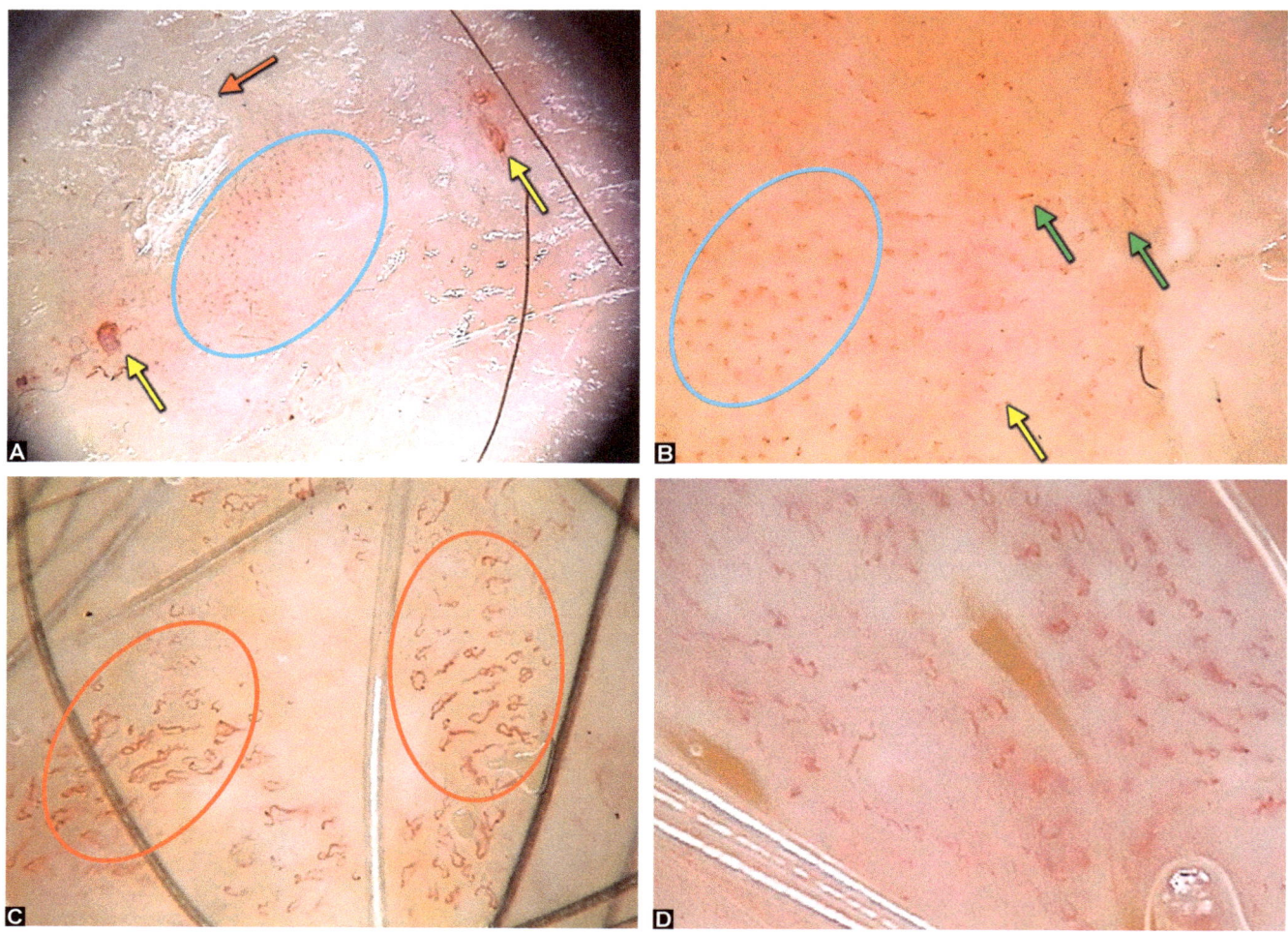

Figs. 11.9A to D: Vascular patterns in pemphigus vulgaris and foliaceus. Presence of vascular abnormalities correlated positively with activity of diseases. (A) Dotted blood vessels (blue oval) are usually seen in patients with pemphigus vulgaris. Note also blood extravasation (yellow arrows) and white scaling (red arrow) (x20). (B) Polymorphic pattern of blood vessels—dotted (blue oval), linear (green arrows), and comma (yellow arrow) blood vessels in a patient with pemphigus vulgaris. In some cases, polymorphic pattern of blood vessels, defined as more than two different patterns of blood vessels, can be seen in one lesion (x70). (C and D) Linear serpentine blood vessels (red oval) are a common finding in early lesions of pemphigus foliaceus (x70).

These yellow dots probably correspond to follicular openings covered by detached epidermis. Also, variable vascular patterns can be seen and they are associated with a poor prognosis. A previous study conducted by Sar-Pomian et al. showed linear, serpentine blood vessels, which was detectable in 77.8% of patients with PV and 30% of patients with PF (Figs. 11.9C and D). A more recent study conducted by the same group showed that the most common vascular patterns were dotted blood vessels, visible in 50% of patients with PV and in 11.8% of patients with PF (Figs. 11.9A and B). Moreover, dotted vessels with a whitish halo and circular vessels were exclusively present in PV.

DERMATITIS HERPETIFORMIS

Dermatitis herpetiformis (DH) is an autoimmune blistering disease often associated with gluten-sensitive enteropathy. Clinically, patients present higly pruritic and excoriated vesicles associated with utricle plaques and papules symmetrically distributed over the buttocks and extensor surface of the limbs. In the course of the disease, scalp is usually affected in 30% of cases. This location can be very rarely a first manifestation of the disease.

Dermoscopy shows clusters of regularly distributed dotted, comma, and linear blood vessels. A recent work of Sar-Pomian et al. showed that dotted vessels arranged in clusters were present in 62.5% of the patients

Autoimmune Bullous Disorders

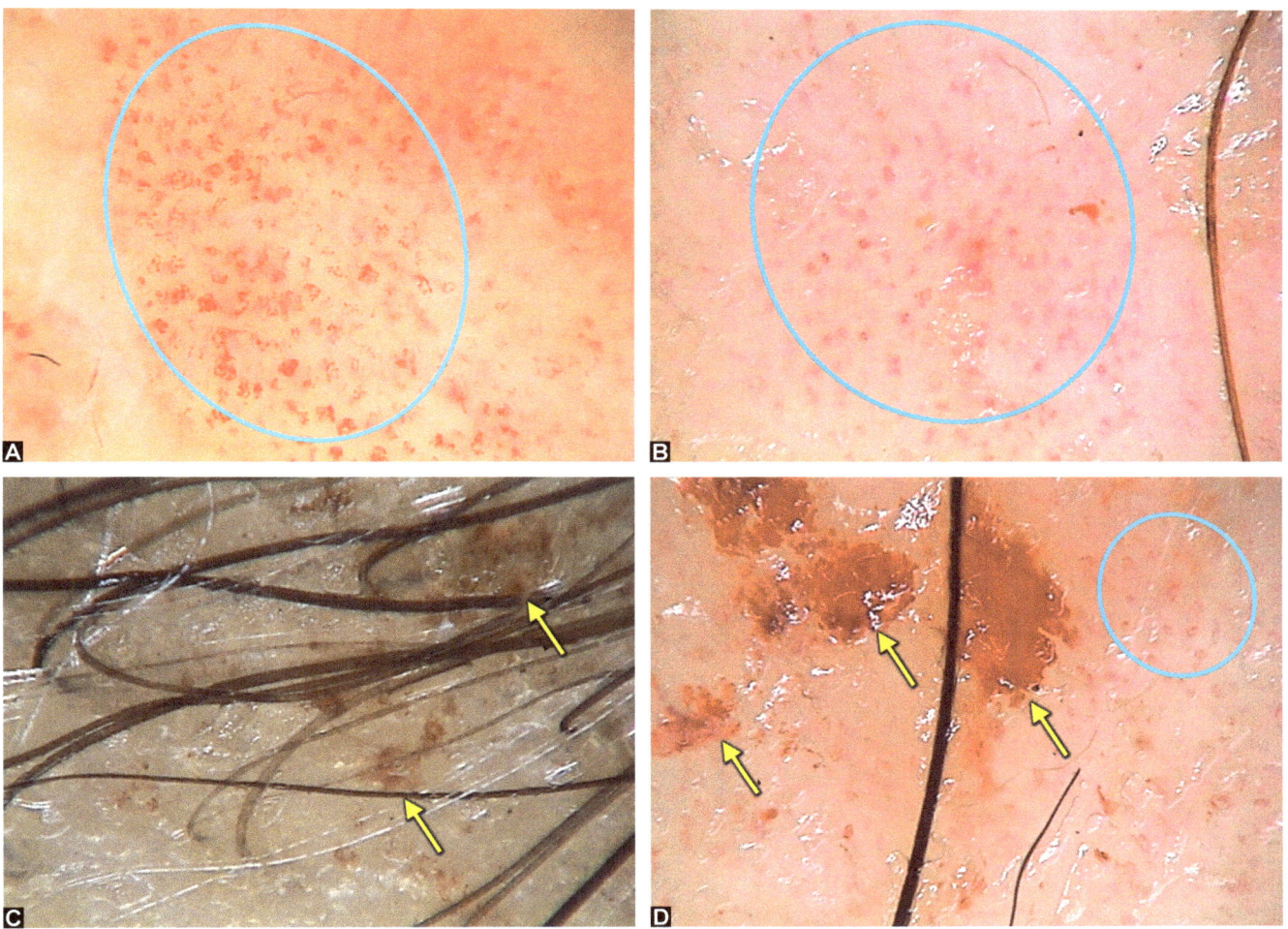

Figs. 11.10A to D: Scalp lesions in dermatitis herpetiformis. (A and B) Dotted vessels arranged in clusters (blue oval)—the vascular hallmark of the disease (x70). (C) White diffuse scaling and blood extravasation (yellow arrows, x70). (D) Dotted vessels arranged in clusters (blue oval) and blood extravasation (yellow arrows, x70).

(Figs.11.10A, B, and D). Moreover, in all cases, blood extravasations (Fig. 11.10D) were present, while white diffuse scaling (Fig. 11.10C) occurred in half of the patients.

PEMPHIGOID

Pemphigoid is a heterogeneous group of autoimmune disorders characterized by distinct clinical and immunological variants with subepidermal blisters. Most frequently, bullous pemphigoid (BP) is clinically characterized by tense blisters on an erythematosus, utricle, or noninflammatory background, which often rupture forming crusted erosions. Bullae and erosions with subsequent scarring could be also observed on the scalp.

The trichoscopic hallmark of BP is sharply demarcated creamy-white oval structures, clinically corresponding to tense blisters on the scalp (Figs. 11.11A and B). As in other autoimmune bullous skin disorders, blood extravasation is the most frequent trichoscopic feature and can be seen in most patients. Another trichoscopic feature is white and yellow scaling. Vascular abnormalities, such as common linear serpentine blood vessels, are also present in highly active diseases. As in PF and PV, yellow dots with a whitish halo can also be present in some patients.

Systemic corticosteroids remain the gold standard in treatment of pemphigus. Initially it should be also added adjuvant steroid-sparing agents such as azathioprine, cyclophosphamide or mycofenolate mofetil. Rituximab, a monoclonal antibody against CD20+B cells is also very effective treatment.

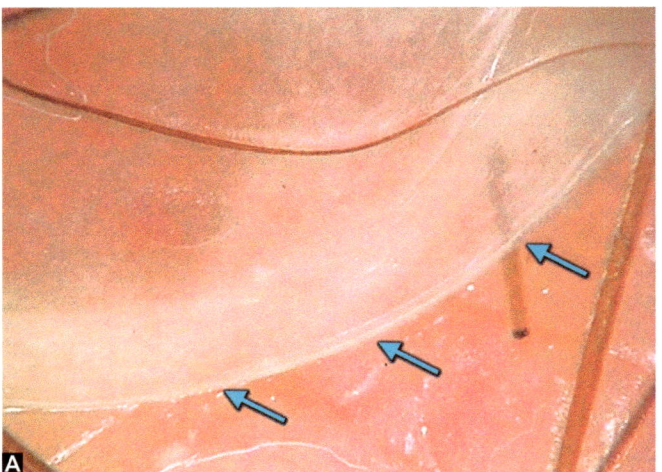 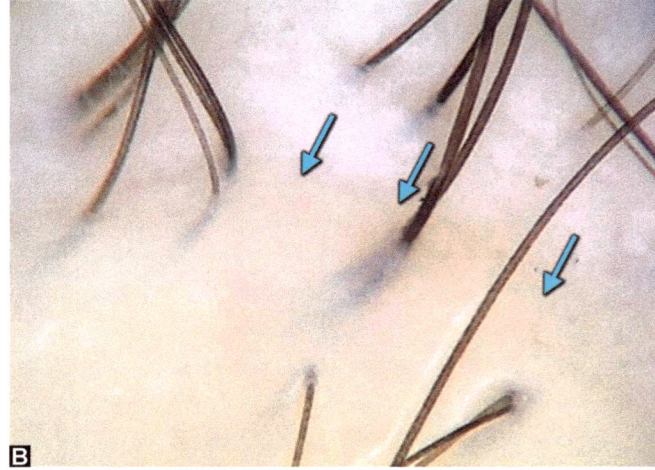

Figs. 11.11A and B: Scalp lesions in bullous pemphigoid. Sharply demarcated creamy-white circular structures (blue arrows) that clinically correspond to blisters. Note that hair shafts can emerge from the blister (A: x70; B: x20).

Take-Home Message
• Blood extravasation is the most frequent dermoscopic feature in the patients with autoimmune blistering diseases. • Large yellow dots with a whitish halo ("fried egg sign") can also be seen in the patient's with autoimmune blistering diseases. • Dotted blood vessels and linear serpentine blood vessels are most frequent vascular patterns in pemphigus scalp lesions. • Dotted blood vessels arranged in clusters are the hallmark of DH. • Sharply demarcated creamy-white oval structures are the hallmark of BP.

SUGGESTED READING

1. Ball S, Walkden V, Wojnarowska F. Cicatricial pemphigoid rarely involves the scalp. Australs J Dermatol. 1998;39(4): 258-60.
2. Bystryn JC, Rudolph JL. Pemphigus. Lancet. 2005;366 (9479):61-73.
3. Daneshpazhooh M, Mahmoudi HR, Rezakhani S, et al. Loss of normal anagen hair in pemphigus vulgaris. Clin Exp Dermatol. 2015;40(5);485-8.
4. Gaitanis G, Patmanidis K, Skandalis K, et al. Scarring alopecia in pemphigus vulgaris: a rare or underdiagnosed presentation? Eur J Dermatol. 2013;23(2):253-5.
5. Gul U, Soylu S, Herper AO. An unusual case of dermatitis herpetiformis presenting with initial scalp localization. Indian J Dermatol Venerol Leprol. 2009;75(6):620-2.
6. Hadayer N, Ramot Y, Maly A, et al. Pemphigus vulgaris with loss of hair on the scalp. Int J Trichology. 2013;5:157-8.
7. Jappe U, Schroder K, Zillikens D, et al. Tufted hair folliculitis associated with pemphigus vulgaris. J Eur Acad Dermatol Venerol. 2003;17(2):223-6.
8. Kneisel A, Hertl M. Autoimmune bullous diseases. Part 1: Clinical manifestation. J Dtsch Dermatol Ges. 2011;9(10):844-956.
9. Ko DK, Chae IS, Chung KH, et al. Persistent pemphigus vulgaris showing features of tufted folliculitis. Ann Dermatol. 2011,23(4):523-5.
10. Kurzeja M, Olszewska M, Rudnicka L. Autoimmune Bullous Diseases. Atlas of Trichoscopy: Dermoscopy in Hair and Scalp Diseases. London: Springer; 2012.
11. Kurzeja M, Rakowska A, Olszewska M, et al. Trichoscopy (dermoscopy of the scalp) in autoimmune bullous skin diseases. Abstract CD. 21st Congress of European Academy of Dermatology and Venerology, Prague;2012.
12. Miteva M, Murrell DF, Tosti A. Hair loss in autoimmune cutaneous bullous disorders. Dermatol Clin. 2011;29(3) 503-9.
13. Mutasim DF. Therapy of autoimmune bullous diseases. Ther Clin Risk Manag. 2007;3(1):29-40.
14. Petronić-Rosić V, JKrunić A, Mijusković M, et al. Tufted hair folliculitis: a pattern of scarring alopecia? J Am Acad Dermatol. 1999;41(1):112-4.
15. Pirmez R. Acantholytic hair casts: a dermoscopic sign of pemphigus vulgaris of the scalp. Int J Trichology. 2012;4(3):172-3.
16. Rose C, Bröcker EB, Zillikens D. Clinical, histological and immunological findings in 32 patients with dermatitis herpetiformis Duhring. J Dtsch Dermatol Ges. 2010;8(4):265-71.
17. Sar-Pomian M, Kolacinska-Straz Z, Labecka H, et al. Scalp lesions in pemphigus. Przegl Dermatol. 2010;97:162-3.
18. Sar-Pomian M, Kurzeja M, Rudnicka L, et al. The value of trichoscopy in differential diagnosis of scalp lesions in pemphigus vulgaris and pemphigus foliaceus. An Bras Dermatol. 2014;89(6):1007-12.
19. Sar-Pomian M, Rudnicka L, Olszewska M. Trichoscopy—a useful tool in the preliminary differential diagnosis of autoimmune bullous diseases. Int J Dermatol. 2017;56(10):996-1002.
20. Veraitch O, Ohyama M, Yamagami J, et al. Alopecia as a rare but distinct manifestation of pemphigus vulgaris. J Eur Acad Dermatol Venerol. 2013;27(1):86-91.

CHAPTER 12

Hair Shaft Disorders

Giselle Martins, Patricia Damasco, Isabella Doche, Neusa Yuriko Sakai Valente

12.1 Monilethrix

Giselle Martins, Patricia Damasco, Isabella Doche

Monilethrix is characterized by regular constrictions along the hair shaft, leading to increased hair fragility and alopecia. Usually, it has an autosomal dominant trait, although a recessive pattern has also been reported. Affected individuals can have normal hair at birth, but develop the disease over the first months of life.

Clinical lesions are variable in affected members of the family, ranging from almost normal hair to near complete alopecia (Fig. 12.1.1). Follicular keratosis lesions are commonly present on the occiput (Fig. 12.1.2). Eyebrows, eyelashes, and axillary and pubic hairs may be also affected, and other associated systemic lesions, such as syndactyly, cataracts, teeth, and nail abnormalities can occur (Fig. 12.1.3).

Dermoscopy shows multiple, regularly beaded hairs that tend to fracture at constriction sites. Nodosities correspond to the normal diameter of hair, whereas the defect is the constriction point (Figs. 12.1.4 to 12.1.6)

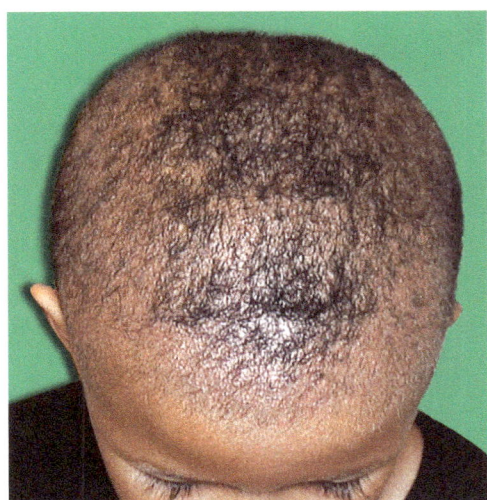

Fig. 12.1.1: Monilethrix. Partial scalp alopecia in a 3-year-old patient.
Source: Hair Department, Division of Sanitary Dermatology of Porto Alegre.

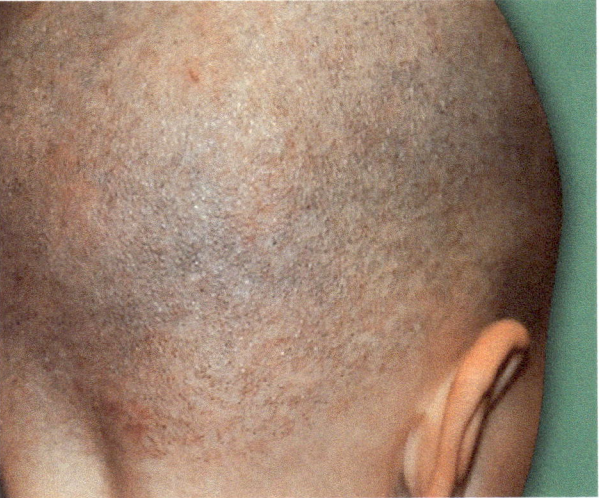

Fig. 12.1.2: Monilethrix. Severe scalp alopecia associated with keratosis follicularis in the occipital area of the scalp.
Source: Hair Department, Division of Sanitary Dermatology of Porto Alegre.

164 Fundamentals of Hair and Scalp Dermoscopy

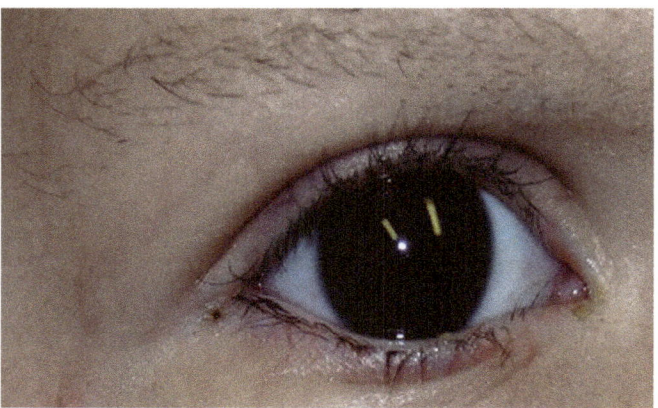

Fig. 12.1.3: Monilethrix. Partial eyebrow and eyelash alopecia in a 2-year-old patient.
Source: Hair Department, Division of Dermatology, Santa Casa of Porto Alegre Hospital.

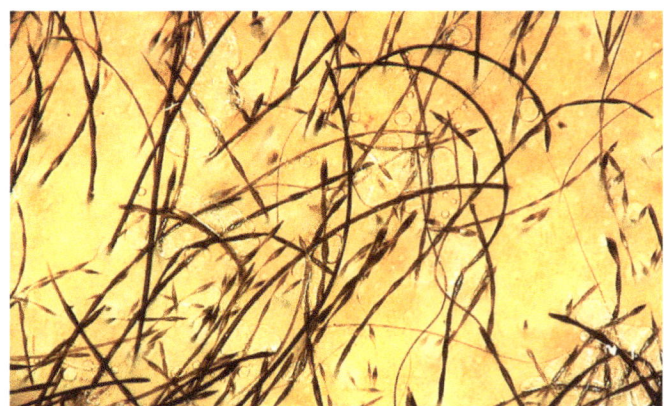

Fig. 12.1.4: Monilethrix. Dermoscopy shows numerous broken hairs, black dots, and beaded hairs. Note that not all hairs are affected.
Source: Hair Department, Division of Sanitary Dermatology of Porto Alegre.

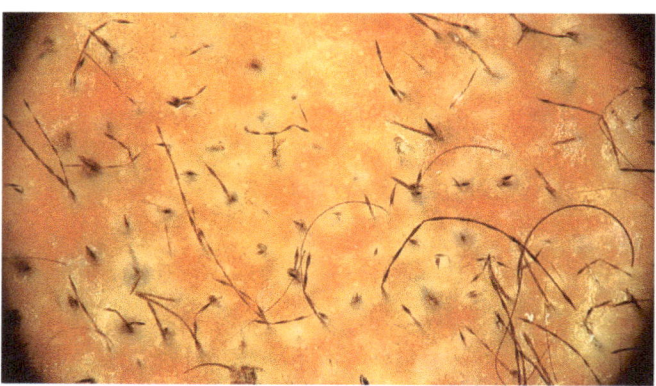

Fig. 12.1.5: Monilethrix. Note severe hair breakage, multiple broken hairs, and black dots. Hair breakage can occur in different levels from scalp emergence.
Source: Hair Department, Division of Dermatology, Santa Casa Hospital of Porto Alegre.

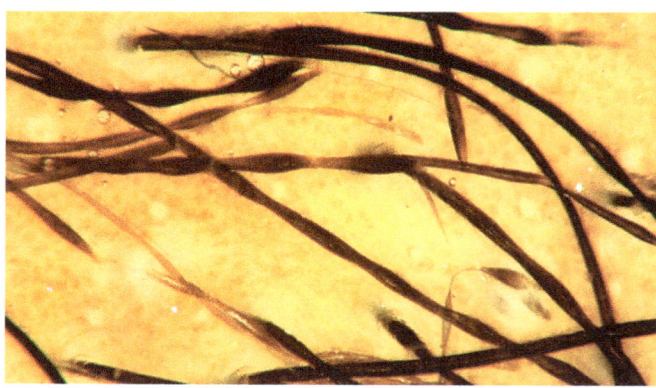

Fig. 12.1.6: Monilethrix. Note the constrictions regularly distributed along the hair shafts.
Source: Hair Department, Division of Sanitary Dermatology of Porto Alegre.

True monilethrix should be distinguished from pseudomonilethrix or monilethrix-like hairs, which have irregularly distributed contrictions along the hair shafts.

There is no specific treatment for monilethrix. Although hair fragility tends to improve with age, reduction friction and traumatic hairdressing may prevent affected hairs from breakage. Oral retinoids and topical minoxidil have been used with limited efficacy.

Take-Home Message

- Monilethrix is a hair shaft disorder characterized by regular constrictions along the hair shafts, hair fragility, and variable alopecia.
- Follicular keratosis in the occiput is usually present.
- Body hairs may be also affected and other systemic conditions may be associated.
- Dermoscopy of the affected hairs shows uniform elliptical nodosities with intermittent regular constrictions, and variable broken hairs.

SUGGESTED READING

1. Avhad G, Ghuge P. Monilethrix. Int J Trichology. 2013;5(4);224-5.
2. Leitner C, Cheung S, de Berker D. Pitfalls and pearls in the diagnosis of monilethrix. Pediatr Dermatol. 2013;30(5):633-5.
3. Lencastre A, Tosti A. Monilethrix. J Pediatr. 2012;161(60):1176.
4. Oliveira EF, Araripe AL. Monilethrix: a typical case report with microscopic and dermatoscopic findings. An Bras Dermatol. 2015;90(1):126-7.
5. Rakowska A, Slowinska M, Kowalska-Oledzka E, et al. Trichoscopy in genetic hair shaft abnormalities. J Dermatol Case Rep. 2008;2(2):14-20.
6. Rudnicka L, Rakowska A, Kurzeja M, et al. Hair shafts in trichoscopy: clues for diagnosis of hair and scalp diseases. Dermatol Clin. 2013;31(4):695-708.
7. Sharma VK, Chiramel MJ, Rao A. Dermoscopy: a rapid bedside tool to assess monilethrix. Indian J Dermatol Venereol Leprol. 2016;82(1):73-4.
8. Sinclair R. Treatment of monilethrix with oral minoxidil. JAAD Case Rep. 2016;2(3):212-5.
9. Singh G, Miteva M. prognosis and management of congenital hair shaft disorders with fragility—part I. Pediatr Dermatol. 2016;33(5):473-80.
10. Vora RV, Anjaneyan G, Mehta MJ. Monilethrix, a rare inherited hair shaft disorder in siblings. Indian Dermatol Online J. 2014;5(3):339-40.

12.2 Pili Torti

Giselle Martins, Patricia Damasco, Isabella Doche

Pili torti is characterized by flattened and irregularly twisted hair shafts as a result of an abnormal inner root sheath. The affected hair is coarse, brittle, and shows a lusterless appearance, due to uneven light reflection on the twisted hair surface (Fig. 12.2.1). Eyebrows and eyelashes may also be affected. Pili torti may be acquired or congenital, as part of many genetic syndromes (Tables 12.2.1 and 12.2.2), although it may also be an occasional finding in healthy subjects.

Dermoscopy with high magnification shows flattened shafts with clusters of narrow twists of 180° at irregular intervals (Figs. 12.2.2A to F). Low magnifications may mimic pseudomonilethrix, which shows hair shafts acutely bended at different angles and irregular intervals.

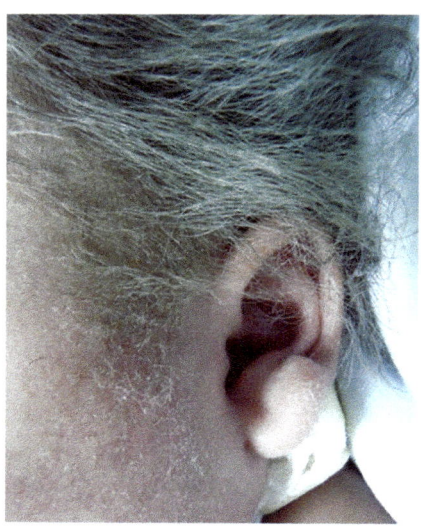

Fig. 12.2.1: Pili torti. Dry, brittle, and lusterless hairs in a child with Menkes syndrome.
Source: Dr Sandra Romero.

There is no specific treatment for this condition. In healthy subjects, it may improve spontaneously after puberty.

Table 12.2.1: Congenital diseases associated with pili torti.

Barre syndrome: Scarce beard and body hair, and alopecia after puberty in African descent individuals
Ronchese syndrome: Leukonychia, ichthyosis, keratosis pilaris, nail dystrophy, and dental abnormalities
Björnstad syndrome: Sensorineural deafness
Menkes syndrome: Growth retardation of early onset, hypotonia, seizures, skin and joint laxity, and focal brain degeneration
Rapp-Hodgkin syndrome: Ectodermal dysplasia, hypohidrosis, cleft lip, cleft palate, hypodontia, nail abnormalities, and genitourinary abnormalities
Trichodysplasia-xeroderma: Skin xerosis, alopecia, hypotrichosis, and trichorrhexis nodosa
Trichothiodystrophy: Ichthyosis, developmental delay, brittle hair, and photosensitivity
Goltz syndrome: Ectodermal dysplasia, asymmetric Blaschko-linear and reticulated atrophy, pigmentary changes, telangiectasias, papillomas, punctate erosions, hypohidrosis, patchy alopecia, diffuse thin hairs, and nail abnormalities
Bazex-Dupré-Christol syndrome: Follicular atrophoderma, multiple basal cell carcinomas, hypotrichosis, and trichorrhexis nodosa

Table 12.2.2: Acquired diseases associated with pili torti.

Scarring alopecias: Frontal fibrosing alopecia, lichen planopilaris, and others
Alopecia areata
Malnutrition
Oral retinoid treatment

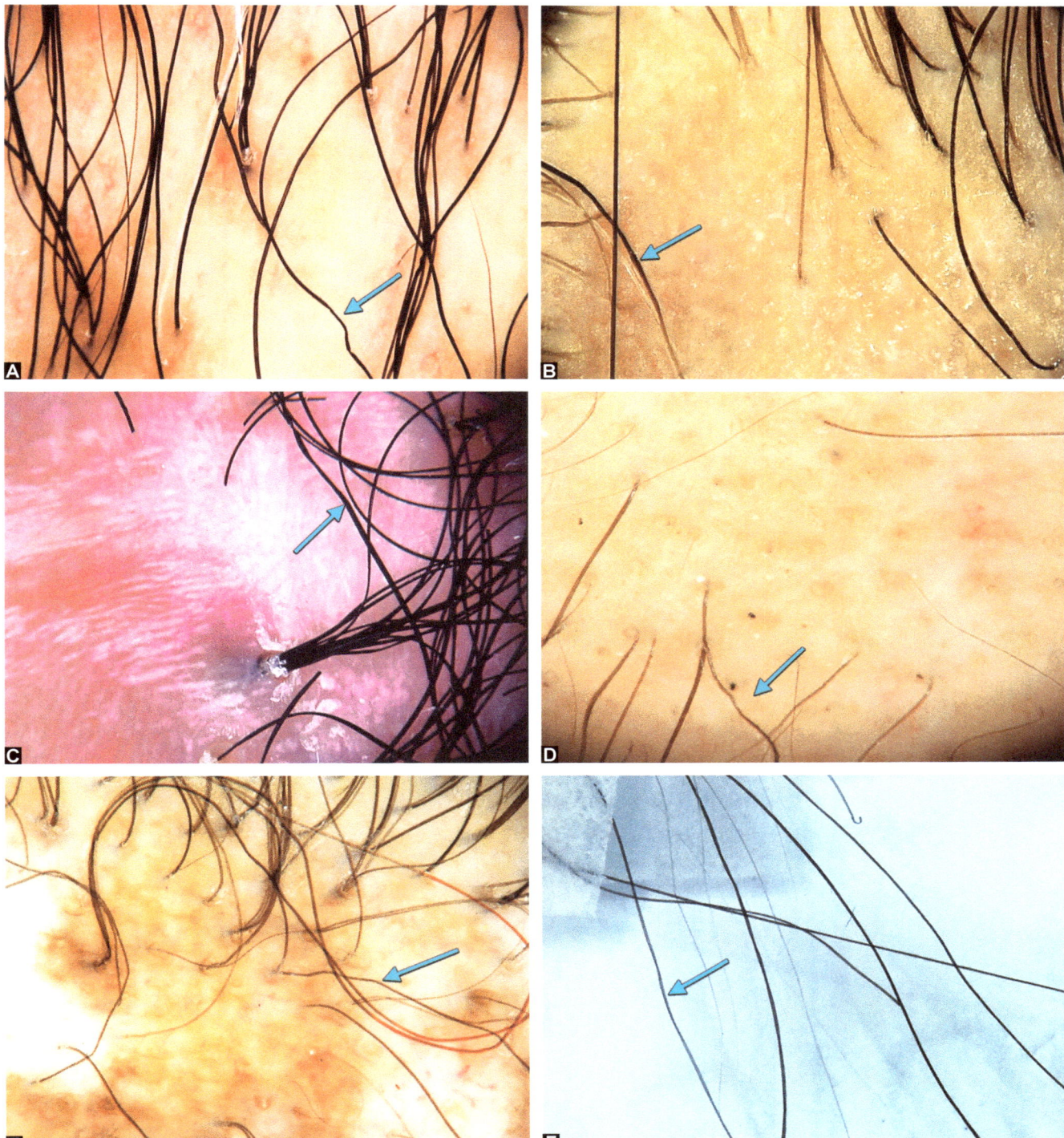

Figs. 12.2.2A to F: Pili torti. Note flattened and irregularly twisted hair shafts (blue arrows) in (A) Frontal fibrosing alopecia, (B) Lichen planopilaris, (C) Folliculitis decalvans, (D) Alopecia areata, (E) Discoid lupus erythematosus, and (F) Menkes syndrome.

Source: (C to E) Division of Dermatology, Hospital das Clínicas, University of São Paulo Medical School. (F) Dr Sandra Romero.

> **Take-Home Message**
> - Pili torti is a rare hair shaft disorder characterized by short and brittle hairs.
> - Pili torti may be an occasional finding in healthy subjects.
> - It is commonly associated with cicatricial alopecias and genetic syndromes.
> - Dermoscopy shows flattened hairs with 180° irregular twists.

SUGGESTED READING

1. Bree AF, Grange DK, Hicks MJ, et al. Dermatologic findings of focal dermal hypoplasia (Goltz syndrome). Am J Med Genet C Semin Med Genet. 2016;172C(1):44-51.
2. Chatterjee M, Neema S, Mukherjee S. Rapp Hodgkin syndrome. Indian Dermatol Online J. 2017;8(3):215-6.
3. Marubashi Y, Yanagishita T, Muto J, et al. Morphological analyses in fragility of pili torti with Björnstad syndrome. J Dermatol. 2017;44(4):455-8.
4. Maruyama T, Toyoda M, Kanei A, et al. Pathogenesis in pili torti: morphological study. J Dermatol Sci. 1994;7(Suppl):S5-12.
5. Mirmirani P, Samimi SS, Mostow E. Pili torti: clinical findings, associated disorders, and new insights into mechanisms of hair twisting. Cutis. 2009;84(3):143-7.
6. Olszewska M, Rakowska A. Pili torti. In: Rudnicka L, Olszewska M, Rakowska A. Atlas of Trichoscopy Dermoscopy. London: Springer-Verlag; 2012. pp. 167-8.
7. Price V. Structural anomalies of the hair shaft: pili torti. In: Orfanos CE, Happle R (Eds). Hair and Hair Diseases. Berlin: Springer-Verlag; 1990. pp. 384-90.
8. Rakowska A, Slowinska M, Kowalska-Oledzka E, et al. Trichoscopy in genetic hair shaft abnormalities. J Dermatol Case Rep. 2008;2(2):14-20.
9. Rossi L, Lombardo MF, Ciriolo MR, et al. Mitochondrial dysfunction in neurodegenerative diseases associated with copper imbalance. Neurochem Res. 2004;29(3):493-504.
10. Smpokou P, Samanta M, Berry GT, et al. Menkes disease in affected females: the clinical disease spectrum. Am J Med Genet A. 2015;167A(2):417-20.
11. Whiting DA. Hair shaft defects. In: Olsen EA (Ed). Disorders of Hair Growth: Diagnosis and Treatment. 2nd edition. New York: McGraw Hill; 2003. pp. 123-75.
12. Yang JJH, Cade KV, Rezende FC, et al. Clinical presentation of pili torti: case report. An Bras Dermatol. 2015;90(3 Suppl 1):29-31.

12.3 Pili Annulati

Giselle Martins, Patricia Damasco, Isabella Doche

Pili annulati is an autosomal-dominant or sporadic hair shaft disorder with variable expression characterized by alternating light and dark bands. The presence of air-filled cavities within the cortex produces a shiny and brilliant appearance to the affected hairs (Fig. 12.3.1). Usually, about 20–80% of hairs can be affected and the same follicle may present intermittent involvement. Although pili annulati is usually not associated with hair fragility, increased breakage secondary to weathering of the abnormal hair shafts can occur (Fig. 12.3.2).

Dermoscopy shows hair shafts with alternating light and dark bands (Fig. 12.3.3). White bands are subtle and cloudy, covering 50–100% of the hair shaft thickness. On light microscopy, hair shafts show a random pattern of intermittent abnormal cavities (Fig. 12.3.4). Light bands appear as dark bands when imaged by light microscopy, reflecting cortical spaces containing air in the light bands and fluid in the dark bands.

Fragmented medulla should not be mistaken for pili annulati. The white bands in fragmented medulla are located centrally in the hair shaft and cover less than 50% of the hair shaft thickness. Other differential diagnoses of pili annulati include inaccurate hair colorization and pseudopili annulati that happens due to incident light being reflected by the flattened segments of the twisted hair shafts.

Pili annulati does not require any treatment. Patients should be aware of possible hair breakage and prefer gentler hair grooming practices.

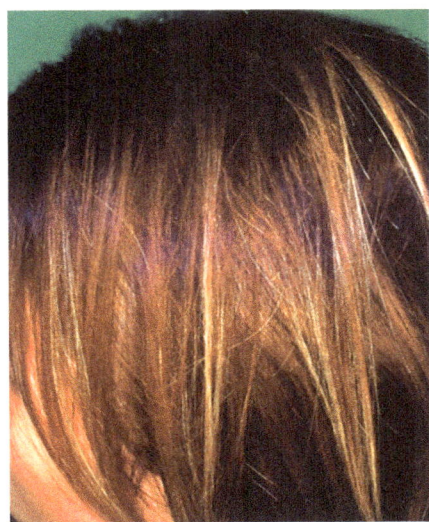

Fig. 12.3.1: Pili annulati. The hair is clinically normal. Alternating white and dark bands can be seen depending on light's incidence.
Source: Division of Dermatology, Hospital das Clínicas, University of São Paulo Medical School.

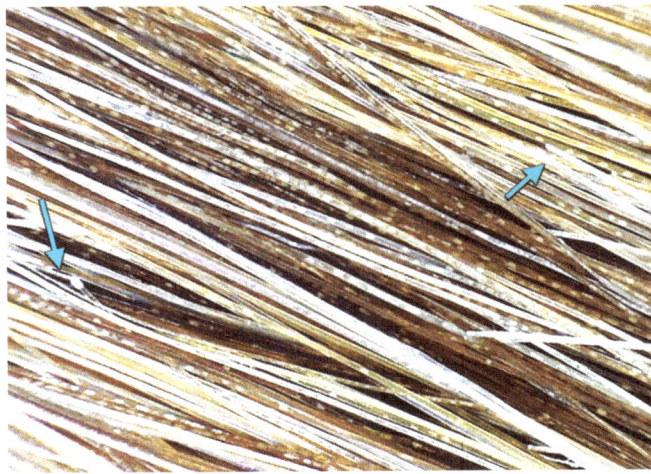

Fig. 12.3.2: Pili annulati. Air-filled cavities within the cortex. Note associated trichorrhexis nodosa and hair breakage (blue arrows).

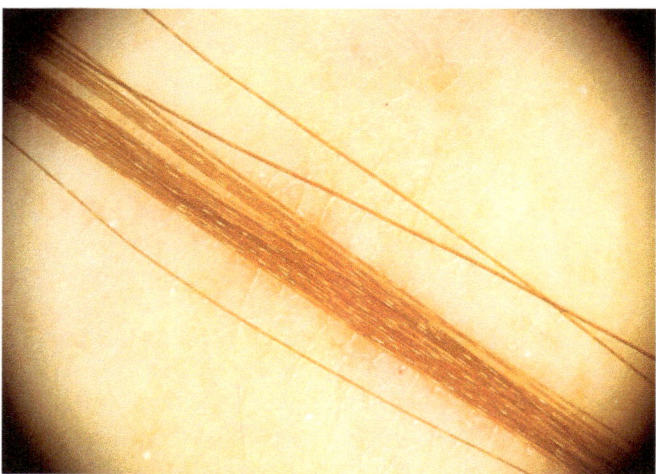 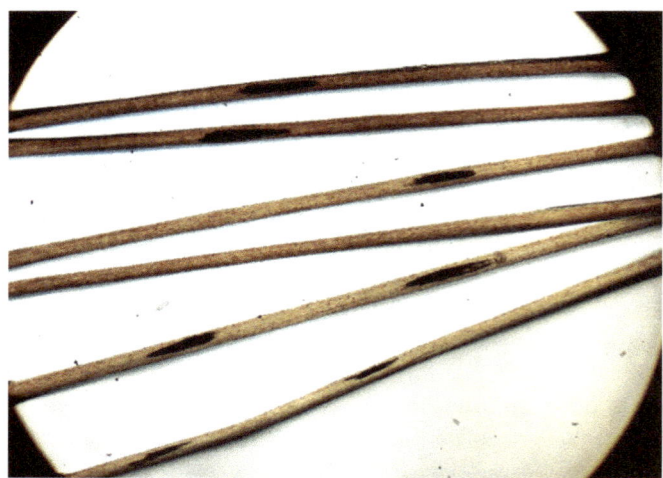

Fig. 12.3.3: Pili annulati. Typical alternating light and dark bands on the hair shafts.

Source: Division of Dermatology, Hospital das Clínicas, University of São Paulo Medical School.

Fig. 12.3.4: Pili annulati. Light microscopy shows intermittent air-filled cavities in black (OM, x100).

Source: Dr Neusa Valente.

> **Take-Home Message**
> - Pili annulati is characterized by alternating white and dark bands along the hair shaft.
> - Secondary hair fragility can occur.
> - Dermoscopy and light microscopy show alternating white and dark bands and air-filled cavities within the cortex.
> - Differential diagnoses are pseudopili annulati, hair colorization, and fragmented medulla.
> - No treatment is required.

SUGGESTED READING

1. Akoglu G, Emre S, Metin A, et al. Pili annulati with fragility: electron microscopic findings of a case. Int J Trichology. 2012;4(2):89-92.
2. Donati A, Andriolo AC, Barletta M, et al. Pili annulati and trichorrhexis nodosa in the same patient: cause or coincidence? Skin Appendage Disord. 2015;1(1):25-7.
3. Feldmann KA, Dawber RP, Pittelkow MR, et al. Newly described weathering pattern in pili annulati hair shafts: a scanning electron microscopic study. J Am Acad Dermatol. 2001;45(4):625-7.
4. Giehl KA, Ferguson DJP, Dawber RP, et al. Update on detection, morphology and fragility in pili annulati in three kindreds. J Eur Acad Dermatol Venereol. 2004;18(6):654-8.
5. Lee SS, Lee YS, Giam YC. Pseudopili annulati in a dark-haired individual: a light and electron microscopic study. Pediatr Dermatol. 2001;18(1):27-30.
6. Osório F, Tosti A. Pili annulati—what about racial distribution? Dermatol Online J. 2012;18(8):10.
7. Streck AP, Moncores M, Sarmento DF, et al. Study of nanomechanical properties of human hair shaft in a case of pili annulati by atomic force microscopy. J Eur Acad Dermatol Venereol. 2007;21(8):1109-10.
8. Werner K, St-Surin-Lord S, Sperling LC. Pili annulati associated with hair fragility: cause or coincidence? Cutis. 2013;91(1):36-8.

12.4 Trichorrhexis Invaginata

Giselle Martins, Patricia Damasco, Isabella Doche

Trichorrhexis invaginata (TI) is a rare hair shaft disorder characterized by multiple points of invagination of the hair shafts, leading to a "bamboo hair" appearance. Affected hairs are sparse, dry, dull, short, and brittle, especially in areas of constant friction. Eyebrows and eyelashes may also be affected. TI is part of Netherton syndrome, an autosomal recessive disorder which includes also ichthyosiform erythroderma and atopic dermatitis (Fig. 12.4.1). Sometimes, other manifestations as neurologic retardation, immune problems, frequent bacterial infections, and aciduria may be present.

Dermoscopy with low magnifications shows multiple small nodules or knots irregularly spaced along the shaft (Fig. 12.4.2). A "ball and cup" or "bamboo hair" appearance can be seen at high magnification, due to intussusception of the distal hair shaft into the proximal portion. When the hair fractures at the site of invagination, the proximal end will appear cupped. This appearance is named "golf-tee hairs." Not all hairs are affected (Figs. 12.4.3A and B).

There is no specific treatment for congenital hair shaft abnormalities. Gentle hair care is the mainstay of care for hair shaft disorders associated with fragility. Oral retinoids can be used with variable results.

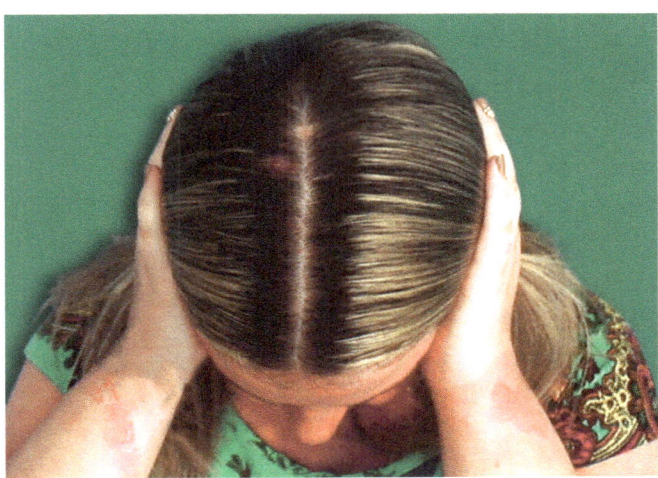

Fig. 12.4.1: Netherton syndrome. Multiple ichthyosiform erythroderma in the arms and small alopecic scalp areas.
Source: Division of Dermatology, Hospital das Clínicas, University of São Paulo Medical School.

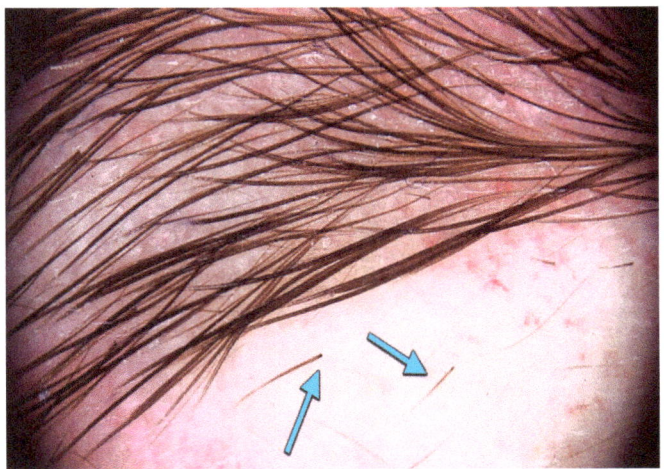

Fig. 12.4.2: Trichorrhexis invaginata in the eyebrow. Dermoscopy with low magnifications shows small black knots or nodules along the hair shafts. Some may mimic dystrophic hairs with a pigmented distal tip (blue arrows).
Source: Division of Dermatology, Hospital das Clínicas, University of São Paulo Medical School.

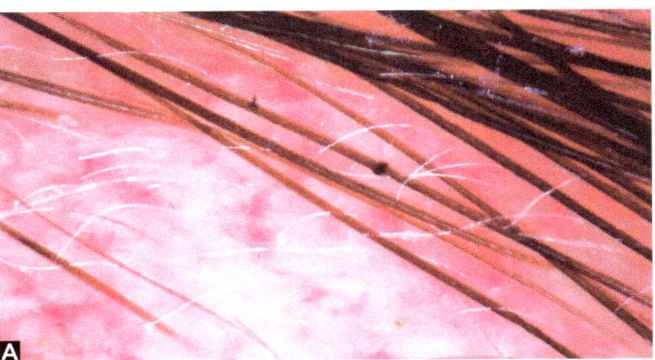

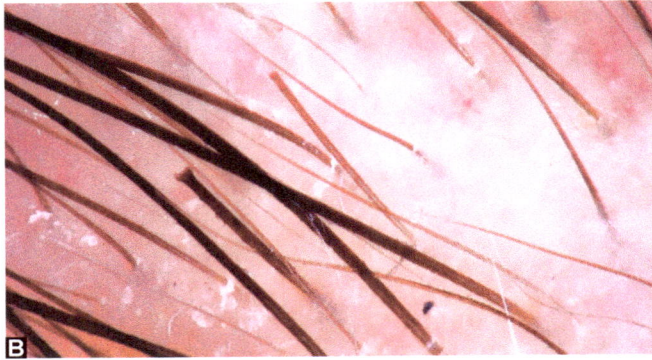

Figs. 12.4.3A and B: Trichorrhexis invaginata. (A) Dermoscopy with high magnifications shows the hair shaft invagination, leading to a "bamboo hair" appearance. (B) The fractured proximal end portion appears with a cupped format, resembling a "golf-tee."
Source: Division of Dermatology, Hospital das Clínicas, University of São Paulo Medical School.

> **Take-Home Message**
> - Trichorrhexis invaginata is a result of hair shaft invagination, causing increased hair fragility, mostly in areas of scalp friction.
> - Pathognomonic feature of Netherton syndrome, which also shows ichthyosis and atopic dermatitis.
> - Eyebrows and eyelashes may be affected.
> - Dermoscopy with low magnifications shows multiple small knots or nodules along the hair shaft and dark pigmented ends.
> - Dermoscopy with high magnifications shows "bamboo hairs." When the hair shaft is fractured, "golf tee hairs" or "ball and cup" can be seen.

SUGGESTED READING

1. Bittencourt MJS, Moure ER, Pies OTC, et al. Trichoscopy as a diagnostic tool in trichorrhexis invaginata and Netherton syndrome. An Bras Dermatol. 2015;90(1):114-6.
2. Haliasos EC, Kerner M, Jaimes-Lopez N, et al. Dermoscopy for the pediatric dermatologist part I: dermoscopy of pediatric infectious and inflammatory skin lesions and hair disorders. Pediatr Dermatol. 2013;30(2):163-71.
3. Melten Akkurt Z, Tuncel T, Ayhan E, et al. Rapid and easy diagnosis of Netherton syndrome with dermoscopy. J Cut Med Surg. 2014;18(4):280-2.
4. NG E, Hale CS, Meehan SA, et al. Netherton syndrome with ichthyosis linearis circumflexa and trichorrhexis invaginatum. Dermatol Online J. 2014;20(12):piii.
5. Rakowska A, Kowalska-Oledzka E, Slowinska M, et al. Hair shaft videodermoscopy in Netherton syndrome. Pediatr Dermatol. 2009;26(3):320-2.
6. Rudnicka L, Olszewska M, Rakowska A, et al. Trichoscopy update 2011. J Dermatol Case Rep. 2011;5(4):82-8.
7. Singh G, Miteva M. Prognosis and management of congenital hair shaft disorders with fragility: part I. Pediatr Dermatol. 2016;33(5):473-80.

12.5 Woolly Hair

Giselle Martins, Patricia Damasco, Isabella Doche

Woolly hair (WH) is a group of hair shaft disorders characterized by fine, tightly curled hair, covering the hole scalp or part of it. The hair shafts wave or curl in 180° longitudinal twisting without an increase in fragility. It is divided into three types—(1) hereditary dominant WH, (2) familial or sporadic recessive WH, and (3) WH nevus. In the autosomal dominant form, a variable degree of tight curling is present in all hairs throughout the scalp. The recessive form is characterized by abnormal, tightly curled, fine short white, or blond hair present from the birth. A WH nevus is a well-circumscribed patch of such tightly coiled hair. Most patients exhibit only WH, without any associated systemic or skin diseases. However, WH has also been associated with Naxos disease, Carvajal syndrome, Noonan syndrome, Costello syndrome, and ichthyosis.

Hair can be normal at birth and becomes coarser with age giving an unsightly appearance. The hairs are sparse, kinked, lighter in color, and smaller in diameter, without an increase in fragility (Fig. 12.5.1). Some cases of diffuse partial woolly hair may show few pigmented and curly affected hair fibers mostly of the top of the hair (Fig. 12.5.2). In this case, acquired kinking hairs may be an early sign of androgenetic alopecia. Trichoscopy is not decisive for diagnosis; however, it typically shows hair shaft with waves at very short intervals, giving a "crawling snake" appearance, and broken hairs (Fig. 12.5.3).

There is no documented effective treatment for WH. The use of minoxidil and tretinoin combined with an oral vitamin D analog may show some improvement. The prognosis is poor in individuals who do not improve with age.

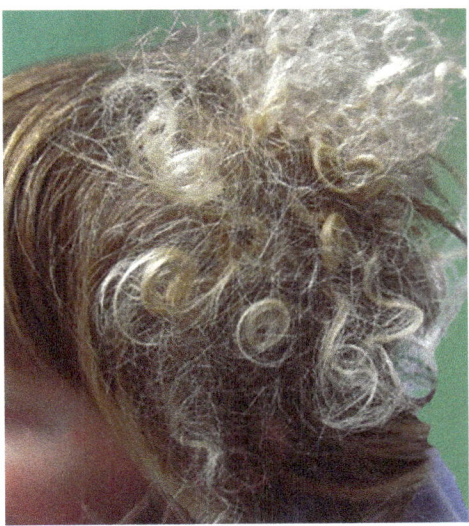

Fig. 12.5.1: Woolly hair nevus. Note localized kinked and lighter hair fibers on the vertex scalp area from a young girl.
Source: Dr Carmen Gloria Gonzalez.

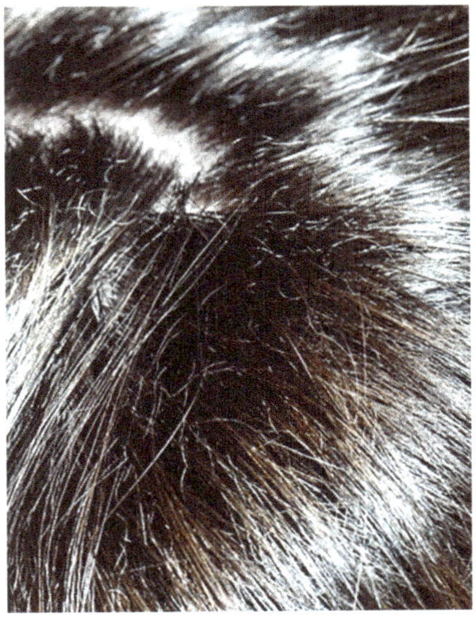

Fig. 12.5.2: Diffuse partial woolly hair. Note some curly hairs over the vertex scalp. Early androgenetic alopecia must be ruled out in this case.
Source: Dr Mariya Miteva and Dr Evgeni Hristozov.

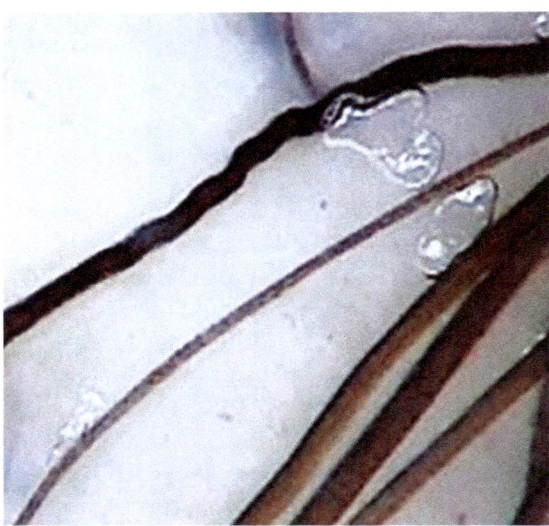

Fig. 12.5.3: Woolly hair syndrome. Hair shafts resembling a "crawling snake," with ondulations placed very closely together (×70).
Source: Gerkowicz A, Rakowska A, Slowinska M, et al. Trichoscopy in genetic hair shaft abnormalities. J Dermatol Case Rep. 2008;2(2):14-20.

Take-Home Message
- Woolly hair is a hair shaft disorder characterized by fine and tightly curled hair.
- Classified into three distinct types—hereditary dominant WH, familial or sporadic recessive WH, and WH nevus.
- Dermoscopy shows hair shafts with waves at very short intervals (crawling snake appearance) and broken hairs.

SUGGESTED READING

1. Choi SY, No YA, Kim BJ, et al. Topical minoxidil and tretinoin combined with an oral vitamin D analog as a treatment for woolly hair. Dermatol Ther. 2016;29(5):4-5.
2. Gerkowicz A, Rakowska A, Slowinska M, et al. Trichoscopy in genetic hair shaft abnormalities. J Dermatol Case Rep. 2008;2(2):14-20.
3. Martínez-Velasco MA, Quaresma MV, Hristozov E, et al. Diffuse partial woolly hair. Dermatología Rev Mex. 2015;59(5):430-3.
4. Rudnicka L, Rakowska A, Kerseja M, et al. Hair shafts in trichoscopy: clues for diagnosis of hair and scalp diseases. Dermatol Clin. 2013;31(4):695-708.
5. Singh G, Miteva M. Prognosis and management of congenital hair shaft disorders without fragility—part II. Pediatr Dermatol. 2016;33(5):481-7.
6. Swamy SS, Ravikumar BC, Vinay KN, et al. Uncombable hair syndrome with a woolly hair nevus. Indian J Dermatol Venereol Leprol. 2017;83(1):87-8.

12.6 Pili Trianguli et Canaliculi

Neusa Yuriko Sakai Valente, Isabella Doche

Pili trianguli et canaliculi (PTC) or uncombable hair syndrome is a rare hair shaft disorder characterized by a premature keratinization of the inner rooth sheat. PTC can have autosomal dominant inheritance or be sporadic. A genetic mutation or causal gene has not been identified.

In most cases, the hair is normal in childhood or at birth and becomes uncombable during the first year of life. Although this syndrome does not cause hair fragility, excessive attempts to comb and style the hair can lead to hair shaft damages, such as trichorrhexis nodosa, trichoptilosis, and hair breakage. PTC usually improves during puberty or later in life.

Affected scalp hairs show an unruly and rough appearance and a silvery-blonde color (Fig. 12.6.1). In some cases, eyebrows and body hairs may be also affected (Figs. 12.6.2A to C). Usually, PTC appears as an isolated finding, although the association with congenital anonychia, wooly hair nevus, and body hypotrichosis was previously reported in the literature.

The diagnosis must be suspected clinically and can be confirmed with microscopy. Dermoscopy and light microscopy can sometimes show subtle features and be alternative tools (Figs. 12.6.3 to 12.6.5). However, scanning electron microscopy can show the typical features of

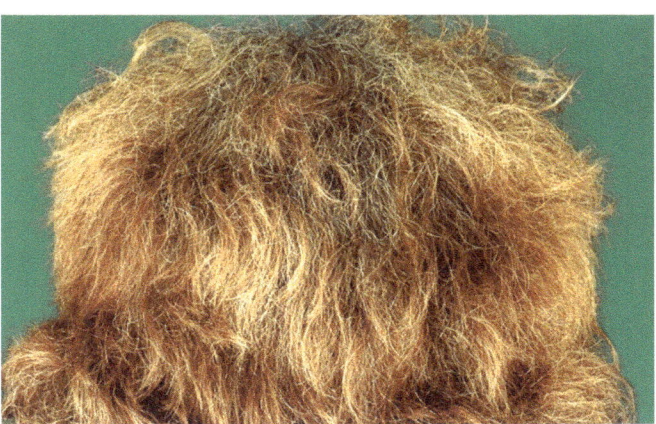

Fig. 12.6.1: Pili trianguli et canaliculi. Dry, frizzy, and disorganized appearance of the hairs even after combing.

PTC—triangular shafts in cross-sections (*pili trianguli*, Figs. 12.6.6A and B) and canal-like longitudinal grooves (*pili canaliculi*, Figs. 12.6.7A and B). Main differentials are pili torti and Woolly hair syndrome. Marie Unna syndrome must be ruled out, if hypotrichosis is present. Treatment is limited. Keeping hair short and avoiding excessive combing can help to prevent hair breakage.

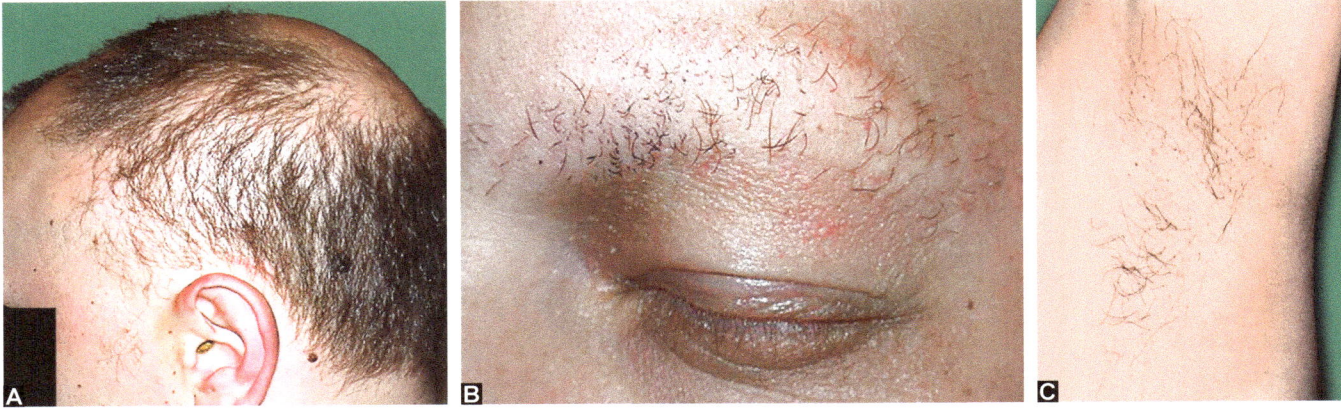

Figs. 12.6.2A to C: Pili trianguli et canaliculi. (A) Unruly and frizzy scalp hairs in a Caucasian young man. Note decreased hair density hypotrichosis in the eyebrow (B) and axillary areas (C).
Source: Dr Hiram Laranjeira Almeida (Junior).

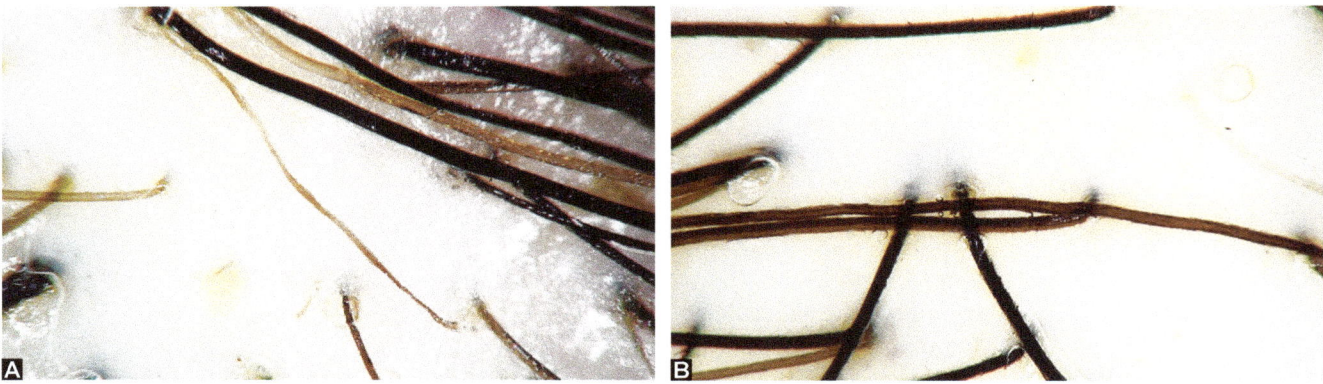

Figs. 12.6.3A and B: Pili trianguli et canaliculi. Dermoscopy shows irregular hair shafts with a longitudinal groove.

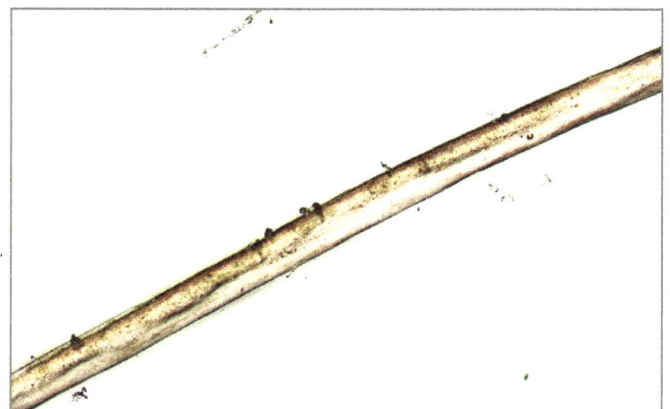

Fig. 12.6.4: Pili trianguli et canaliculi. Canal-like longitudinal grooves on light microscopy (OM, x 200).

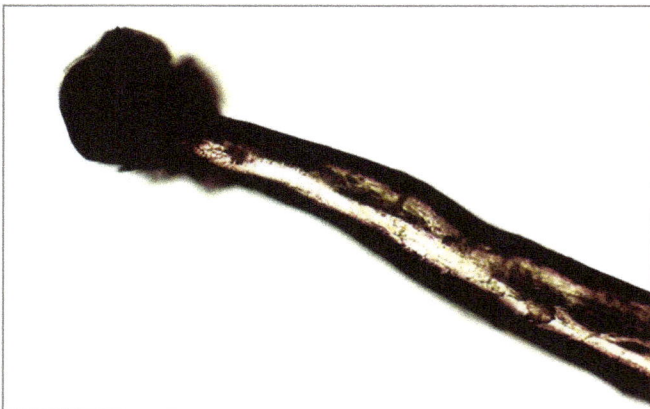

Fig. 12.6.5: Pili trianguli et canaliculi. Anagen hair with a longitudinal groove and flattening appearance on light microscopy (OM, x 400).

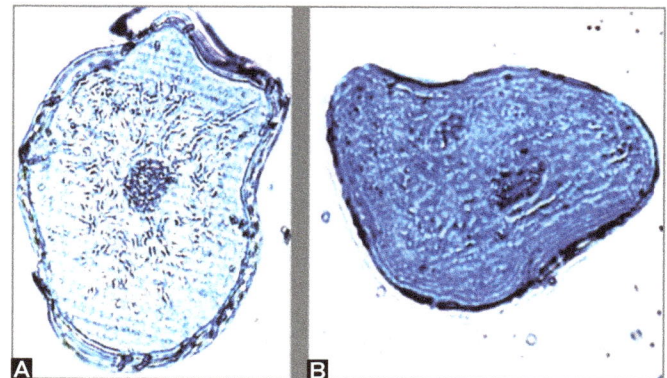

Figs. 12.6.6A and B: Pili trianguli et canaliculi. Transversal sections show triangular-like hair shafts in scalp hairs (A) and body hairs (B). Scanning electron microscopy with methylene blue dye (OM, x 180).
Source: Dr Hiram Laranjeira Almeida (Junior).

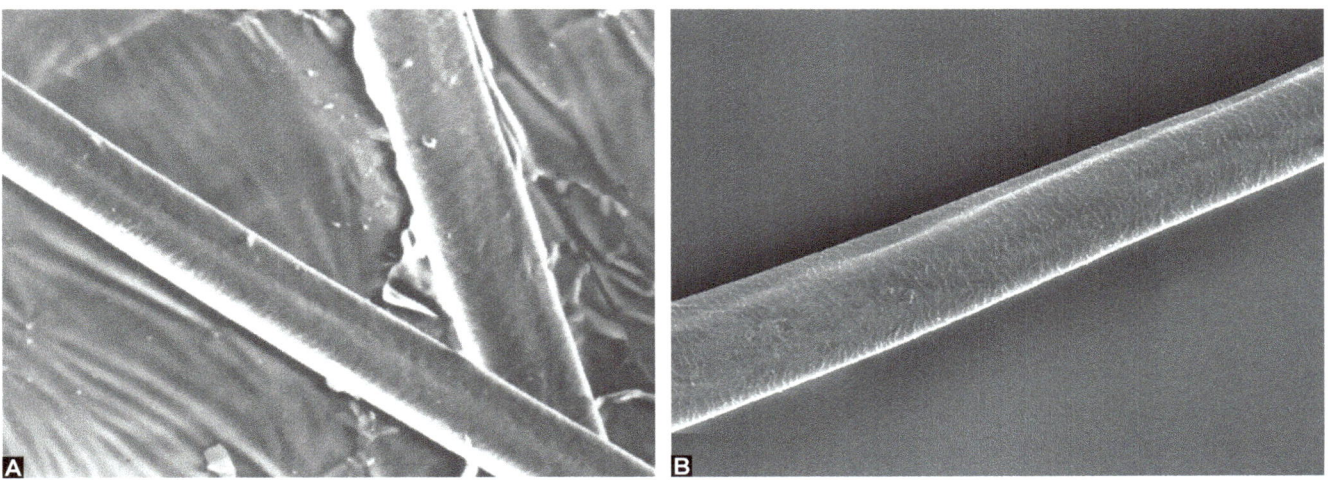

Figs. 12.6.7A and B: Pili trianguli et canaliculi. Longitudinal sections show canal-like grooves on the scalp (A, OM, x 500) and axillary hair shaft (B, OM, x 300) on scanning electron microscopy.
Source: (B) Dr Hiram Laranjeira Almeida (Junior).

Take-Home Message

- Frizzy, dry, and unruly hairs can be observed in pili trianguli et canaliculi, pili torti, and wooly hair syndrome.
- Scanning electron microscopy or cross sections of the hair shafts seen on light microscopy are the best diagnostic tools.
- Dermoscopy can sometimes show triangular shafts with longitudinal grooving.
- Pili trianguli et canaliculi does not cause hair fragility, but excessive hair combing may lead to hair breakage.
- Spontaneous improvement with aging.

SUGGESTED READING

1. Calderon P, Otberg N, Shapiro J. Uncombable hair syndrome. J Am Acad Dermatol. 2009;61(3):512-5.
2. Cunha Filho RR, Almeida Jr HL, Rocha NM, et al. Uncombable hair syndrome (pili trianguli et canaliculi): clinical variation in 12 members of one family. An Bras Dermatol. 2008;83(1):53-5.
3. Dupré A, Bonafé JL, Litoux F, et al. Uncombable hair syndrome. Pili trianguli et canaliculi. Ann Dermatol Venereol. 1978;105(6-7):627-30.
4. Hsu CK, Romano MT, Nanda A, et al. Congenital anonychia and uncombable hair syndrome. Coinheritance of homozygous mutations in RSPO4 and PADI3. J Invest Dermatol. 2017;137(5):1176-9.
5. Jarell AD, Hall MA, Sperling LC. Uncombable hair syndrome. Pediatr Dermatol. 2007;24(4):436-8.
6. Swamy SS, Ravikumar BC, Vinay KN, et al. Uncombable hair syndrome with a wooly hair nevus. Indian J Dermatol Venereol Leprol. 2017;83(1):87-8.

12.7 Trichothiodystrophy

Neusa Yuriko Sakai Valente, Isabella Doche

Trichothiodystrophy (TTD) is a rare inherited condition characterized by sparse and brittle hairs with sulfur (cysteine) deficiency. The signs and symptoms of TTD vary widely (Box 12.7.1). Mild cases may involve few hairs, while severe presentations of the disease can cause delayed development, significant intellectual disability, and recurrent respiratory infections. Death may occur during childhood in severely affected individuals.

The inheritance pattern is autosomal recessive. The hallmark of the disorder is brittle hair and nails. The scalp hairs are thin, sparse, lightly pigmented, and fragile. Cycling shedding of hairs may occur and often there is alopecia (Fig. 12.7.1). Eyebrows and eyelashes may be absent. Nails are hypoplastic. About half patients present associated photosensitivity, but have no apparent predisposition for UV damage or skin cancer.

Dermoscopy is not very useful and can show very subtle features of the disease. Light microscopy can show fine and short hairs with waving appearance and absence of cuticle (Fig. 12.7.2). Trichoschisis, a "clean" transverse fracture of the shaft can also be seen (Fig. 12.7.3). Diagnosis is made with polarizing microscopy, which shows hair shafts with alternating light and dark bands ("tiger tail" pattern), highly suggestive of TTD (Figs. 12.7.4 and 12.7.5). "Tiger tail hairs" can be also observed on confocal laser scanning microscopy (Fig. 12.7.6). Low sulfur and cystine content is characteristic of TTD. Raman test is useful for TTD hairs microspectroscopic analysis. DNA testing in fibroblast culture is diagnostic.

Main differentials include xeroderma pigmentosum, Cockayne syndrome, other hair shaft disorders presented with hair fragility, and congenital ichthyosis. There is no specific treatment for TTD. Fragile hairs need to be manipulated very gently. Systemic symptoms have to be handled by proper specialists.

Box 12.7.1	Syndromes associated with trichothiodystrophy.

- **PIBIDS, SIBIDS, IBIDS, BIDS**, (**P**hotosensitivity, **I**chthyosis, **B**rittle hair, **I**ntelligence impairment, **D**ecreased fertility, **S**hort stature, and osteo**S**clerosis)
- **KID** (**K**eratitis, **I**chthyosis, and **D**eafness)
- **ONMR** (**O**nychotrichodysplasia, **N**eutropenia, and **M**ental **R**etardation)
- **Tay** (ichthyosiform erythroderma and trichothiodystrophy)
- **Pollit** (trichothiodystrophy, trichorrhexis nodosa, and physical and mental retardation)
- **Sabinas** (trichothiodystrophy, mental retardation, and ungual dysplasia)

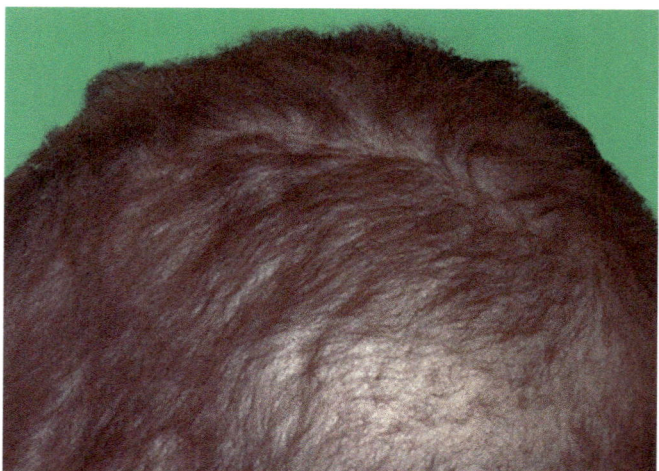

Fig. 12.7.1: Trichothiodystrophy. Child with thin, brightless, fragile, and short hairs forming an alopecic patch in the occipital scalp area.

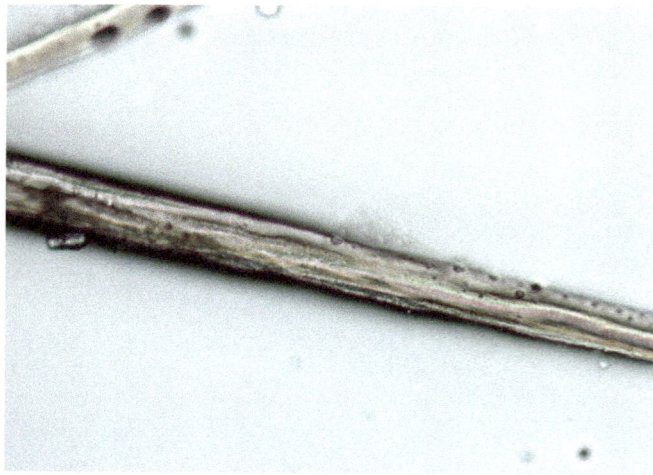

Fig. 12.7.2: Trichothiodystrophy. Slightly wavy and undulating contour of the hair shaft with a nonhomogeneous appearance (resembling grain of sands within the hair shaft) on light microscopy (OM, x 200).

Hair Shaft Disorders

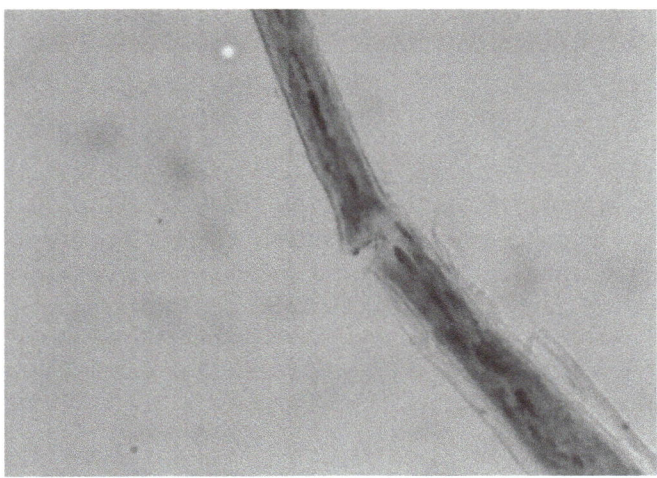

Fig. 12.7.3: Trichothiodystrophy. Trichoschisis ("clean" transverse fracture) of the hair shaft on light microscopy. Differently from trichorrhexis nodosa, no frayed fibers can be noted (OM, x 200).

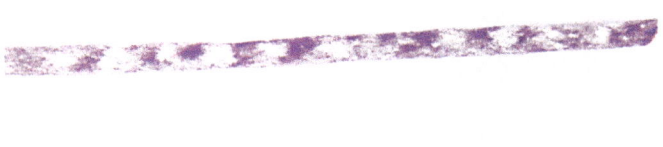

Fig. 12.7.4: Trichothiodystrophy. "Tiger tail" hairs on polarized light microscopy. Note alternate dark and light bands (OM, x100).

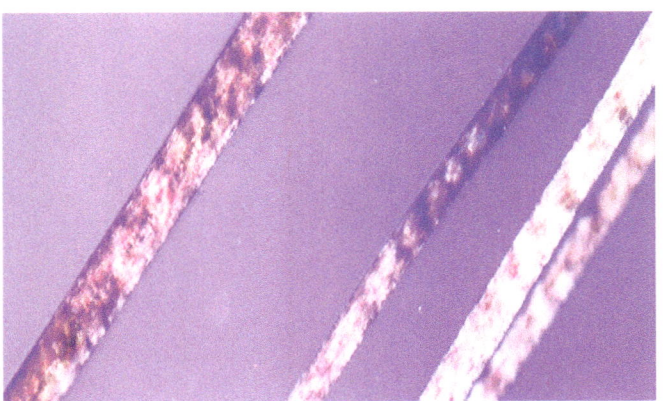

Fig. 12.7.5: Trichothiodystrophy. "Tiger tail" hairs on polarized light microscopy (OM, x 100).

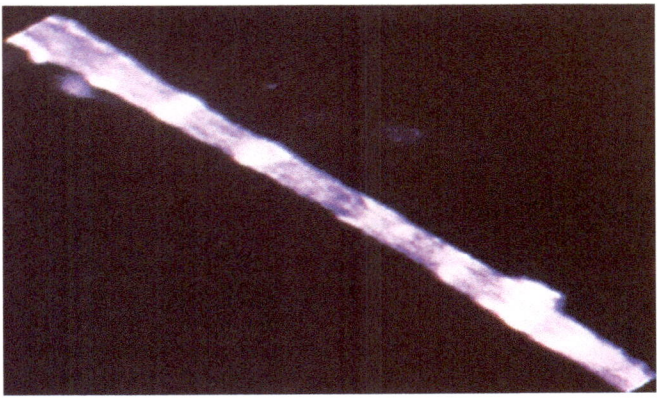

Fig. 12.7.6: Trichothiodystrophy. "Tiger tail" hairs on confocal laser scanning microscopy/emission of coherent and polarized light (OM, x 200).

Take-Home Message
- Short, fragile, and brittle hairs.
- Associated syndromes usually present.
- Polarized light microscopy can show "tiger tail" appearance hairs, highly suggestive of TTD.

SUGGESTED READING

1. Cheng AS, Bayliss SJ. The genetics of hair shaft disorders. J Am Acad Dermatol. 2008;59(1):1-22.
2. Hashimoto S, Egly JM. Trichothiodystrophy view from the molecular basis of DNA repair/transcription factor TFIIH. Human Mol Genet. 2009;18(R2):R224-30.
3. Itin PH, Sarasin A, Pittelkow MR. Trichothiodystrophy: update on the sulfur-deficient brittle hair syndromes. J Am Acad Dermatol. 2001;44(6):891-920.
4. Kraemer KH, Patronas NJ, Schiffmann R, et al. Xeroderma pigmentosum, Trichothiodystrophy and Cockayne syndrome: a complex genotype-phenotype relationship. Neuroscience. 2007;145(4):1388-96.
5. Schlücker S, Liang C, Strehle KR, et al. Conformational differences in protein disulfide linkages between normal hair and hair from subjects with trichothiodystrophy: a quantitative analysis by Raman microspectroscopy. Biopolymers. 2006;82(6):615-22.
6. Sung P, Bailly V, Weber C, et al. Xeroderma pigmentosum group D gene encodes a DNA helicase. Nature. 1993;365(6449):852-5.

12.8 Silvery Hair Syndromes

Neusa Yuriko Sakai Valente, Isabella Doche

Silvery hair is a common presentation of a rare group of autosomal recessive disorders caused by a genetic disturbance in the transference of melanosomes from melanocytes to keratinocytes. This group includes Chediak-Higashi syndrome, Griscelli-Prunieras syndrome, and Elejalde disease, now considered a Griscelli-Prunieras syndrome type 1.

Affected children present with a silvery hair color and skin hypopigmentation (Figs. 12.8.1 and 12.8.2). In most cases, immune, hematological, and nervous systems are also affected (Table 12.8.1). Dermoscopy is not very useful. However, light microscopy with high magnification and polarized light microscopy can help to distinguish the silvery hair syndromes (Figs. 12.8.3 to 12.8.7).

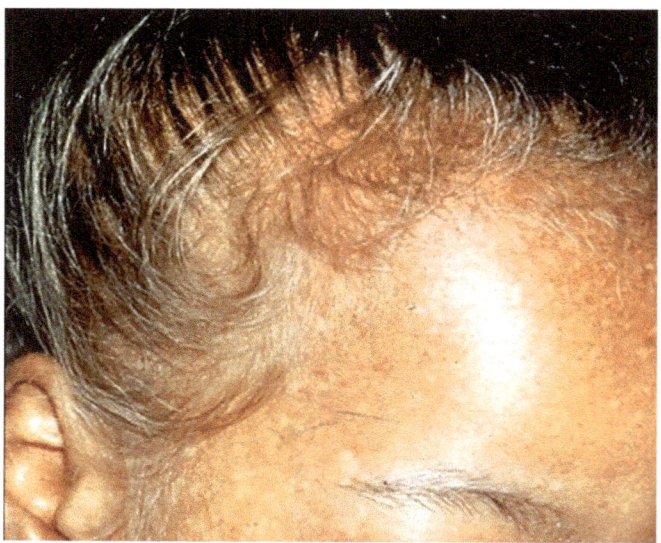

Fig. 12.8.1: Chediak-Higashi syndrome. Girl with brown-gray hairs and hypopigmented lesions on the face. Note tanned skin after sunbathing.

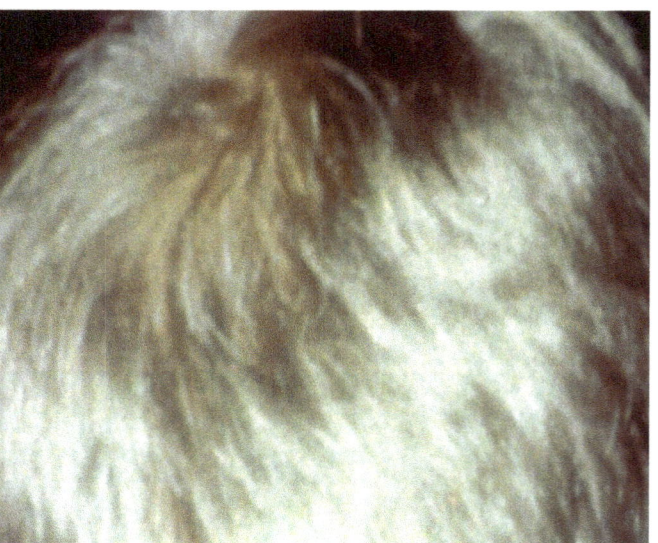

Fig. 12.8.2: Griscelli-Prunieras syndrome. Silvery blond hair in a 4-year-old child.

Table 12.8.1: Main differences in silvery hair syndromes.

Disease/typical features	Chediak-Higashi syndrome	Griscelli-Prunieras syndrome	Elejalde disease
Genetic mutation	LYST	MYO5A	MYO5A
Clinical lesions	Skin and nail hypopigmented lesions, immunodeficiency, and neural deterioration usually fatal at early ages	Skin and nail hypopigmented lesions, variable immunodeficiency, neurological impairment, occasional retinal pigmentation, usually fatal in the first years. Type 1 or Elejalde disease, type 2 (immunodeficiency), type 3 (restricted to skin and hair, good prognosis)	GPS type 1 (skin and nail hypopigmented lesions, severe neurological impairment with no immunodeficiency), fatal
Light microscopy	Small clumps of melanin regularly distributed inside the hair shaft	Small and large irregular clumps of melanin close to the medulla area	Small and large irregular clumps of melanin close to the medulla area
Polarized light microscopy	Polychromatic birefringence	Monochromatic birefringence	Monochromatic birefringence

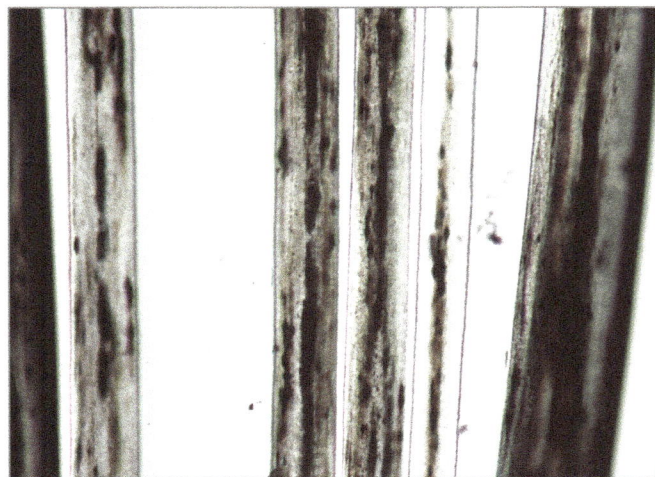

Fig. 12.8.3: Elejalde disease (Griscelli-Prunieras syndrome type 1). Larger melanin granules irregularly distributed on the medullar zone can be noted in all hair shafts. Light microscopy (OM, x 200).

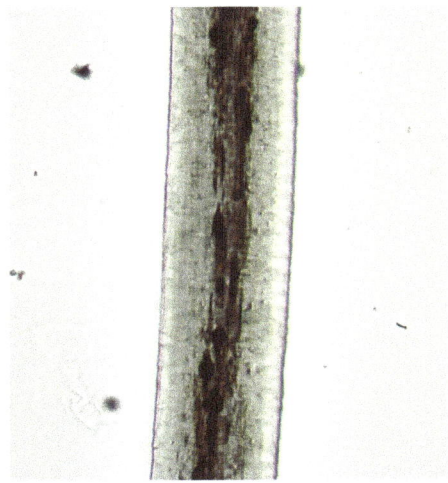

Fig. 12.8.4: Griscelli-Prunieras syndrome type 2. Larger melanin granules near the medullar zone (similar to type 1). Light microscopy (OM, x 400).

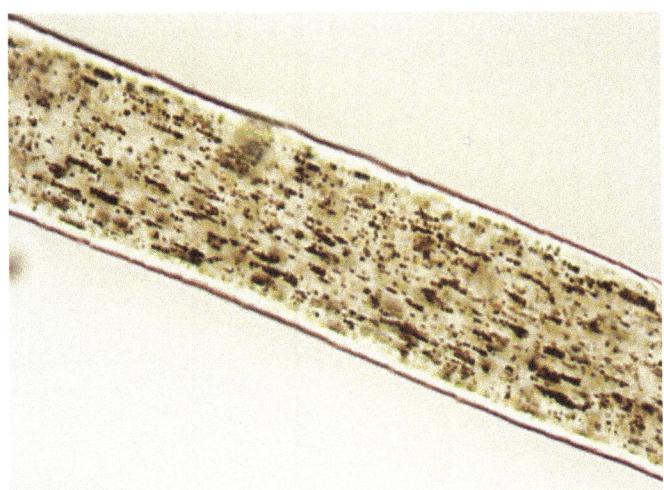

Fig. 12.8.5: Chediak-Higashi syndrome. Larger melanin granules diffusely distributed inside the hair shaft. These granules are smaller than those found in Griscelli-Prunieras syndrome. Light microscopy (OM, x 400).

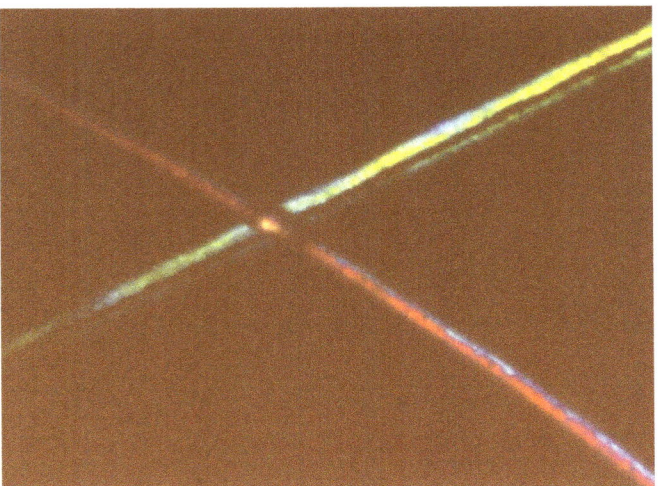

Fig. 12.8.6: Chediak-Higashi syndrome. Polarized light microscopy shows polychromatic birefringence of the hairs (OM, x100).

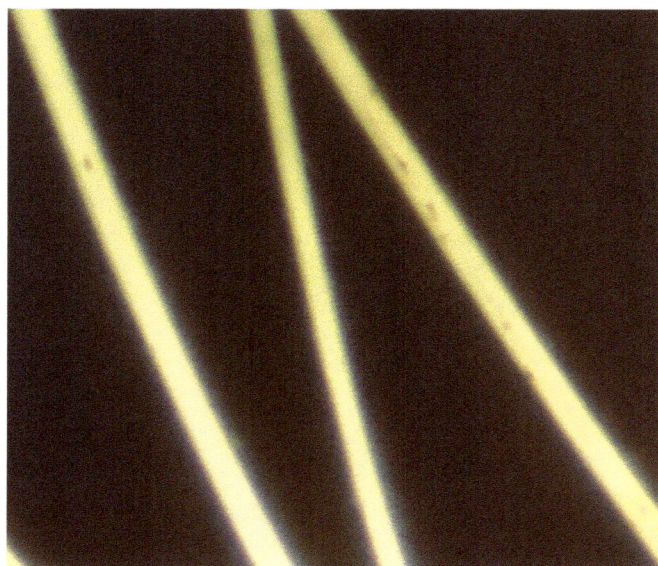

Fig. 12.8.7: Griscelli-Prunieras syndrome. Polarized light microscopy shows hairs with whitish birefringence (OM, × 100).

Take-Home Message

- Silvery hair syndromes include Chediak-Higashi, Griscelli-Prunieras, and Elejalde disease.
- Silver hair, partial albinism (hair and skin), variable immunodeficiency, and neural impairment lead frequently to death.
- Dermoscopy is not very useful. Light microscopy with high magnifications shows abnormal deposition of larger melanin granules or clumps inside the hair.

SUGGESTED READING

1. Cahali JB, Fernandez SA, Oliveira ZN, et al. Elejalde syndrome: report of a case and review of the literature. Pediatr Dermatol. 2004;21(4):479-82.
2. Kaplan J, De Domenico I, Ward DM. Chediak-Higashi syndrome. Current Opin Hematol. 2008;15(1):22-9.
3. Najmuddin F, Rai R, Lahiri K, et al. Elejalde syndrome: the silvery hair syndrome. SOJ Genet Sci. 2015;2(1):1-2.
4. Shanehsaz SM, Rezazadeh A, Dandashli A. Elejalde syndrome: case presentation. J Pakistan Assoc Dermatol. 2014;24(4):351-4.
5. Valente NYS, Machado MCR, Boggio P, et al. Polarized light microscopy of hair shafts aids in the differential diagnosis of Chédiak-Higashi and Griscelli-Prunieras syndromes. Clinics. 2006;61(4):327-32.
6. Yamada T, Chen-Yoshikawa TF, Oh S, et al. Living-donor lung transplantation after bone marrow transplantation for Chediak-Higashi syndrome. Ann Thorac Surg. 2017;103(3):e281-3.

12.9 Trichorrhexis Nodosa

Patricia Damasco, Giselle Martins, Isabella Doche

Trichorrhexis nodosa (TN) is a disorder of the hair shaft characterized by nodes along the hair shaft and hair breakage. The hair appears lusterless and dry, and the patients may complain of increased hair breakage. The underlying pathogenic mechanism is a cuticular cell disruption, which allows the underlying cortical fibers to separate and fray. As a result, weak points called nodes lead to partial or complete hair breakage.

TN may be congenital or acquired and can be associated with many syndromes (Table 12.9.1). Acquired TN is the most common hair shaft disorder and occurs as a response to physical or chemical trauma. Several external factors are described including application of heat, repeated ultraviolet radiation, excessive hair combing, traction-producing hair styles, and chemical hair procedures, as bleaching, perming, and dyeing of hair. African descent patients are more prone to develop acquired TN due to structural differences in the hair fiber and the combination of various hair care and styling practices that contribute to the hair damage. It may also be related to malnutrition or endocrinopathy, especially iron deficiency and hypothyroidism.

Congenital TN becomes apparent at a young age and is the most common congenital defect of the hair shaft. TN may be part of many syndromes with variable clinical symptoms, such as mental retardation, motor and growth defects, seizures, infertility, nails and skin lesions, and photosensitivity. A family history of a similar condition may indicate a congenital cause for TN. Fractured hairs are found mainly in the scalp, but they also may involve body or public hairs.

Clinically, affected hairs contain multiple and small white nodes at irregular intervals throughout the length of the shaft. Dermoscopy shows white areas along the hair shaft (Fig. 12.9.1). Sometimes these areas may mimic hair casts on low magnifications (Fig. 12.9.2). High magnifications can identify the frayed cortical layers and hair fracturing into brush-like ends at the distal end of the hair shaft (Figs. 12.9.3 to 12.9.5). Acquired TN usually affects the distal shaft, but proximal TN can be seen as a consequence of many scratching processes affecting the scalp (Fig. 12.9.6).

Managing TN includes cutting hair tips and avoiding physical and chemical trauma to the hair shafts. The use of moisturizers and heat-protection products can help to decrease hair damage.

Table 12.9.1: Conditions associated with trichorrhexis nodosa.

- Trichothiodystrophy
- Tay syndrome
- Bazex-Dupré-Christol syndrome
- Laron syndrome
- Kabuki syndrome
- Menkes disease
- Pollitt syndrome
- Ectodermal dysplasia
- Ichthyosis
- Monilethrix-like congenital hypotrichosis
- Biotin and zinc deficiency
- Iron deficiency
- Argininosuccinic aciduria
- Hypothyroidism
- External factors (physical and chemical trauma)
- Conditions with scalp pruritus

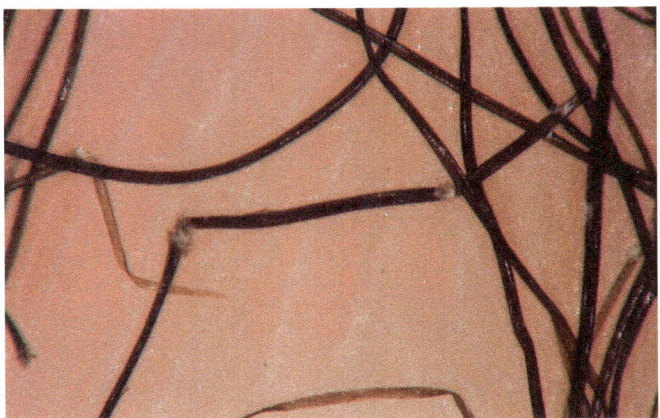

Fig. 12.9.1: Trichorrhexis nodosa. Multiple white nodes along the hair shaft in an African descent patient.

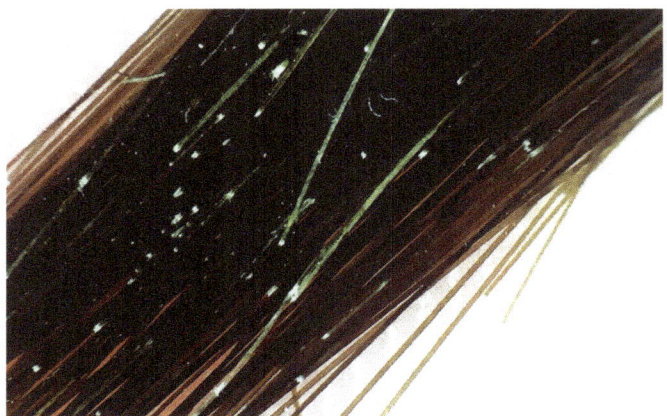

Fig. 12.9.2: Trichorrhexis nodosa. On lower magnifications, multiple white areas along the hair shafts can mimic hair casts.

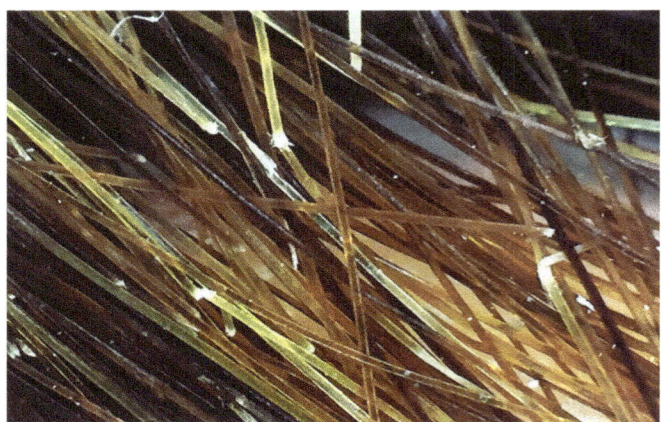

Fig. 12.9.3: Trichorrhexis nodosa. Multiple white nodes along the hair shafts. The hair shafts have the tendency to break, leaving brush-like ends.

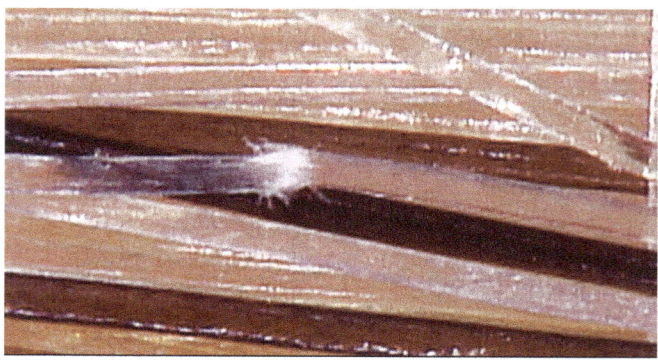

Fig. 12.9.4: Trichorrhexis nodosa. Brush-like hair fracturing. The image was obtained with dry trichoscopy, in a higher magnification, to better visualize the frayed fibers.

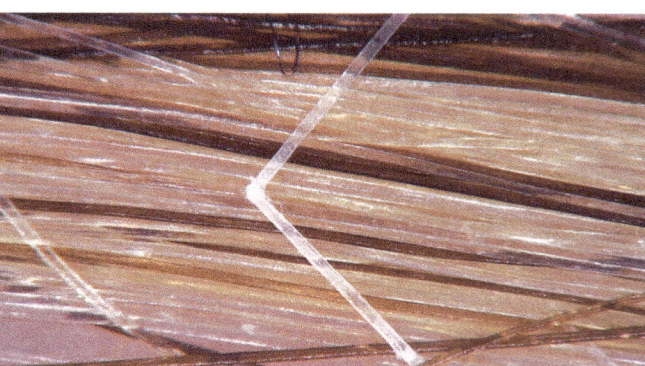

Fig. 12.9.5: Trichorrhexis nodosa. Brush-like hair fracturing developed after hairstyling procedure. At the level of the nodular thickening, the hair bends with a rounded edge.

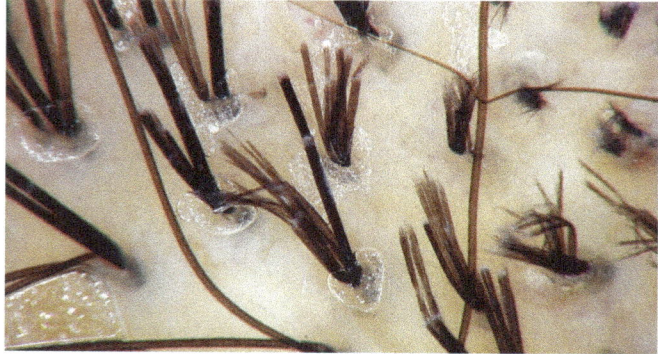

Fig. 12.9.6: Trichorrhexis nodosa. Proximal (trichoteiromania) hair breakage as a result of scalp scratching.

Take-Home Message

- The most common hair shaft disorder.
- Acquired and congenital causes.
- Hair breakage and white small nodes along the hair shafts.
- On low magnifications, dermoscopy shows small white nodes, mimicking hair casts.
- High magnifications can show frayed corticals fibers and hair breakage brush-like endings.

SUGGESTED READING

1. Abdel-Salam GM, Afifi HH, Eid MM, et al. Ectodermal abnormalities in patients with Kabuki syndrome. Pediatr Dermatol. 2011;28(5):507-11.

2. Bartels NG, Blume-Peytavi U. Hair loss in children. In: Blume-Peytavi U, Tosti A, Whiting D, Trueb R (Eds). Hair Growth and Disorders. Leipzig: Springer; 2008. pp. 293-4.
3. Colomb D, Ducros B, Boussuge N. Bazex, Dupré and Christol syndrome. Apropos of a case with prolymphocytic leukemia. Ann Dermatol Venereol. 1989;116(5):381-7.
4. Fichtel JC, Richards JA, Davis LS. Trichorrhexis nodosa secondary to argininosuccinic aciduria. Pediatr Dermatol. 2007;24(1):25-7.
5. Haskin A, Kwatra SG, Aquh C. Breaking the cycle of hair breakage: pearls for the management of acquired trichorrhexis nodosa. J Dermatolog Treat. 2017;28(4):322-6.
6. Lawson CN, Hollinger J, Sethi S, et al. Updates in the understanding and treatments of skin and hair disorders in women of color. Int J Womens Dermatol. 2015;1(2):59-75.
7. Lindsey SF, Tosti A. Ethnic hair disorders. Curr Probl Dematol. 2015;47:139-49.
8. Lurie R, Ben-Amitai D, Laron Z. Laron syndrome (primary growth hormone insensitivity): a unique model to explore the effect of insulin-like growth factor 1 deficiency in human hair. Dermatology. 2004:208(4):314-8.
9. Lurie R, Hodak E, Ginzburg A, et al. Trichorrhexis nodosa: a manifestation of hypothyroidism. Cutis. 1996;57(5):358-9.
10. Martin AM, Sugathan P. Localised acquired trichorrhexis nodosa of the scalp hair induced by a specific comb and combing habit: a report of three cases. Int J Trichol. 2011;3(1):34-7.
11. Mirmirani P. Ceramic flat irons: improper use leading to acquired trichorrhexis nodosa. J Am Acad Dermatol. 2010;62(1):145-7.
12. Ogunbiyi A, Ogun O, Enechukwu N. Recurrent hair loss resulting from a generalized proximal trichorrhexis nodosa in a Nigerian female. Int J Trichology. 2014;6(2):83-4.
13. Pollitt RJ, Jenner FA, Davies M. Sibs with mental and physical retardation and trichorrhexis nodosa with abnormal amino acid composition of the hair. Arch Dis Child. 1968;43(228):211-6.
14. Rakowska A, Górska R, Rudnicka L, et al. Trichoscopic hair evaluation in patients with ectodermal dysplasia. J Pediatr. 2015;167(1):193-5.
15. Rodney IJ, Onwudiwe OC, Callender VD, et al. Hair and scalp disorders in ethnic populations. J Drugs Dermatol. 2013;12(4):420-7.

12.10 Bubble Hair

Patricia Damasco, Giselle Martins, Isabella Doche

Bubble hair is an acquired hair shaft abnormality characterized by cavity or bubble areas inside the hair shaft due to the exposure of wet hair to very high temperature from flat irons and blow dryers. When the hair is wet, the hair fiber becomes filled with water. The use of high heat causes sudden evaporation of the water and distension of the hair shaft. These damaged hairs are weak and brittle as the bubbles destroy the integrity of the fiber. Fragile and chemical-treated hairs are more susceptible to develop bubble hairs.

Dermoscopy shows white oval spaces similar to a spongy "Swiss-cheese" that correspond to air-filled spaces of different sizes within the hair shafts (Figs. 12.10.1 and 12.10.2).

Bubble hair can be prevented by avoiding excessive heat and chemicals on the hair. Damaged hairs must be cutted off.

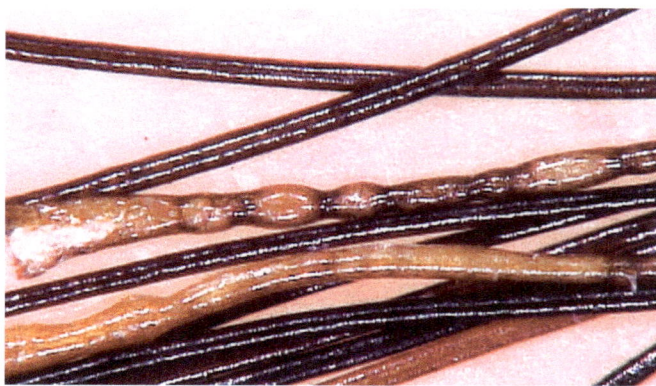

Fig. 12.10.2: Bubble hairs. Note the spongy appearance as a consequence of air cavities.

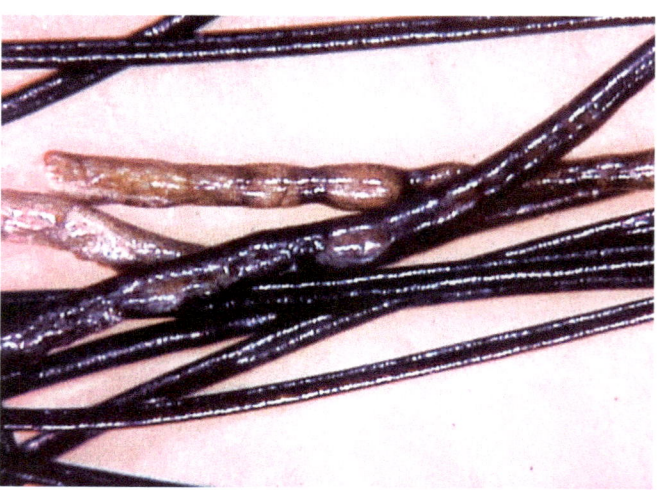

Fig. 12.10.1: Bubble hairs. White enlarged tips, with irregular air cavities distributed along the hair shaft similar to a spongy "Swiss cheese appearance." Note that the damage does not affect all the hairs.

Take-Home Message
- Cavities of air inside the hair shaft formed by sudden air evaporation after very high temperature.
- Dermoscopy shows multiple and irregular white spaces inside the hair shaft, with a spongy "Swiss-cheese" appearance.

SUGGESTED READING

1. Elston DM, Bergfeld WF, Whiting DA, et al. Bubble hair. J Cutan Pathol. 1992;19(5):439-44.
2. Mehregan D, Sayoc L, Ramos DR, et al. Bubble hair, a report of two cases. Int J Dermatol. 2006;45(11):1319-20.
3. Savitha AS, Sacchidanand S, Revathy TN. Bubble hair and other acquired hair shaft anomalies due to hot ironing on wet hair. Int J Trichol. 2011;3(2):118-20.
4. Wallace MP, de Berker DA. Hair Diagnosis and signs: the use of dermatoscopy. Clin Exp Dermatol. 2010;35(1):41-6.

12.11 Trichoptilosis

Patricia Damasco, Giselle Martins, Isabella Doche

Trichoptilosis is an acquired hair shaft disorder characterized by a longitudinal splitting of the hair shaft due to cumulative effects of chemical and physical trauma. The distal end of the hair shaft splits longitudinally into two or more divisions.

Trichoptilosis can be found in normal and weathered hair. African descent patients are more commonly affected as the hair is more fragile and often exposed to various hair care and styling practices. It can be associated with other signs of hair weathering like trichorrhexis nodosa, trichonodosis, and bubble hair, and in congenital brittle hair syndromes, such as trichothiodystrophy, trichorrhexis invaginata, monilethrix, and pili torti.

Dermoscopy shows a longitudinal splitting of the hair shaft with two or several divisions (Figs. 12.11.1 and 12.11.2). Central trichoptilosis is rare and mostly affects African descent patients (Fig. 12.11.3).

It can be prevented and treated by careful handling of the hair, especially when washing and combing, and by cutting off the damaged hair.

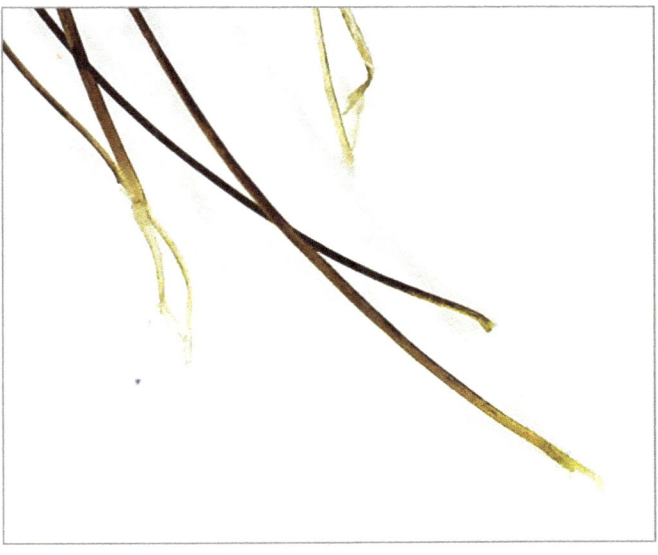

Fig. 12.11.2: Trichoptilosis. Several splittings with a paintbrush appearance of the distal tips. Note the lightened shafts by chemical treatment.

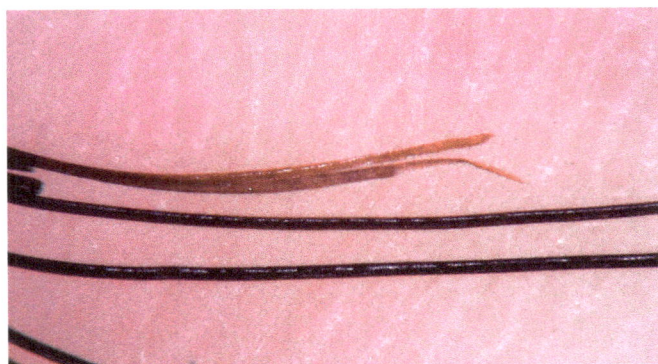

Fig. 12.11.1: Trichoptilosis. Longitudinal splitting of the distal hair shaft in a Caucasian patient. Bifurcated hairs are usually not surrounded by the cuticle.

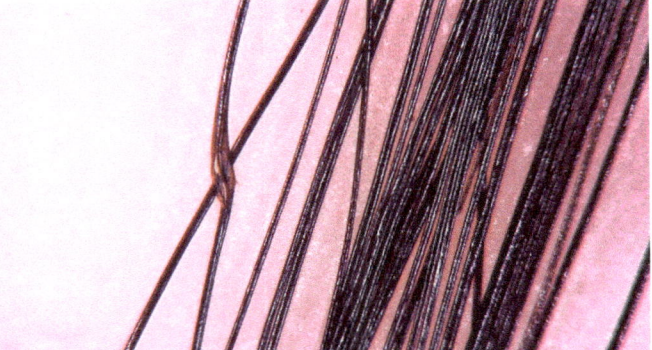

Fig. 12.11.3: Central trichoptilosis. The presence of fissure in the central hair shaft, not reaching the proximal and distal endings in an African descent female patient.

> **Take-Home Message**
> - Trichoptilosis is an acquired hair shaft abnormality, characterized by a longitudinal splitting of the hair tip.
> - It is caused by cumulative physical and chemical trauma to the hair shaft.
> - Broken tips can show a paintbrush appearance on dermoscopy.
> - Central trichoptilosis is rare and affects mostly African descent patients.

SUGGESTED READING

1. Im M, Kye KC, Seo YJ, et al. Central trichoptilosis with onycholysis. Int J Dermatol. 2006;45(10):1187-8.
2. Lee HW, Choi JH, Moon KC, et al. Trichoptilosis developing after first exposure to hair gels. Pediatr Dermatol. 2008;25(1):139-40.
3. Rudnicka L, Rakowska A, Kerzeja M, et al. Hair shafts in trichoscopy: clues for diagnosis of hair and scalp diseases. Dermatol Clin. 2013;31(4):695-708.
4. Savitha A, Sacchidanand S, Revathy T. Bubble hair and other acquired hair shaft anomalies due to hot ironing on wet hair. Int J Trichology. 2011;3(2):118-20.

12.12 Trichonodosis

Patricia Damasco, Giselle Martins, Isabella Doche

Trichonodosis is an acquired hair shaft disorder characterized by knots usually on the distal hair shaft. This can be spontaneous or secondary to mechanical factors like vigorous scratching or combing the hair.

Trichonodosis mostly affects long and kinky hairs, as they tend to recoil into spirals when gently pulled and released. This recoiling may lead to an entanglement, which can form a knot. Friction may also produce tangling and knotting. In this case, the most frequently regions involved are the pubic and thigh, since the curviliness of the hairs in those areas predisposes them to knotting.

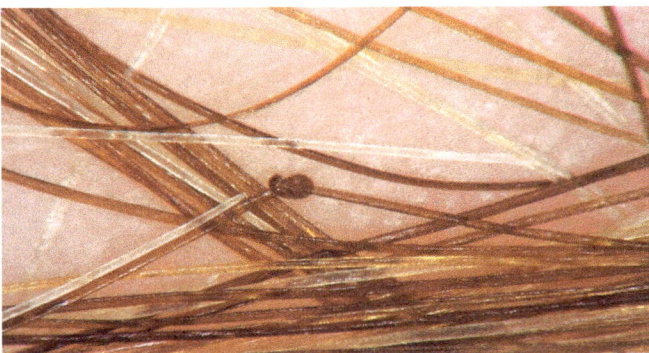

Fig. 12.12.1: Trichonodosis. A single knot in the hair shaft can be seen in a patient with a long hair.

Dermoscopy may show single or double knots in the hair shaft (Fig. 12.12.1). The knots may mimic nits on low magnifications, a sign of lice infection. Differently from nits, the nodules in trichonodosis are located on the distal hair shafts.

Treatment for the acquired type is proper hair care practices.

Take-Home Message

- Trichonodosis is an acquired condition in which single or double knots are formed in the hair shaft.
- Usually, it affects people with long hair, African descent patients, and body hairs exposed to constant friction.
- Usually, it is an accidental finding without clinical significance.
- Dermoscopy may mimic nits on low magnifications.

SUGGESTED READING

1. McCarthy L. Diagnosis and treatment of diseases of the hair. St Louis: CV Mosby Co; 1940. pp. 103-4.
2. Kumaresan M, Deepa MS. Trichonodosis. Int J Trichology. 2014;6(1):31-3.
3. Rudnicka L, Rakowska A, Kurzeja M, et al. Hair shafts in trichoscopy: clues for diagnosis of hair and scalp diseases. Dermatol Clin. 2013;31(4):695-708.

CHAPTER 13

Eyebrows and Eyelashes Disorders

Patricia Damasco, Giselle Martins, Isabella Doche

INTRODUCTION

Dermoscopy of the eyelashes and the eyebrows area is scarce in the literature. Eyebrow hair follicles share the same basic structure as other hair follicles, except that they have a shorter anagen (growing) phase. Although eyelid skin also harbors some vellus hair follicles, eyelash hair follicles are terminal hairs and, as such, produce fully pigmented and medullated hair shafts. Eyelashes tend to be the darkest hairs in the human body, and are the last ones to undergo greying. Eyelash follicles are free of arrector pili muscle and, due to a shorter hair cycle, eyelash fibers are much shorter than those on the scalp. Regarding ethnic differences, the Asian female's eyelashes show a reduced curl angle, an increased hair shaft diameter, and more cuticle layers compared to eyelashes from Caucasian females.

Partial or complete madarosis, loss of eyebrows and eyelashes, can occur in various diseases, ranging from dermatological disorders to systemic diseases (Table 13.1). Besides aesthetic reasons, the absence of eyelashes and eyebrows can be very concerning as it may be a sign of a scarring or nonscarring process affecting the hair follicles.

It is important to remember that cosmetics and camouflage products used on the eyebrows and eyelashes can complicate the examination and lead to a misdiagnosis. The exact diagnosis is essential for the correct management of the condition.

COSMETICS AND CAMOUFLAGE PRODUCTS

Cosmetics, tattoos, and other camouflage products such as powders and mascara are frequently used to darken, thicken, and lengthen existing eyelashes and eyebrows. Dermoscopy of tattoo areas shows large blue-gray dots, pigment discoloration, and blotched areas (Figs. 13.1 and 13.2). Makeup can show irregular residues of dark pigment on the skin, which may be similar to dirty and black dots (Figs. 13.3 to 13.5).

SEBORRHEIC DERMATITIS

Seborrheic dermatitis may induce partial madarosis due to persistent inflammation and scratching. Perifollicular and interfollicular yellow scales with hair casts are usually present (Fig. 13.6). Mild erythema can also be seen (Figs. 13.7A to C).

ALOPECIA AREATA

Alopecia areata may affect the eyebrows or eyelashes as an isolated finding, or be associated with patchy scalp alopecia or alopecia universalis. Dermoscopy shows the same features as in the scalp like black dots, yellow dots, broken hairs, exclamation mark hairs, and circle hairs (Figs. 13.8 and 13.9).

TRICHOTILLOMANIA

Trichotillomania is a result of the repetitive pulling of the hairs. Isolated eyebrow and eyelash lesions can occur (Fig. 13.10A). Dermoscopy shows black dots, broken hairs of different lengths, and dystrophic hairs (Fig. 13.10B).

Eyebrows and Eyelashes Disorders

Table 13.1: Diseases associated with madarosis.

Skin disease	Alopecia areata Psoriasis Seborrheic dermatitis/blepharitis Scleroderma Epidermolysis bullosa Ichthyosis Vogt-Koyanagi-Harada syndrome Telogen effluvium Anagen effluvium Stevens-Johnson syndrome Folliculitis decalvans Dissecting folliculitis Frontal fibrosing alopecia Acquired hair shaft disorders
Infectious disease	Infective blepharitis (e.g. staphylococcal blepharitis) Herpes zoster Herpes simplex Leprosy Secondary and tertiary syphilis Fungal infection HIV infection Paracoccidioidomycosis Lupus vulgaris
Endocrine disease	Hyperthyroidism Hypothyroidism Hyperparathyroidism Hypoparathyroidism Hypopituitarism Pituitary necrosis syndrome
Drugs	Cholinergics (Miotics) Anticoagulants Antithyroid drugs (e.g. thiouracil) Antimetabolites (e.g. doxorubicin, cyclophosphamide, methotrexate, colchicine) Propranolol Valproic acid Barbiturates Vitamin A
Trauma	Radiation Post eyelid surgery Physical or chemical trauma Trichotillomania
Neoplasm	Basal cell carcinoma Squamous cell carcinoma Sebaceous gland carcinoma Cutaneous T cell lymphoma Malignant melanoma Follicular mucinosis
Congenital	Anhidrotic ectodermal dysplasia Oculomandibular dysostosis Oculovertebral dysplasia Progeria Atrichia congenital Ehlers-Danlos syndrome Lid coloboma Rothmund-Thomson syndrome Hereditary hypotrichosis Congenital hair shaft disorders Erythrokeratodermia variabilis Atrichia with popular lesions Vitamin D-dependent rickets type IIA Keratitis-ichthyosis-deafness (KID) syndrome

FRONTAL FIBROSING ALOPECIA

Frontal fibrosing alopecia is a scarring hair loss that results in the loss of frontotemporal hairline and eyebrow alopecia (Figs. 13.11 and 13.12). In some cases, the eyebrow involvement can precede scalp lesions. Dermoscopy of follicular yellow and red dots, mild perifollicular scale, hair casts, pili torti and broken hairs (Figs. 13.13 and 13.14). Eyebrow tattoo can help to accentuate follicular openings (Fig. 13.15).

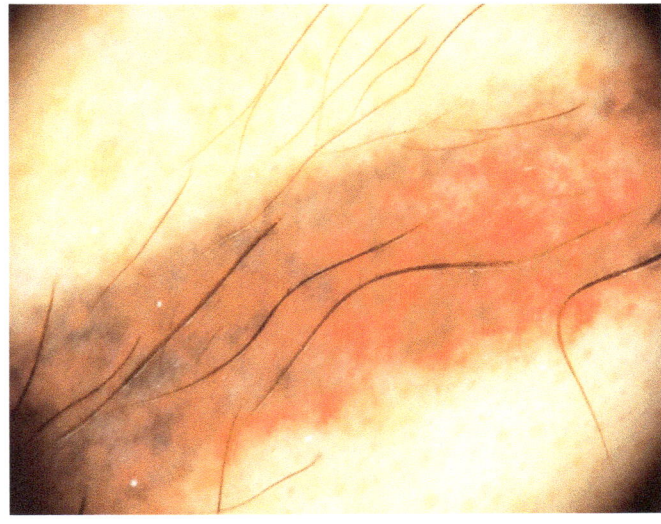

Fig. 13.1: Eyebrow tattoo. Blue-gray dots, pigment discoloration with blotchy appearance. Bluish coloration can appear over time due to deep insertion of the pigment in the skin.

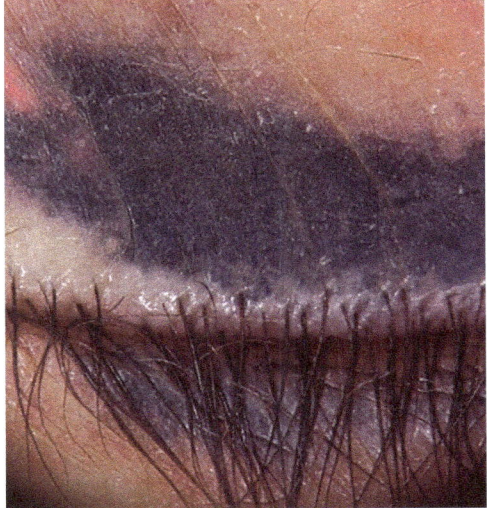

Fig. 13.2: Eyelid tattoo—note the blue-gray discoloration with a blotchy appearance of the tattoo pigment on the upper and lower eyelids.

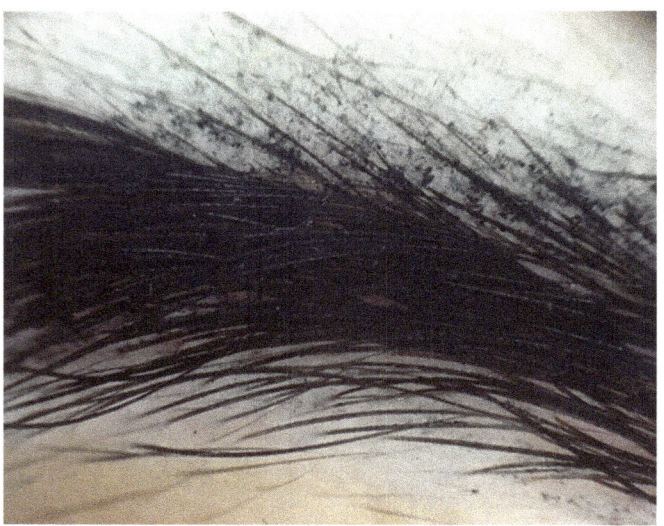

Fig. 13.3: Eyebrow makeup. Irregular residues of pigment makeup on the eyebrow.

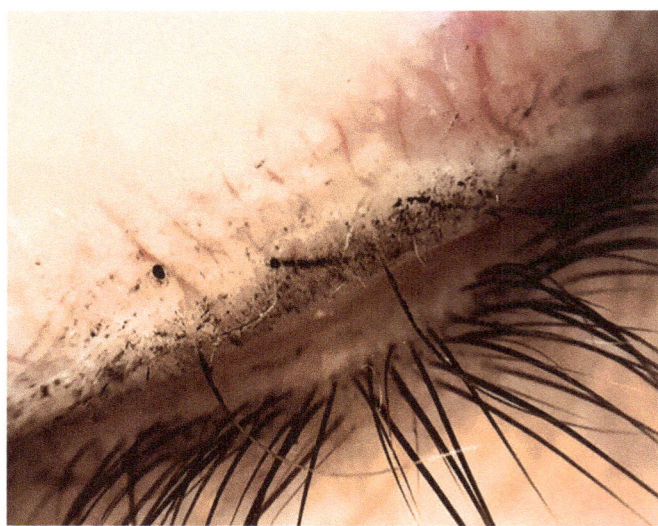

Fig. 13.4: Eyelash makeup. Irregular residues of pigment makeup on the eyelashes.

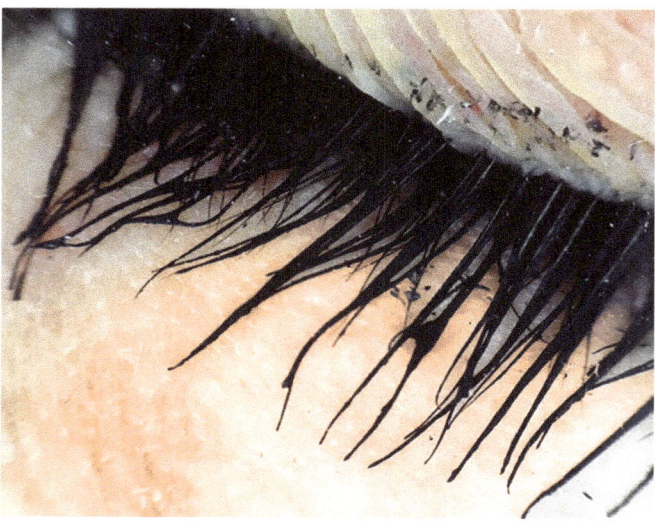

Fig. 13.5: Eyelash makeup. Residues of mascara surrounding the shafts and in the adjacent skin.

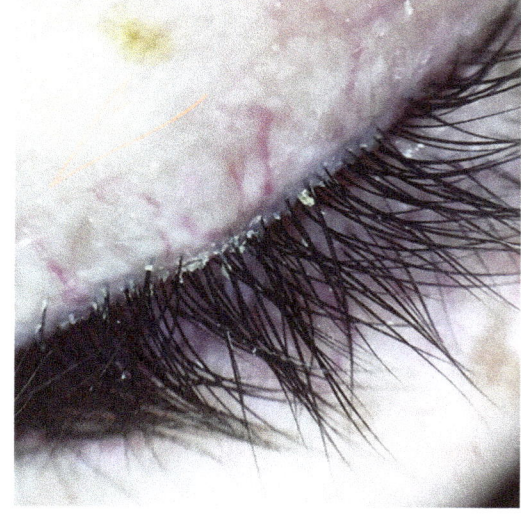

Fig. 13.6: Seborrheic dermatitis of the eyelashes. Note the perifollicular yellowish scales with some hair casts.

DISCOID LUPUS ERYTHEMATOSUS

Discoid lupus may present with scarring alopecia, scales and depigmentation of any hair-bearing site (Fig. 13.16). Dermoscopy shows thick arborizing vessels, loss of pigment, peripilar casts and loss of follicular openings (Figs. 13.17A and B).

MONILETHRIX

Monilethrix is a rare congenital hair shaft disorder characterized by alopecia due to hair fragility and breakage. Usually it is inherited as an autosomal dominant trait with variable penetrance, although rare and severe presentations are related to a recessive

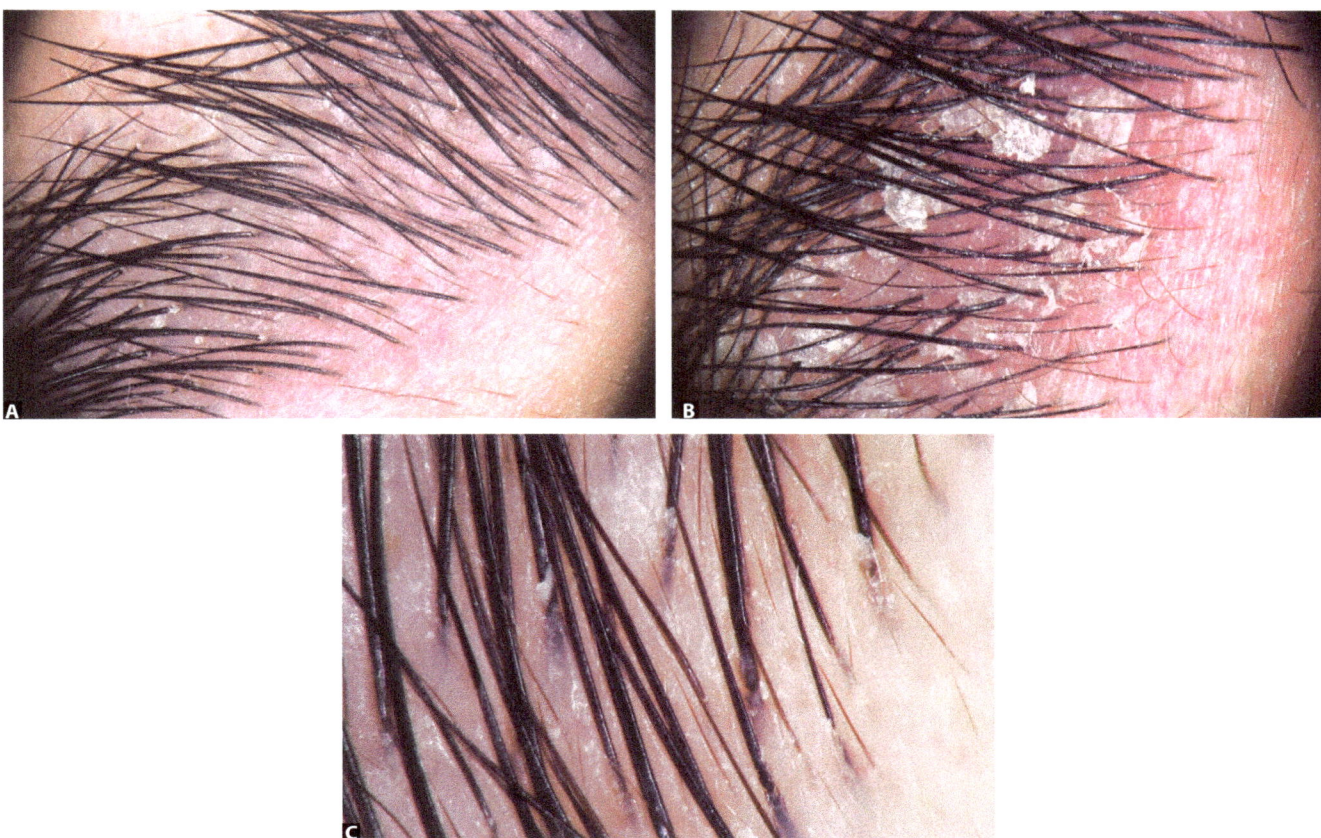

Figs. 13.7A to C: Seborrheic dermatitis of the eyebrow. (A) Scales on a slightly erythematous background. (B) Perifollicular and interfollicular scales on the eyebrow seen in a higher magnification. (C) Note the scales do not completely involve the hair shaft.

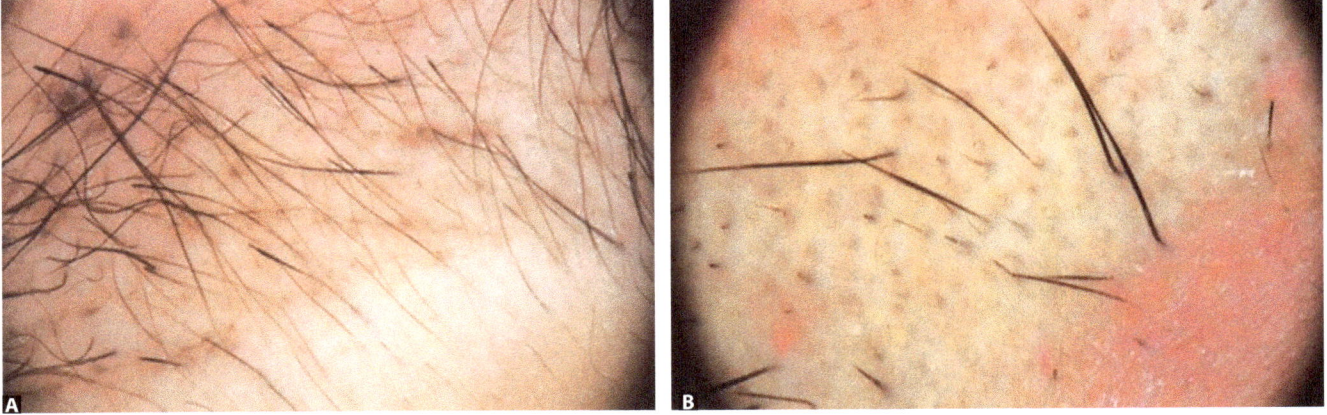

Figs. 13.8A and B: Alopecia areata of the eyebrows. (A) Exclamation mark hairs and broken hairs. (B) Black dots, broken hair and yellow dots.

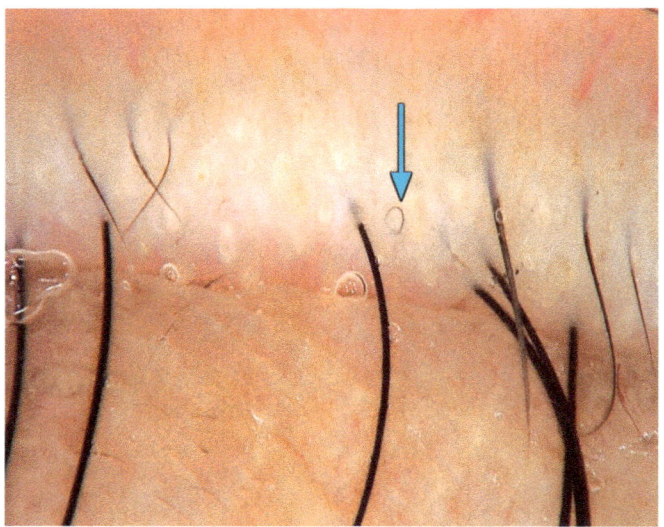

Fig. 13.9: Alopecia areata of the eyelashes. Note multiple yellow dots and one circle hair (blue arrow).

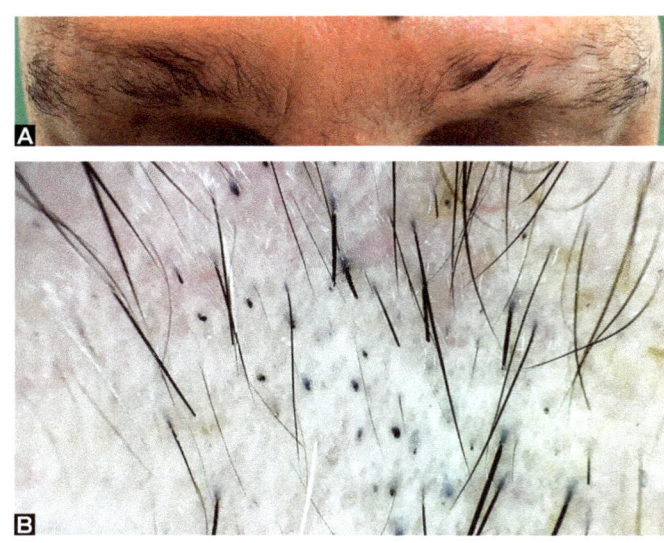

Figs. 13.10A and B: Eyebrow trichotillomania. (A) Partial madarosis. (B) Black dots, and broken hairs of different lengths.

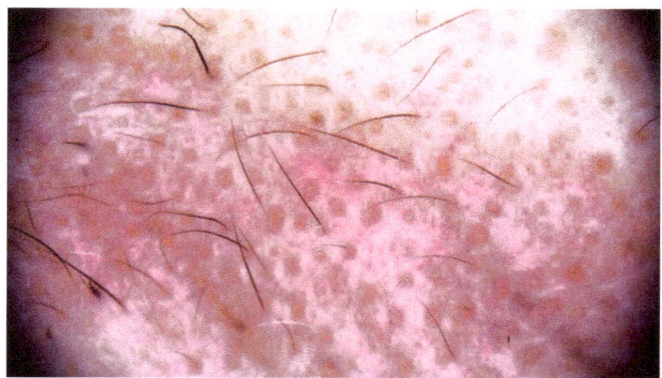

Fig. 13.11: Follicular yellow and red dots in the eyebrow from a patient with frontal fibrosing alopecia. Note broken and dystrophic hairs.
Source: Division of Dermatology, Hospital das Clínicas, University of São Paulo Medical School.

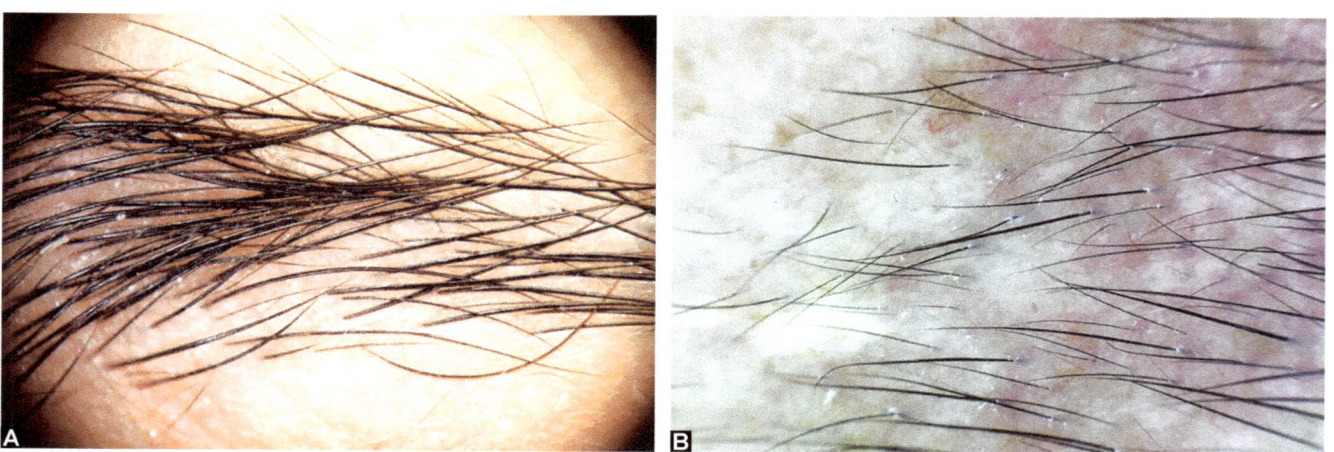

Figs. 13.12A and B: (A) Mild perifollicular scales, hair casts and eyebrow alopecia in an early case of frontal fibrosing alopecia. (B) Note erythema, pigmentation, and decreased hair loss in the eyebrows from a patient with a long-standing disease.
Source: (A) Division of Dermatology, Hospital das Clínicas, University of São Paulo Medical School.

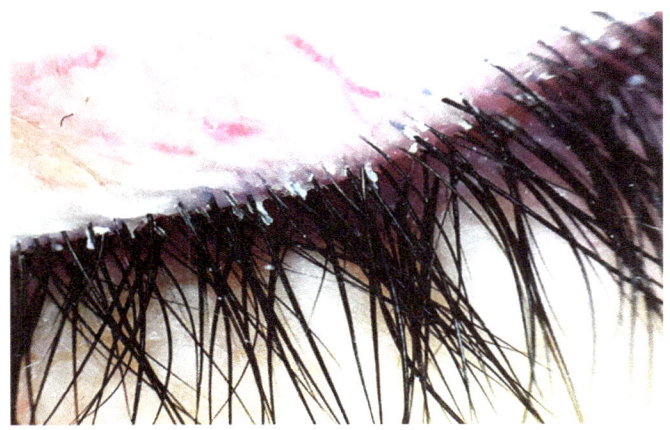

Fig. 13.13: Perifollicular scaling on the eyelashes in a patient with frontal fibrosing alopecia. Differently from seborrheic dermatitis, the scales completely involve the hair shaft.

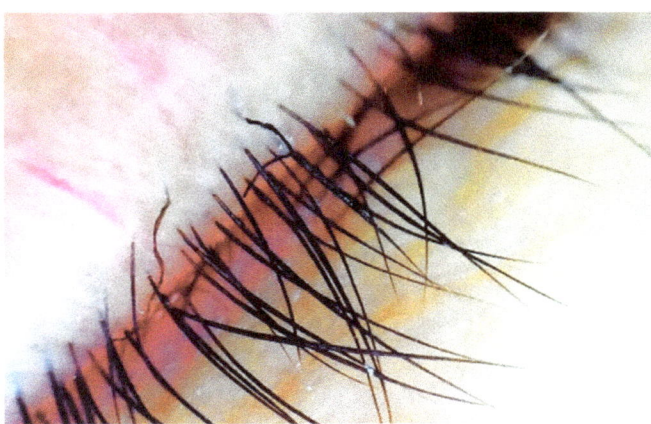

Fig. 13.14: Pili torti on the eyelashes from a patient with frontal fibrosing alopecia.

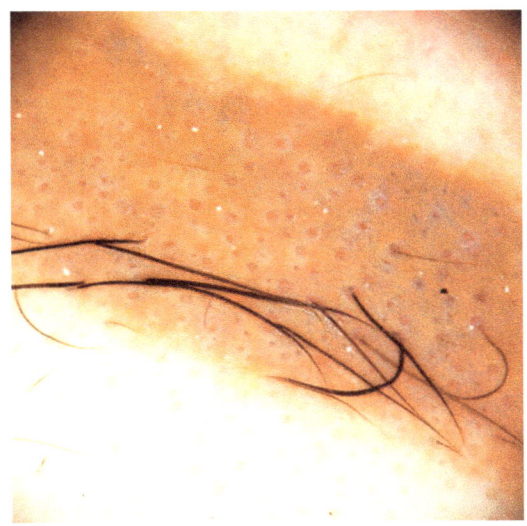

Fig. 13.15: Eyebrow tattoo in a patient with frontal fibrosing alopecia. Note the follicular opening accentuation.
Source: Division of Dermatology, Hospital das Clínicas, University of São Paulo Medical School.

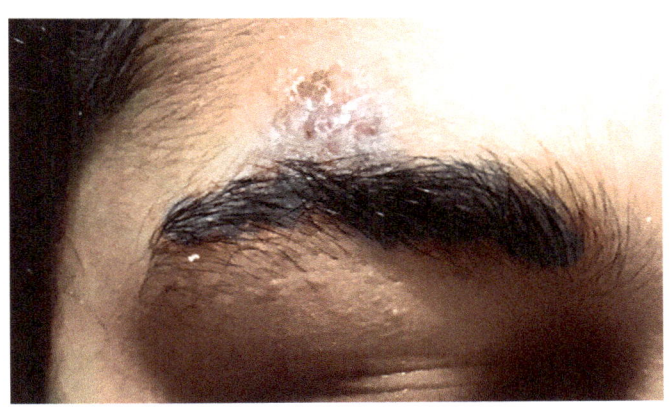

Fig. 13.16: Discoid lupus erythematosus presenting with erythema, scales and dyschromia affecting the upper part of the eyebrow.

inheritance pattern. Affected hairs shafts present a beaded appearance with regular intervals of narrowings. These hairs have the tendency to bend and fracture at constriction sites leading to alopecia. Occipital scalp hairs are more often affected, but the eyebrows, eyelashes, axilla, and pubis may be involved as well. Monilethrix can improve with age and the features depend on the severity of the disease. Dermoscopy shows uniform elliptical nodes and regular intermittent constrictions along the hair shaft (Fig. 13.18).

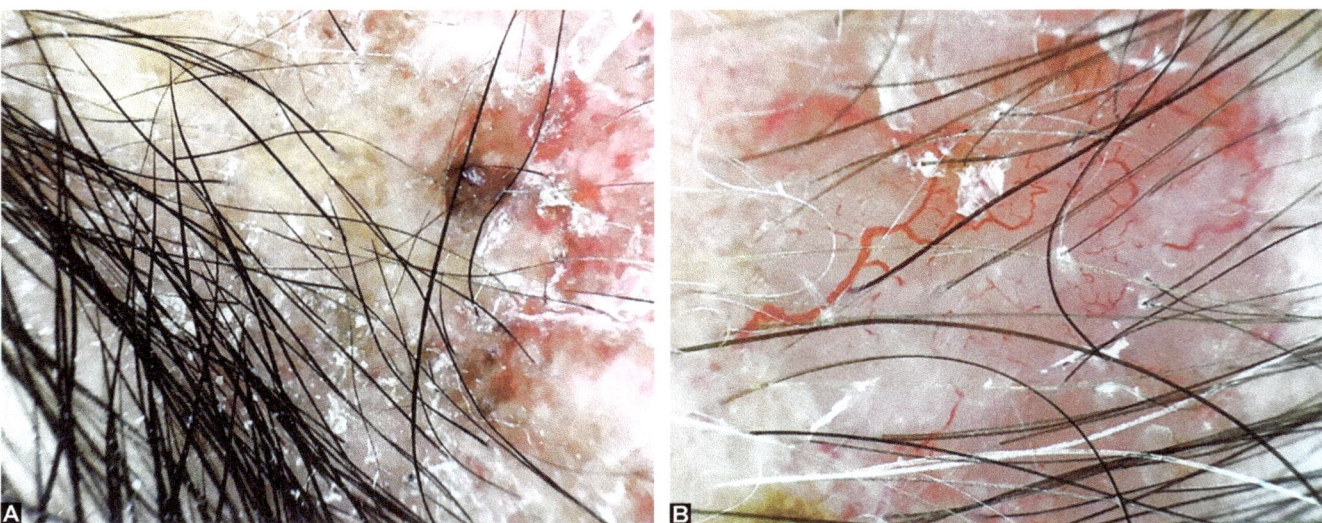

Figs. 13.17A and B: Discoid lupus erythematosus in the eyebrow. (A) Thick interfollicular and follicular scales, dyschromia, keratin plugs, scarring areas with loss of follicular openings, and enlarged vessels. (B) Note the thick arborizing vessels.

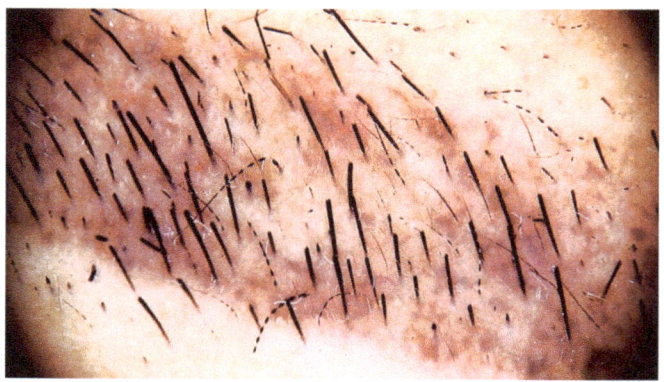

Fig. 13.18: Monilethrix in the eyebrows. Hair beading and breakage at different levels from skin emergence. Note the regular intervals of constrictions. Internode areas are devoid of medulla.

Source: Division of Dermatology, Hospital das Clínicas, University of São Paulo Medical School.

TRICHORRHEXIS INVAGINATA

Trichorrhexis invaginata is a rare congenital hair shaft disorder characterized by multiple knots along the hair shaft and hair breakage. It is considered a typical feature of Netherton disease, a rare genodermatosis presenting with ichthyosis, atopic dermatitis, and bamboo-like hairs. This disease can affect eyebrow and eyelashes hairs even when scalp hairs are normal. Dermoscopy shows single or knots irregularly distributed along the hair shafts on lower magnifications. Higher magnifications can show hair shaft invagination at several points along the shaft, similar to the bamboo appearance (Fig. 13.19A). When the breakage occurs in that point, a golf-tee sign appears (Fig. 13.19B).

LEPROSY

Leprosy is an important cause of madarosis in epidemic countries. It usually occurs in half of the patients with advanced cases of multibacillary leprosy as a result of histiocytic infiltration of the hair follicles. However, in paucibacillary cases, skin lesions over the eyebrows may cause unilateral madarosis due to follicle destruction caused by the granulomatous inflammation (Fig. 13.20). The absence of madarosis in long-standing cases of leprosy indicates a good prognostic sign. Dermoscopy shows decreased hair density, empty follicles and thinned hairs (Fig. 13.21). As leprosy leads to a nonscarring form of madarosis, proper management requires the treatment of the underlying condition.

EYELASHES TRICHOMEGALY

Trichomegaly is defined as an increase in the length, curling, pigmentation, or thickness of the eyelashes (Fig. 13.22). Many congenital, pharmacological and acquired conditions have been associated with eyelashes trichomegaly (Table 13.2). However, in some cases it may be an isolated finding. The pathophysiology of this disorder is unknown. Some immune factors, such as prostaglandins and epidermal growth factor appear to be involved as both mediators increase the duration of the anagen phase. The treatment is symptomatic and sometimes requires the use of artificial tears to prevent associated meibomitis.

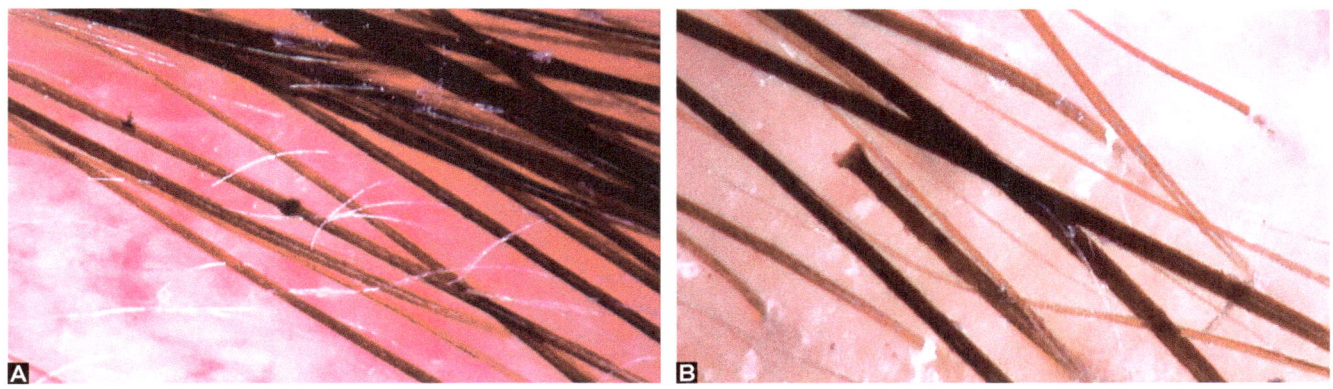

Figs. 13.19A and B: Trichorrhexis invaginata in the eyebrows. (A) Bamboo hairs. (B) Golf-tee sign.
Source: Division of Dermatology, Hospital das Clínicas, University of São Paulo Medical School.

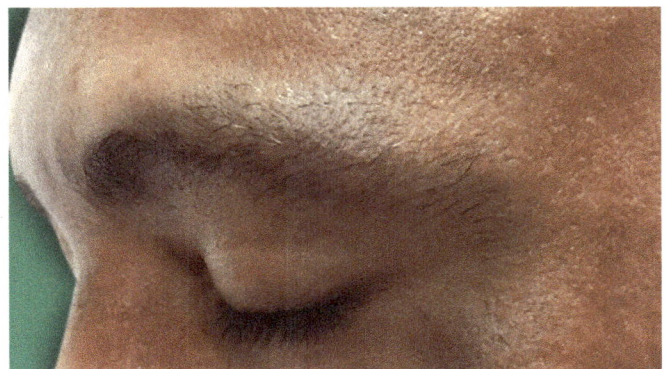

Fig. 13.20: Madarosis in leprosy. Note the unilateral partial eyebrow hair loss in a patient with multibacillary leprosy.
Source: Dr João Avancini.

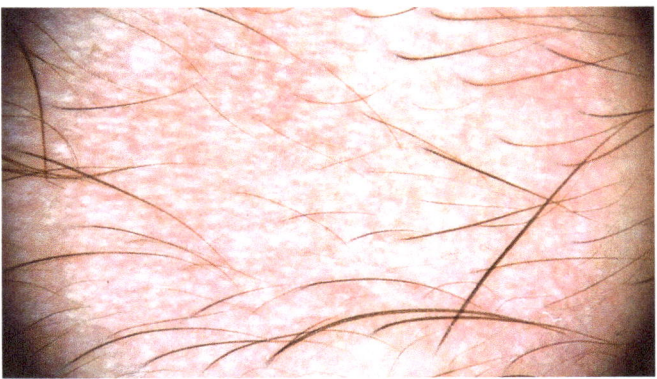

Fig. 13.21: Madarosis in leprosy. Dermoscopy shows a nonscarring process with decreased hair density, thinned hairs, and empty follicles, some surrounded by a whitish halo.
Source: Dr João Avancini.

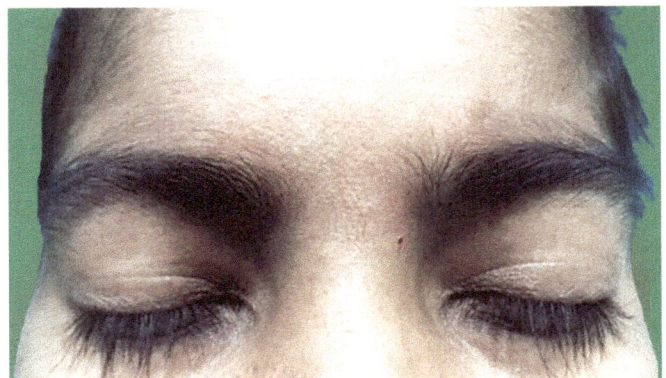

Fig. 13.22: Eyelash trichomegaly. Note the increased hair length in a patient with systemic lupus erythematosus.
Source: Dalal A, et al. Eyelash trichomegaly: a rare presenting feature of systemic lupus erythematosus. Int J Trichology. 2017;9(2):79-81

Table 13.2: Congenital, pharmacological and acquired conditions in eyelashes trichomegaly.

Congenital syndromes	Acquired disorders	Drug associations
Oliver McFarlane syndrome	Areata alopecia	Prostaglandin analogs
Cornelia de Lange syndrome	Connective tissue disorders	Bimatoprost, latanoprost
Cone rod dystrophy	Lupus, dermatomyositis, hen fever, atopic dermatitis	Cetuximab
Fallot tetralogy	HIV infection	Zidovudine
Hermansky-Pudlak syndrome	Renal metastatic adenocarcinoma	Phenytoin
Familial trichomegaly	Eating disorders (anorexia nerviosa)	Minoxidil
Goldstein Hutt syndrome	Pregnancy	Cyclosporine
Phylloid hypomelanosis		Topiramate, systemic corticosteroids, Streptomycin, Penicillamine

Source: Fernández-Crehuet P, Ruiz-Villaverde R. Essential trichomegaly of the eyelashes. Int J Trichology. 2016;8(3):153-4.

Take-Home Message

- Loss of eyebrows and eyelashes can occur in various diseases.
- Cosmetics and camouflage products can confuse the examination and lead to a misdiagnosis.
- Seborrheic dermatitis can affect eyebrows and eyelashes with perifollicular scales and diffuse erythema.
- Alopecia areata of the eyebrows and eyelashes can be an isolated finding and may be distinguished from other causes of madarosis.
- Trichotillomania of the eyebrow can be an isolated presentation of the disease.
- In frontal fibrosing alopecia, partial eyebrow alopecia may be the first sign of the disease. Dermoscopy shows mild perifollicular scale and follicular yellow and red dots.
- Discoid lupus erythematosus can affect any hair-bearing area, leading to scarring alopecia.
- Some congenital hair shaft disorders, as monilethrix and trichorrhexis invaginata may affect eyebrows and eyelashes despite hair scalp lesions.

SUGGESTED READING

1. Ankad BS, Sakhare PS. Dermoscopy of borderline tuberculoid leprosy. Int J Dermatol. 2017;57(1):74-6.
2. Avhad G, Ghuge P. Monilethrix. Int J Trichology. 2013;5(4):224-5.
3. Dalal A, Sharma S, Kumar A, et al. Eyelash trichomegaly: a rare presenting feature of systemic lupus erythematosus. Int J Trichology. 2017;9(2):79-81.
4. Fernández-Crehuet P, Ruiz-Villaverde R. Essential trichomegaly of the eyelashes. Int J Trichology. 2016;8(3): 153-4.
5. Jain N, Khopkar U. Monilethrix in pattern distribution in siblings: diagnosis by trichoscopy. Int J Trichology. 2010;2(1):56-9.
6. Kaur S, Mahajan BB. Eyelash trichomegaly. Indian J Dermatol. 2015;60(4):378-80.
7. Khong JJ, Casson RJ, Huilgol SC, et al. Madarosis. Surv Ophthalmol. 2006;51(6):550-60.
8. Krishnan A, Kar S. Bilateral madarosis as the solitary presenting feature of multibacillary leprosy. Int J Trichology. 2012;4(3):179-80.
9. Kumar A, Karthikeyan K. Madarosis: a marker of many maladies. Int J Trichology. 2012;4(1):3-18.
10. Miteva M, Tosti A. Dermatoscopy of hair shaft disorders. J Am Acad Dermatol. 2013;68(3):473-81.
11. Na JI, Kwon OS, Kim BJ, et al. Ethnic characteristics of eyelashes: a comparative analysis in Asian and Caucasian females. Br J Dermatol. 2006;155(6):1170-6.
12. Pirmez R, Donati A, Valente NS, et al. Glabellar red dots in frontal fibrosing alopecia: a further clinical sign of vellus follicle involvement. Br J Dermatol. 2014;170(3):745-6.
13. Rudnicka L, Olszewska M, Rakowska A, et al. Trichoscopy update 2011. J Dermatol Case Rep. 2011;5(4):82-8.
14. Rudnicka L, Rakowska A, Kurzeja M, et al. Hair shafts in trichoscopy: clues for diagnosis of hair and scalp diseases. Dermatol Clin. 2013;31(4):695-708.
15. Sharma VK, Chiramel MJ, Rao A. Dermoscopy: a rapid bedside tool to assess monilethrix. Indian J Dermatol Venereol Leprol. 2016;82(1):73-4.
16. Thibaut S, De Becker E, Caisey L, et al. Human eyelash characterization. Br J Dermatol. 2010;162(2):304-10.
17. Vij A, Bergfeld WF. Madarosis, milphosis, eyelash trichomegaly, and dermatochalasis. Clin Dermatol. 2015;33(2):217-26.

CHAPTER 14

Cosmetic Hair Products

Patricia Damasco, Giselle Martins, Isabella Doche

14.1 Camouflage

Patricia Damasco, Giselle Martins, Isabella Doche

Camouflage products can be used to conceal thinning hair. Options include topical hair fibers, powder cakes, camouflage lotions, and sprays. Topical hair fibers are positively charged particles that adhere to the negatively charged terminal and vellus hair on the scalp. The hair-bonding property is a major benefit over other camouflaging techniques but has limited utility in areas of complete hair loss. It must be applied daily and requires existing hairs to bind.

Pigmented concealing powder, lotions, and sprays are applied to the scalp to limit color contrast between the existing hair and the scalp. They can be easily removed with shampoo and need daily application.

Dermoscopy shows regular fragments of similar lengths and deposits of products on the surface of the scalp (Fig. 14.1.1). The presence of those products may resemble short regrowing hairs, broken hairs, and black dots (Figs. 14.1.2 to 14.1.4). The camouflage products may hinder diagnosis as they cover the surface of the scalp. It is important to ask patients about the use of camouflage products before performing the exam.

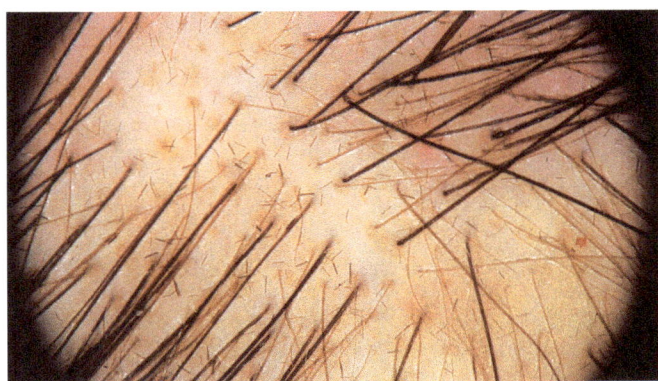

Fig. 14.1.1: Hair fibers. Fragments of similar lengths are seen on the scalp and adhered to some hair shafts.

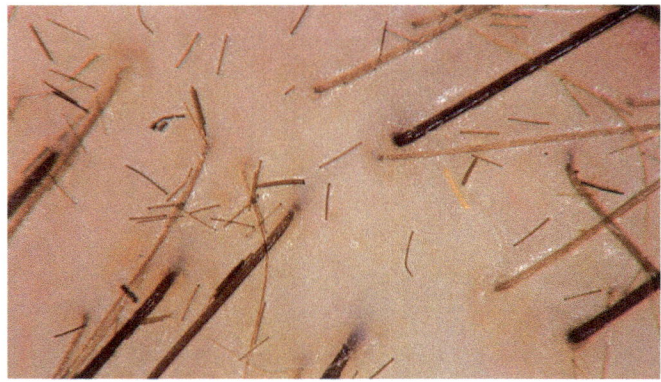

Fig. 14.1.2: Hair fibers. Note the small, pigmented, and regular fragments. These fragments are thinner than the normal hair shaft and should be distinguished from broken hairs.

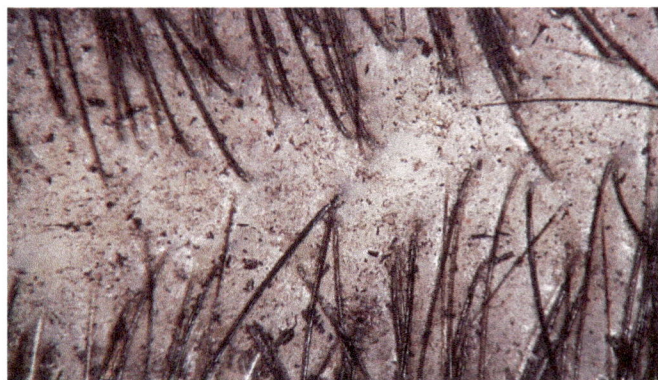

Fig. 14.1.3: Hair spray. Pigmented residues irregularly deposited on the scalp surface and hair shafts may mimic black dots.

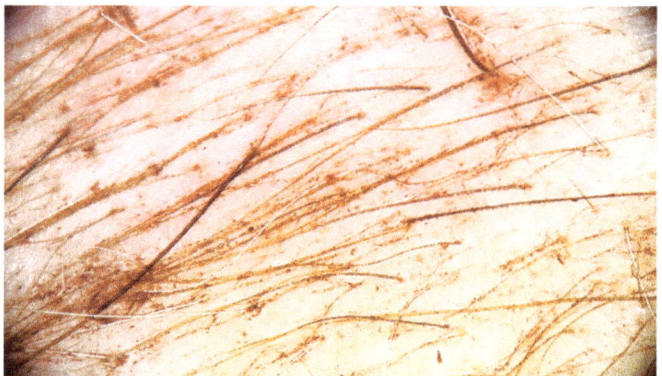

Fig. 14.1.4: Hair powder. Pigmented powder residues on the scalp surface and hair shafts.

> **Take-Home Message**
> - Hair fibers, powder cakes, camouflage lotions, and sprays are options of temporary concealers for thinning hairs.
> - Dermoscopy shows regular fragments irregularly distributed in the scalp surface that are easily removed after shampooing.
> - Product residues may mimic other scalp disorders and hinder the correct diagnosis.

SUGGESTED READING

1. Cossman JP, Ladizinski B, Lee KC. Pigmented concealing powders for the hair loss patient. J Cosmet Dermatol. 2013;12(4):322-4.
2. Donovan JC, Shapiro RL, Shapiro P, et al. A review of scalp camouflaging agents and prostheses for individuals with hair loss. Dermatol Online J. 2012;18(8):1.
3. Draelos ZD. Shampoos, conditioners, and camouflage techniques. Dermatol Clin. 2013;31(1):173-8.
4. Harris AG, Kim M, Murrell DF. Pigmented hair-thickening fibers: a camouflage technique for alopecia in patients with epidermolysis bullosa. Skin Appendage Disord. 2016;1(3):153-5.
5. Saed S, Ibrahim O, Bergfeld WF. Hair camouflage: a comprehensive review. Int J Womens Dermatol. 2017;3(1 Suppl):S75-80.

14.2 Extensions

Patricia Damasco, Giselle Martins, Isabella Doche

Hair extensions or hair additions are strands of synthetic or human hair that are attached to existing hair fibers utilizing glue, braids, sewing, or clips. The attachment method selected depends on the amount of natural hair and the number or length of fibers to be added (Figs. 14.2.1 and 14.2.2).

Hair extensions must be changed every 2 months in order to avoid hygiene problems, traction alopecia, or excessive hair breakage due to the glues and clips required to affix the hairpiece.

Dermoscopy shows multiple white dots, which correspond to telogen roots entrapped by the glue, can be seen within the tangled area (Figs. 14.2.3 and 14.2.4).

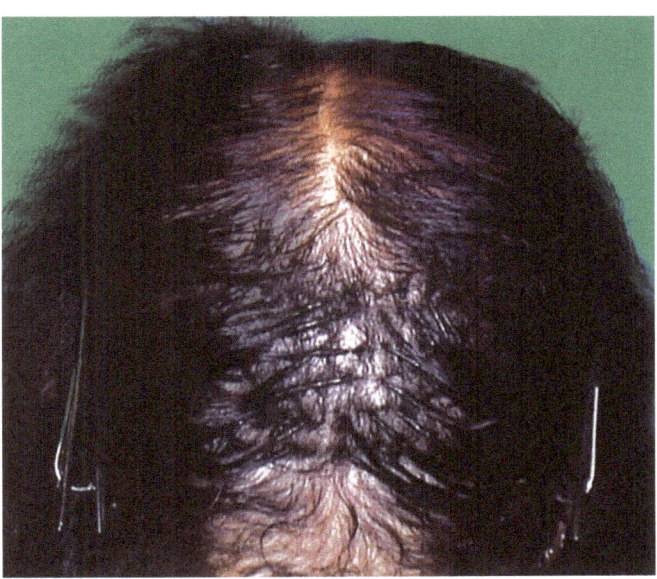

Fig. 14.2.2: Hair extension. Extensions with a glue bond are attached to small pieces of hairs in strand by strand technique.

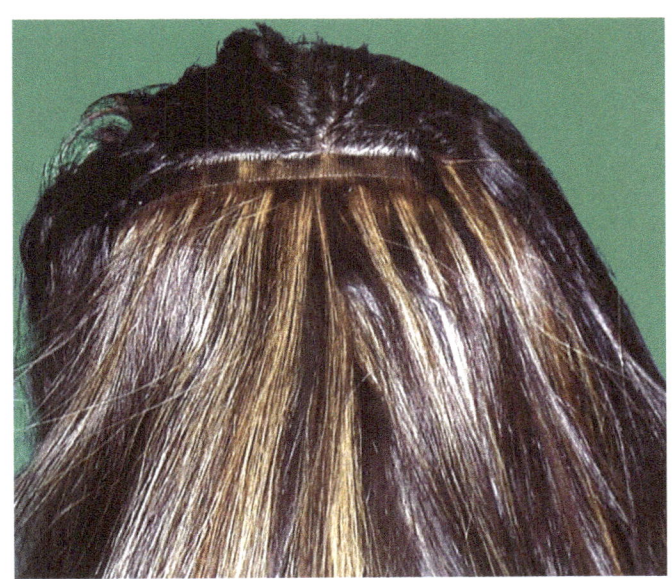

Fig. 14.2.1: Hair extension. The weight of the panel is spread out over a larger area, causing less damage to the hair in glue-in extension technique.

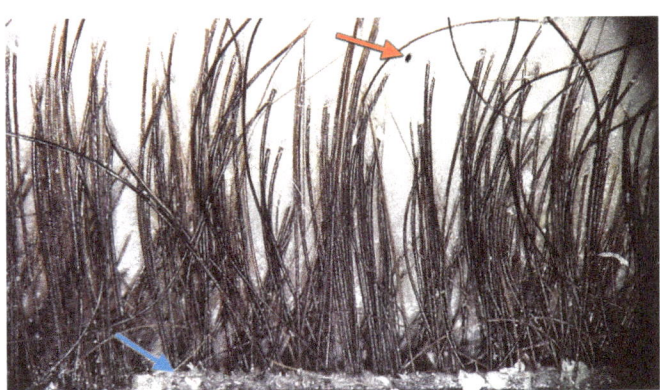

Fig. 14.2.3: Hair extension (glue-in technique). Perifollicular seborrheic scales, entrapped telogen hair within the glue (blue arrow), and one black dot (red arrow).

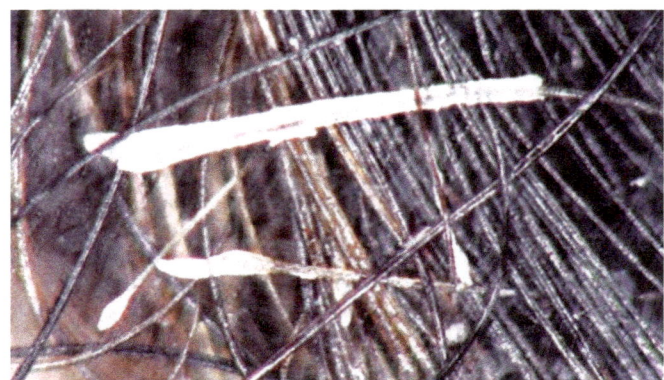

Fig. 14.2.4: Hair extension. Telogen roots entrapped by the glue and hair cast.

Take-Home Message
- Hair extensions are an option for camouflage.
- It can cause traction alopecia, making the hair loss worse.
- Dermoscopy shows broken hairs, perifollicular seborrheic scale, hair casts, and entrapped telogen roots.

SUGGESTED READING

1. Ahdout J, Mirmirani P. Weft hair extensions causing a distinctive horseshoe pattern of traction alopecia. J Am Acad Dermatol. 2012;67(6):e294-5.
2. Donovan JC, Shapiro RL, Shapiro P, et al. A review of scalp camouflaging agents and prostheses for individuals with hair loss. Dermatol Online J. 2012;18(8):1.
3. Draelos ZD. Camouflage technique for alopecia areata: What is a patient to do? Dermatol Ther. 2011;24(3):305-10.
4. Saed S, Ibrahim O, Bergfeld WF. Hair camouflage: a comprehensive review. Int J Womens Dermatol. 2016;2(4):122-7.

14.3 Micropigmentation and Tattoo

Patricia Damasco, Giselle Martins, Isabella Doche

Micropigmentation (MP) is a form of semipermanent cosmetic make-up for scalp and body areas with scars and hair loss. The principle of MP is similar to tattooing. However, in MP, the pigmentation tends to last less than that in conventional tattoo. In MP, the pigment is deposited more superficially in the upper dermis by a delicate needle, creating a more natural-looking appearance and the illusion of texture and fullness (Figs. 14.3.1A and B). In conventional tattooing, the pigment is deposited more deeply in the skin, resulting in blue-gray dots, discoloration, and blotched areas over time (Fig. 14.3.2).

Dermoscopy of skin tattoo shows black structures with dotted and round shapes, irregularly distributed on the skin surface. Pigment botches can also be seen (Figs. 14.3.3 to 14.3.5). MP shows smaller dotted pigments on the skin (Figs. 14.3.6A and B). The main differential diagnosis is black dots. In black dots, residues of hairs are located inside the follicular ostium and are a sign of many hair and scalp inflammatory disorders.

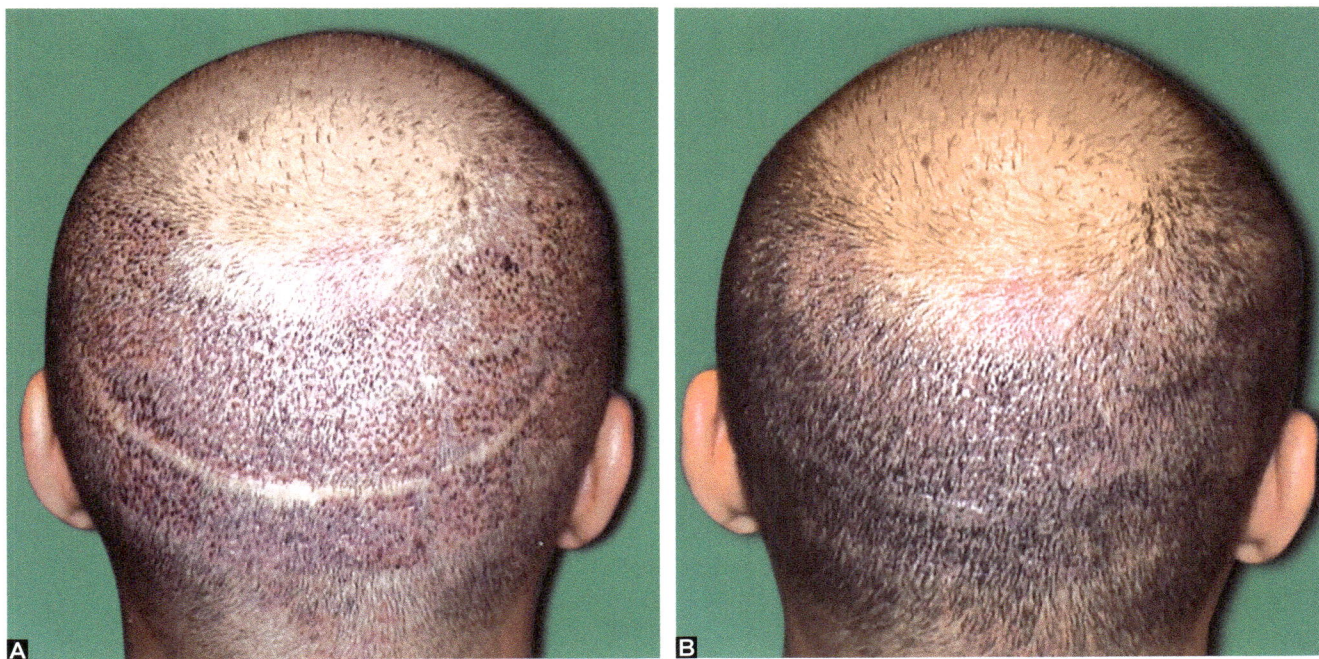

Figs. 14.3.1A and B: Patient with a wide scar from hair transplant with strip harvesting. (A) Before scalp micropigmentation. (B) After scalp micropigmentation.
Source: Dr Alessandra Juliano.

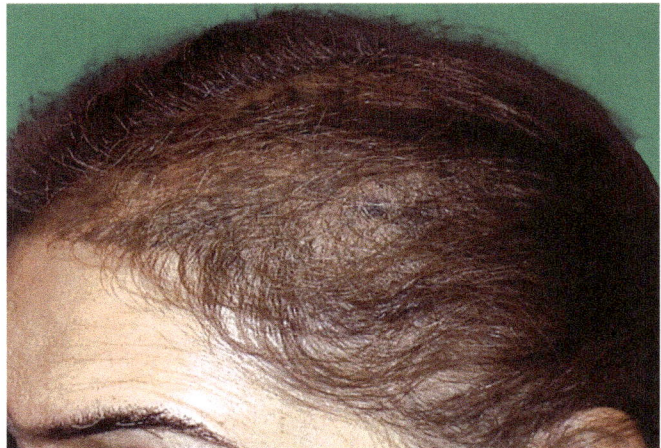

Fig. 14.3.2: Scalp tattoo. Note some bluish irregular areas.
Source: Dr Alessandra Juliano.

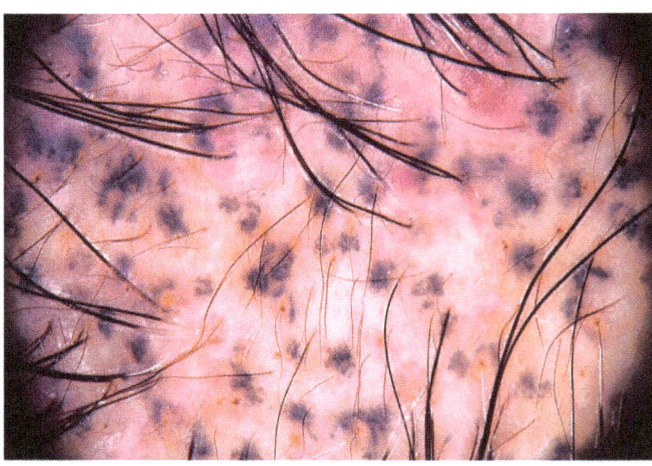

Fig. 14.3.3: Scalp tattoo. Note the irregular distribution of the black-blue structures, with variable shape and size.

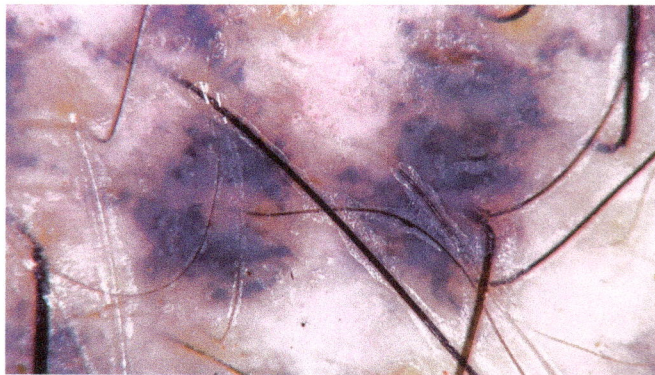

Fig. 14.3.4: Scalp tattoo. Note that the pigment has different shapes, sizes, and shades of black. They are not associated with follicular openings, diverging from the black dots.

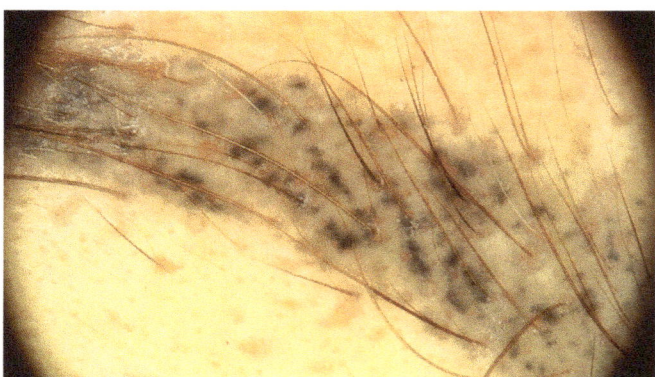

Fig. 14.3.5: Eyebrow tattoo. Blue-gray dots and blotched pigmented areas in a patient with eyebrow hair loss.

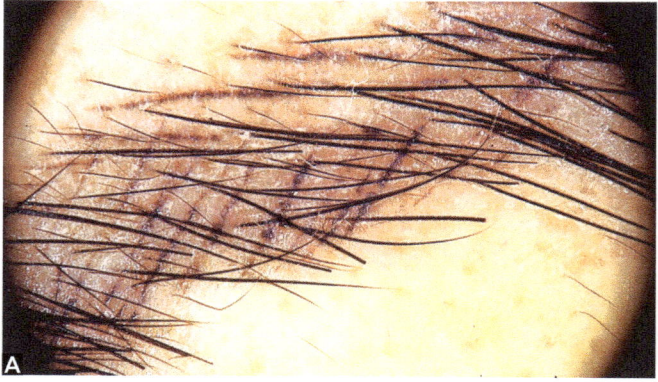
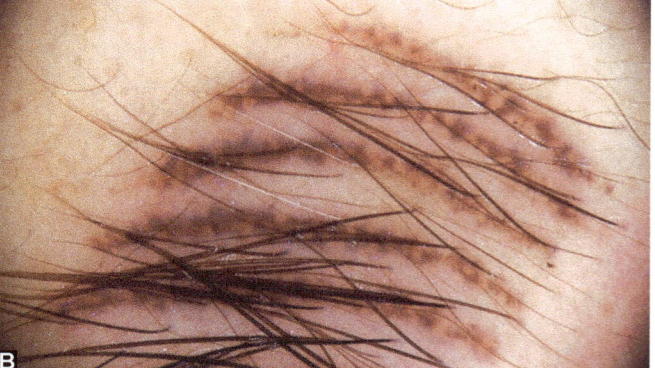

Figs. 14.3.6A and B: Eyebrow micropigmentation. Note small pigments deposited in fine lines in the skin.

> **Take-Home Message**
> - Micropigmentation and tattoo are semipermanent and permanent techniques for hair loss.
> - In micropigmentation, the pigment is deposited more superficially in the upper dermis; in tattoo, the pigment reaches the deep dermis.
> - Dermoscopy shows large and irregular blue-gray dots not restricted to hair follicles, pigment discoloration, and blotched areas.
> - Both techniques may mimic black dots and camouflage products.

SUGGESTED READING

1. Garg G, Thami GP. Micropigmentation: tattooing for medical purposes. Dermatol Surg. 2005;31(8 Pt 1):928-31.
2. Kim EK, Chang TJ, Hong JP, et al. Use of tattooing to camouflage various scars. Aesthetic Plast Surg. 2011;35(3):392-5.
3. Kowalska-Oledzka E, Slowinska M, Rakowska A, et al. "Black dots" seen under trichoscopy are not specific for alopecia areata. Clin Exp Dermatol. 2012;37(6):615-9.
4. Park JH, Moh JS, Lee SY, et al. Micropigmentation: camouflaging scalp alopecia and scars in Korean patients. Aesthetic Plast Surg. 2014;38(1):199-204.
5. Rassman WR, Pak JP, Kim J, Estrin NF. Scalp micropigmentation: a concealer for hair and scalp deformities. J Clin Aesthet Dermatol. 2015;8(3):35-42.
6. Saed S, Ibrahim O, Bergfeld WF. Hair camouflage: a comprehensive review. Int J Womens Dermatol. 2017;3(1 Suppl):S75-80.

14.4 Dry Shampoos, Hair Sprays, and Others

Patricia Damasco, Giselle Martins, Isabella Doche

Cosmetic hair sprays, deodorants, and dry shampoos can leave residues on the hair shaft, producing pseudocasts. Pseudocasts may mimic "true" hair casts, nits, white piedra, and trichorrhexis nodosa on low magnifications. Differently from these other conditions, residues of hair care products can be easily removed with shampooing.

Dermoscopy shows concretions with variable length, thickness, and surface, distributed along the hair shafts at irregular intervals (Figs. 14.4.1 to 14.4.5). The main differential diagnoses are "true" hair casts, mostly related to inflammatory disorders and nits, a sign of lice infection. Differently from the casts, nits have oval shape and attach to the shaft, but do not encircle it. Purple shampoos used to keep blond tone can also leave residues on the scalp and proximal hair hafts (Fig. 14.4.6).

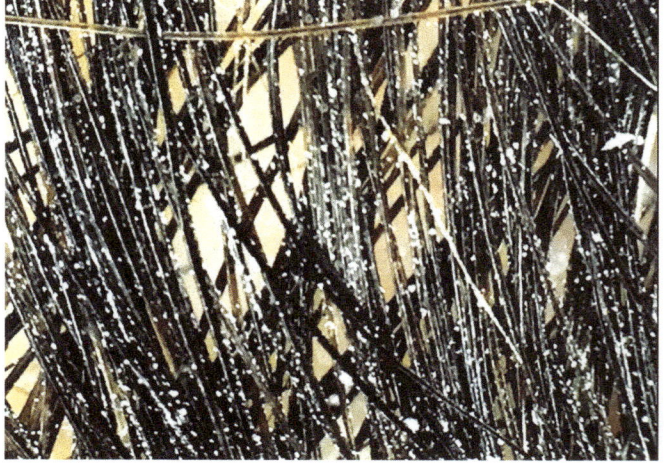

Fig. 14.4.1: Pseudocasts. Multiple residues of leave-in products on the hair shaft.

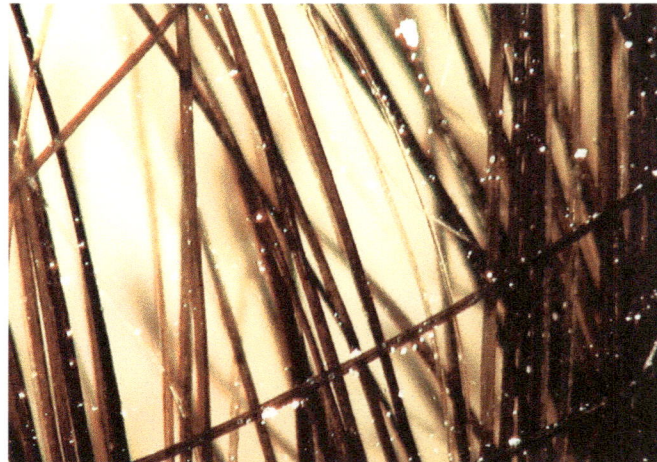

Fig. 14.4.3: Pseudocasts. Residues of dry shampoo on the hair shaft. Small concretions irregularly attached to the hair shaft surface.

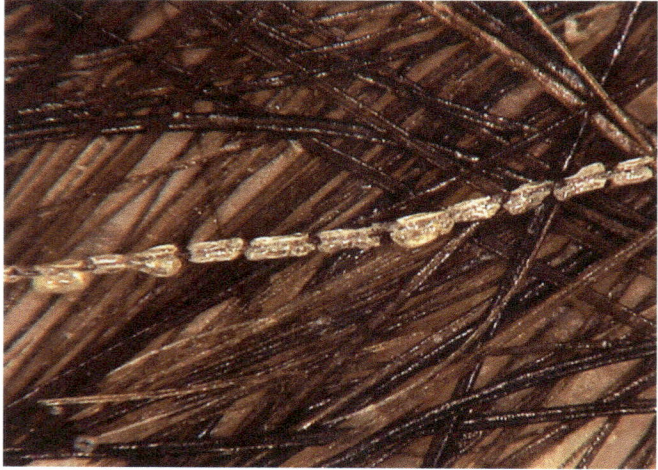

Fig. 14.4.2: Pseudocasts. Note irregular concretions, with variable length, thickness, and surface, surrounding the hair shaft after hair spray use.
Source: Dr Antonella Tosti.

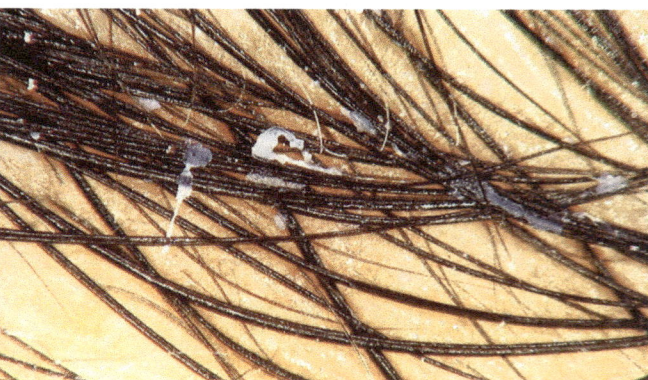

Fig. 14.4.4: Pseudocasts. Eyebrow hair shafts with white residues of sunscreen lotion.

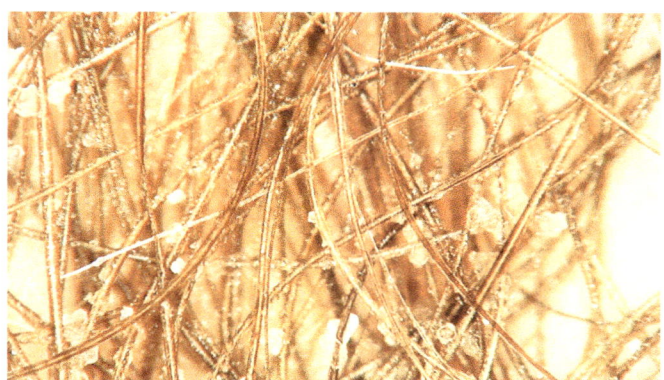

Fig. 14.4.5: Pseudocasts. Irregular residues of deodorant spray in the axillary hairs shafts.

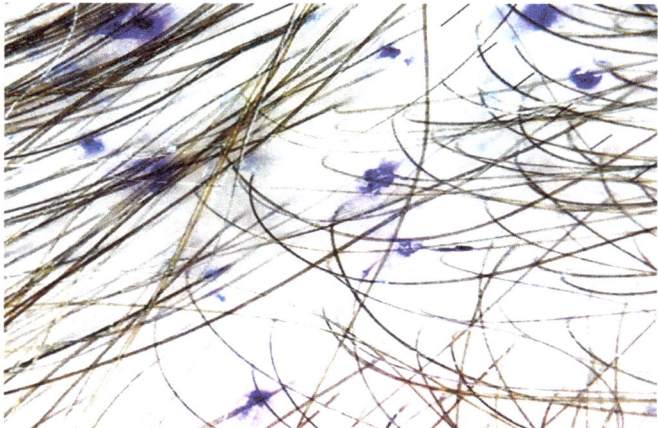

Fig. 14.4.6: Shampoo residues. Multiple bluish oval structures located within the follicular units are residues of the purple shampoo used in a patient with blonde hair.
Source: Dr Rodrigo Vettoratto.

Take-Home Message

- Hair care products, such as dry shampoo, deodorants, and hair sprays can leave residues on the hair shaft, mimicking true hair casts and nits.
- Pseudocasts have irregular shape, thickness, and surface and are irregularly attached to the hair shafts.

SUGGESTED READING

1. Albayrak H, Yanik ME. Dermoscopic appearance of hair casts. J Dermatol. 2017;44(8):e182-3.
2. Doche I, Vincenzi C, Tosti A. Casts and pseudocasts. J Am Acad Dermatol. 2016;75(4):e147-8.
3. Ena P, Mazzarello V, Chiarolini F. Hair casts due to a deodorant spray. Australas J Dermatol. 2005;46(4):274-7.
4. França K, Villa RT, Silva IR, et al. Hair casts or pseudonits. Int J Trichology. 2011;3(2):121-2.
5. Parmar SS, Parmar KS, Shah BJ. Hair casts. Indian Dermatol Online J. 2014;5(4):554-5.
6. Tosti A, Miteva M, Torres F, et al. Hair casts are a dermoscopic clue for the diagnosis of traction alopecia. Br J Dermatol. 2010;163(6):1353-5.

14.5 Hair Matting

Patricia Damasco, Giselle Martins, Isabella Doche

Acute hair matting (AHM), first reported as "plica neuropathica," is a rare condition presenting as a compact mass with irregular twists and severely entangled hairs, abruptly formed in the scalp (Fig. 14.5.1). Although its etiology still remains ascertained, excessive friction and compression in a liquid medium are believed to cause the conglomeration of contiguous hair fibers.

Dermoscopy shows 180° twisted hairs, bended and fractured hair shafts, retained telogen hairs, and trichorrhexis nodosa (Figs. 14.5.2A and B).

Treatment of AHM involves cutting the matted hair. Manual separation using organic solvent can be tried in early and mild cases.

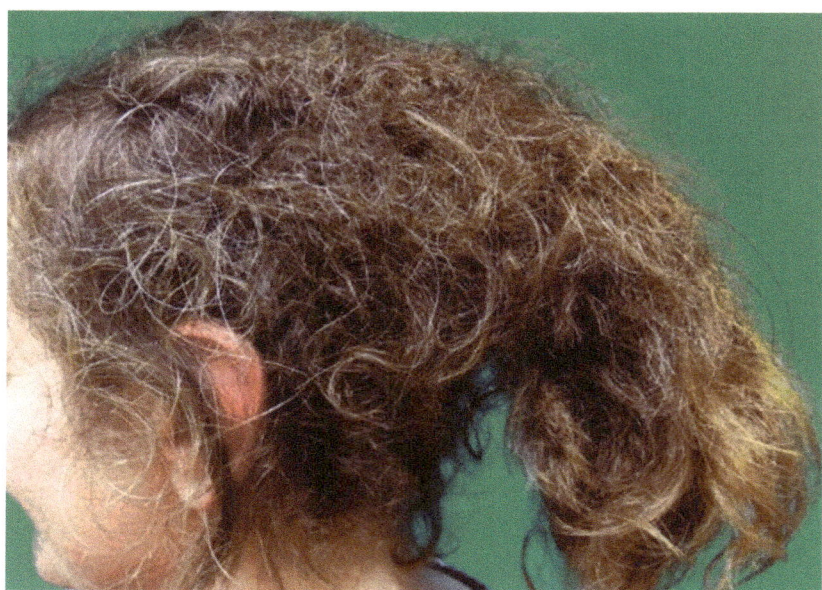

Fig. 14.5.1: Acute hair matting. Woman presenting with curly hairs arranged in a dense matted mass affecting mainly the centered scalp area.

Source: Dr Antonella Tosti. Martins SS, Abraham LS, Doche I, et al. Acute hair matting: case report and trichoscopy findings. J Eur Acad Dermatol Venereol. 2017;31(3):e163-4.

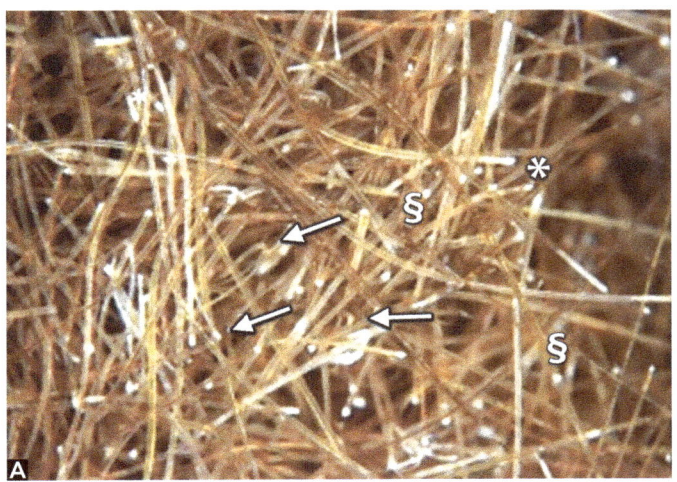 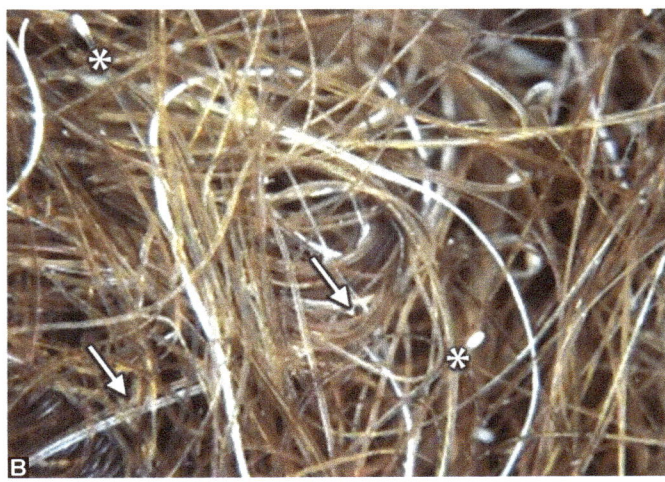

Figs. 14.5.2A and B: Acute hair matting. (A) Note the presence of trichorrhexis nodosa (§), fractured hairs (*), and twisted hairs (arrows). (B) The arrow points to the bending hair shafts. Note the telogen roots embedded in the mass (*).

Source: Dr Antonella Tosti. Martins SS, Abraham LS, Doche I, et al. Acute hair matting: case report and trichoscopy findings. J Eur Acad Dermatol Venereol. 2017;31(3):e163-4.

Take-Home Message
- Abrupt formation of a compact mass and severely entangled in the scalp.
- Probably related to excessive friction in wet hairs.
- Dermoscopy shows 180° twisted hairs, fractured hair shafts, retained telogen hairs, and trichorrhexis nodosa.

SUGGESTED READING

1. Al Ghani Al MA, Geilen CC, Blume-Peytavi U, et al. Matting of hair: a multifactorial enigma. Dermatology. 2000;201(2):101-4.
2. Bogaty H, Dunlap FE. Matting of hair. Arch Dermatol. 1970;101(3):348-51.
3. Ghodake NB, Singh N, Thappa DM. Plica neuropathica (polonica): clinical and dermoscopic features. Indian J Dermatol Venereol Leprol. 2013;79(2):269.
4. Le Page JF. On Neuropathic Plica. Br Med J. 1884;1(1204):160.
5. Marshall J, Parker C. Felted hair untangled. J Am Acad Dermatol. 1989;20(4):688-90.
6. Martins SS, Abraham LS, Doche I, et al. Acute hair matting: case report and trichoscopy findings. J Eur Acad Dermatol Venereol. 2017;31(3):e163-4.
7. Palwade PK, Malik AA. Plica neuropathica: different etiologies in two cases. Indian J Dermatol Venereol Leprol. 2008;74(6):655-6.
8. Pereira JM. Acute matting of hair. An Bras Dermatol. 2002;77(3):353-64.

CHAPTER 15

Nonmelanocytic Scalp Tumors

Jade Cury Martins, José Antonio Sanches, Cyro Festa Neto

INTRODUCTION

Scalp tumors are rare neoplasms accounting for 2% of all skin tumors. They may arise from the epidermis or dermis and from the eccrine, apocrine, hair follicle or sebaceous unit. There is a very broad differential diagnosis for scalp nodules, including different types of cysts, hamartomas, benign, or malignant neoplasms and also metastases from tumors at distant sites.

The use of dermoscopy for nonmelanocytic tumors other than basal cell carcinomas and squamous cell carcinomas is relatively new, with only a few published reports, with descriptions being even rarer for scalp tumors. Therefore, the aim of this chapter is to give a brief description of the clinical characteristics and trichoscopic findings of these infrequent neoplasms reported in the literature.

BASAL CELL CARCINOMA

It is the most common type of skin cancer, representing around 65% of all cases. They are slow-growing tumors, but can cause local destruction and invasion. Metastasis occurs very rarely (<0.1%).

Clinically, basal cell carcinoma (BCC) presents as a translucent papule or nodule, with telangiectasias. Pigmentation and ulceration might be present. Typical dermoscopy findings include arborizing telangiectasias, blue–gray ovoid nests, brown–black dots/globules, and leaf-like and spoke wheel areas.

A recent review of 501 BCC cases tried to identify the most common dermoscopy findings according to tumor location, and described scalp lesions as having blue–gray ovoid nests, leaf-like areas, multiple brown–black dots/globules, blue–white veil-like structures, and greater than or equal to 1 melanocytic pattern more frequently than in other body sites. The presence of greater than or equal to 1 vascular pattern was significantly less frequent on the scalp (Figs. 15.1A and B to 15.3A and B).

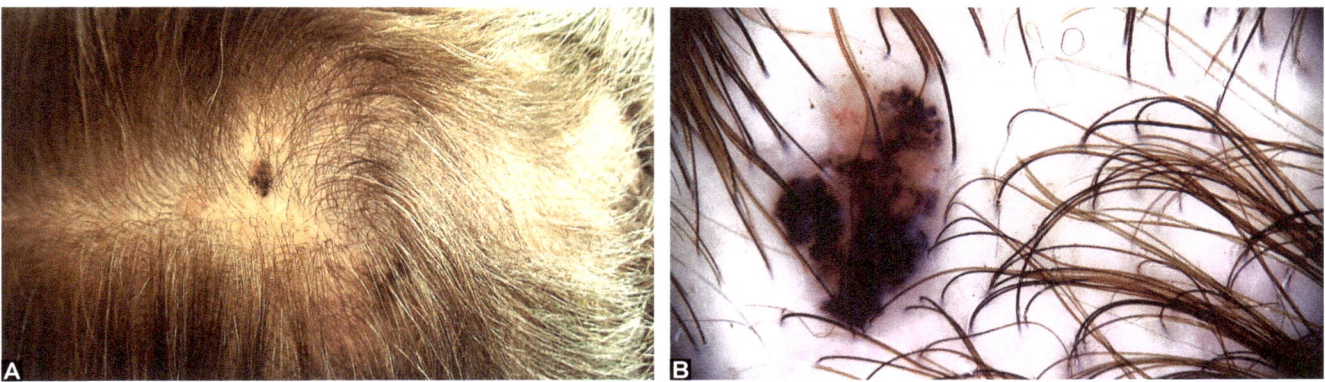

Figs. 15.1A and B: (A) Pigmented basal cell carcinoma on the scalp. (B) Dermoscopy shows multiple pigmented structures, leaf-like areas and brown–black dots. Telangiectasias are also present on the upper left portion (20X).
Source: Dr Paula Ferreira.

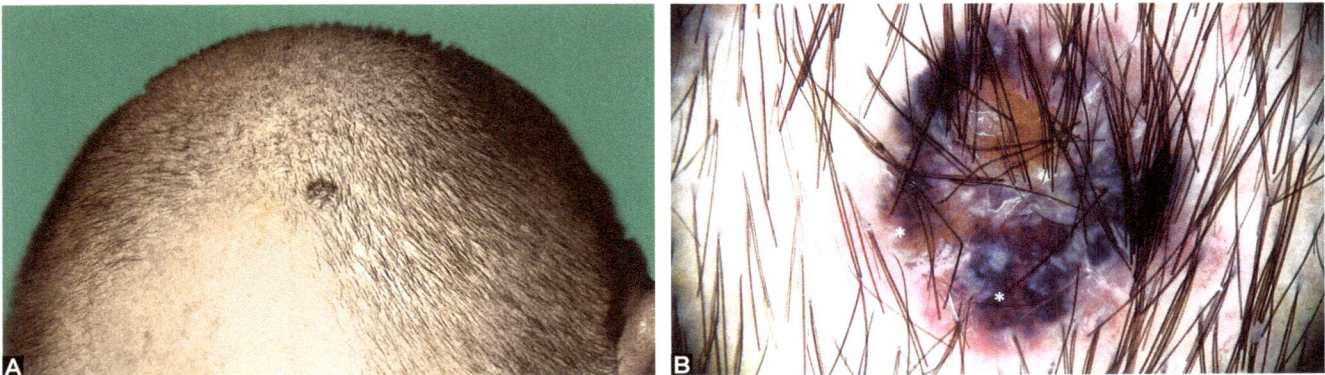

Figs. 15.2A and B: (A) Pigmented basal cell carcinoma on the scalp. (B) Dermoscopy shows structureless pigmented areas, brown globules and blue–white veil-like structures resembling melanoma. Telangiectasias can also be seen (*) (20X).
Source: Dr João Avancini.

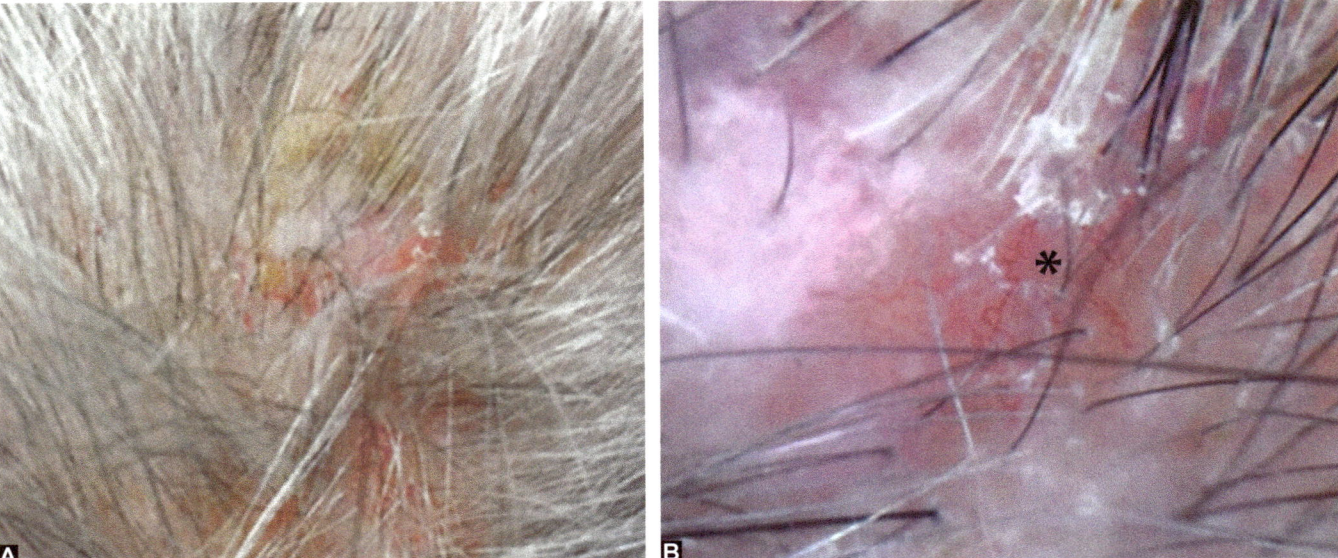

Figs. 15.3A and B: Nonpigmented basal cell carcinoma on the scalp. (A) Clinically note an erythematous, keratotic papule resembling actinic keratosis. (B) Dermoscopy shows multiple arborizing telangiectasias in sharp focus (10X).

Take-Home Message

- The most common cancer in humans representing 65% of all skin cancers.
- Indolent, with rare occurrence of metastasis, but may cause local destruction/invasion.
- Dermoscopy shows arborizing telangiectasias, blue–gray ovoid nests, leaf-like and spoke wheel areas.
- Pigmentation features seem to be more frequent on scalp lesions.

SQUAMOUS CELL CARCINOMA

Cutaneous squamous cell carcinoma (SCC) is the second most common type of skin cancer. It can develop from precursor lesions such as actinic keratosis. Also, SCC can range from superficially invasive to highly infiltrative, metastasizing tumors that can lead to death.

Clinically the most common presentations are erythematous, keratotic papules or plaques, usually on chronically sun-exposed areas. Other characteristics include ulceration, pigmentation and verrucous lesions.

Dermoscopy shows intraepidermal lesions with two main vascular patterns—small dotted vessels and glomerular vessels. In invasive cases, a more polymorphic vascular pattern with irregular vessels is frequent. Other findings include a scaly surface, small brown globules (on pigmented lesions), irregular groups of white perifollicular circles, erosion, and crusting. Regarding lesions on the scalp, on a review of fifteen SCC cases, the most common vascular pattern found was linear-irregular vessels (Figs. 15.4 and 15.5A and B).

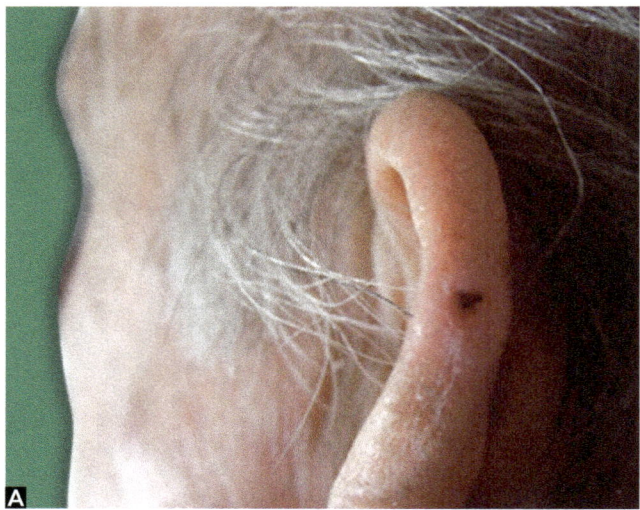

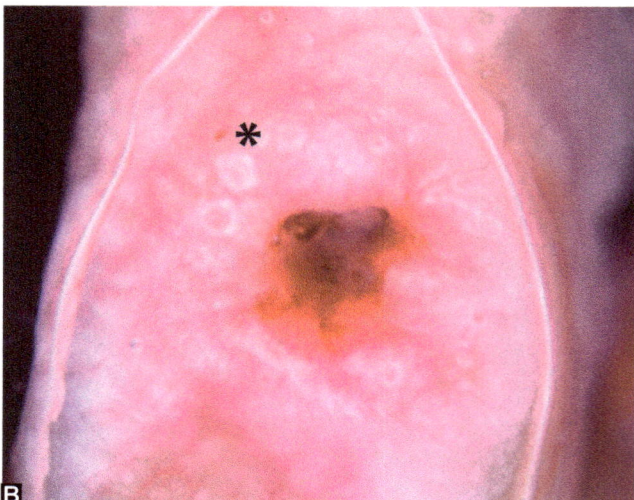

Figs. 15.5A and B: (A) Invasive squamous cell carcinoma on the ear. (B) Dermoscopy shows central erosion with irregular groups of yellow dots surrounded by white circles (*).
Source: Dr Louise Lovatto.

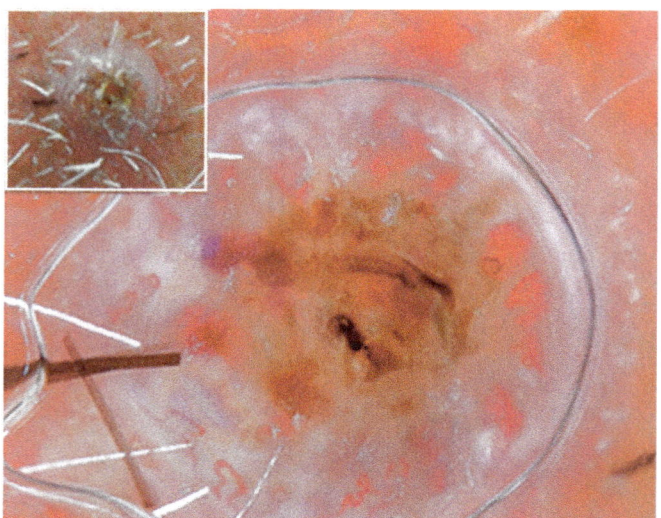

Fig. 15.4: Invasive squamous cell carcinoma. Dermoscopy shows a central keratin mass surrounded by radially-oriented linear irregular vessels and hemorrhagic areas.
Source: Lin MJ, Pan Y, Jalilian C, et al. Dermoscopic characteristics of nodular squamous cell carcinoma and keratoacanthoma. Dermatol Pract Concept. 2014;4(2):2.

Take-Home Message

- It is characterized by erythematous, keratotic papules or plaques.
- It can range from superficially invasive to metastasizing tumors that can lead to death.
- Dermoscopy shows scaly surface, small brown globules, white perifollicular circles, erosion and crusting. Irregular clusters of glomerular and/or globular vessels are found in intraepidermal lesions, with a greater vascular polymorphism in the invasive cases.

ADNEXAL TUMORS

Adnexal tumors differentiate from the normal components of normal appendages into eccrine, apocrine, hair follicle units or sebaceous tumors. They may occur as single or multiple lesions (frequently in association with inherited disorders). The main diagnostic tool is histopathology. The risk of malignant transformation varies between the different types of tumors.

On dermoscopy, these tumors can be mistaken for BCCs as both might show arborizing telangiectasias. Another differential diagnosis includes melanoma, as it may also present a highly polymorphous vascular pattern.

Sebaceous Nevus

Sebaceous nevus (SN), also known as nevus sebaceous of Jadassohn, is a common congenital hamartoma composed of immature sebaceous glands and malformed pilosebaceous units. It presents as a linear or oval, hairless, yellow, waxy, or verrucous plaque on the scalp. Sometimes it can be flat right after birth, with differential diagnosis including aplasia cutis (AC) and congenital triangular alopecia. Tumors can arise within an SN, such as trichoblastomas or syringocystadenoma papilliferum (SP).

Dermoscopy reports describe features such as comedo-like openings and milia-like cysts (as seen in seborrheic keratosis), whitish structures with irregular shapes and sizes covering the lesion on a pale to red colored skin. In early lesions, bright yellow dots not associated with hair follicles may help differentiate from AC, which lacks skin appendages (Figs. 15.6 to 15.8).

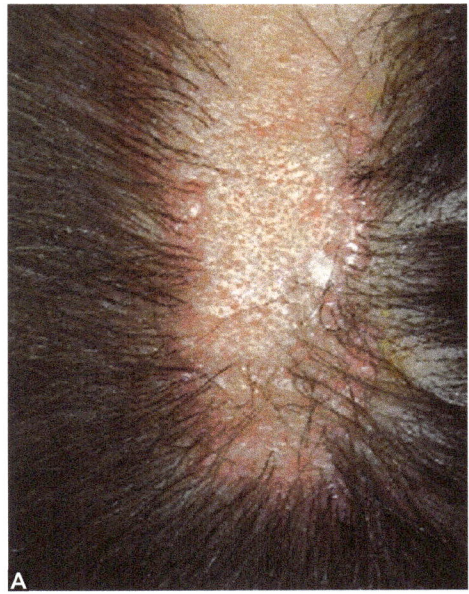

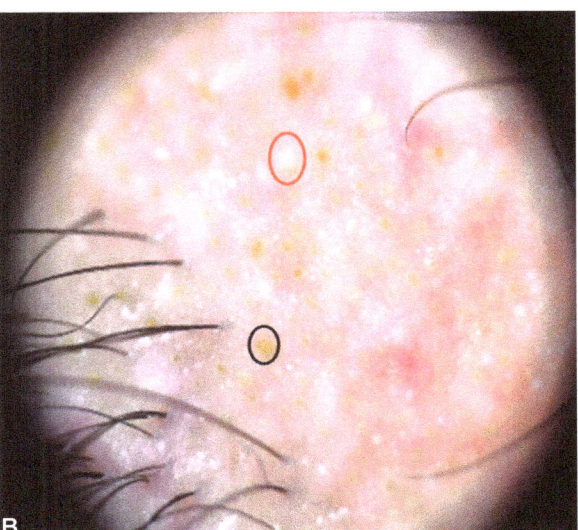

Figs. 15.7A and B: (A) Congenital hairless plaque with a smooth, flesh-colored surface on the scalp. (B) Dermoscopy shows comedo-like openings (black circle), milia-like structures (red circle), and multiple whitish dots (10X).

Source: Dr Aline Donati.

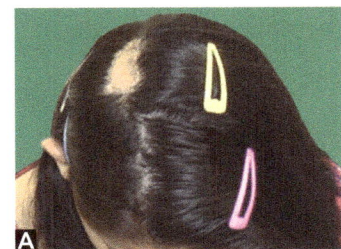

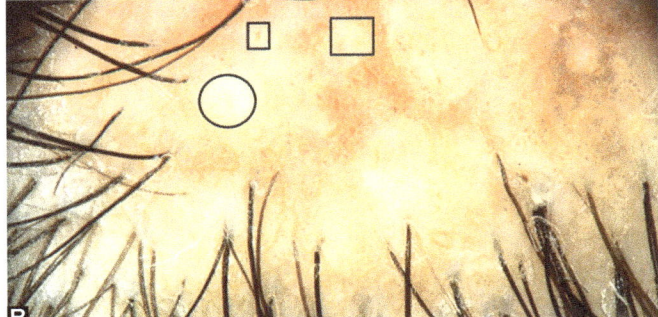

Figs. 15.6A and B: (A) Congenital hairless plaque with a smooth, flesh-colored surface. (B) Dermoscopy shows comedo-like openings (black square), milia-like structures, and yellow–whitish structures with irregular shapes (circled).

Source: Dr Giselle Martins.

Take-Home Message
• Sebaceous nevi are common congenital hamartomas characterized by linear or oval, hairless, yellow, waxy, or verrucous plaque on the scalp. • Most common tumors arising on a SN are trichoblastomas and SP. • Rapidly growing lesions require histology to rule out malignancy. • Dermoscopy shows bright yellow dots not associated with hair follicles.

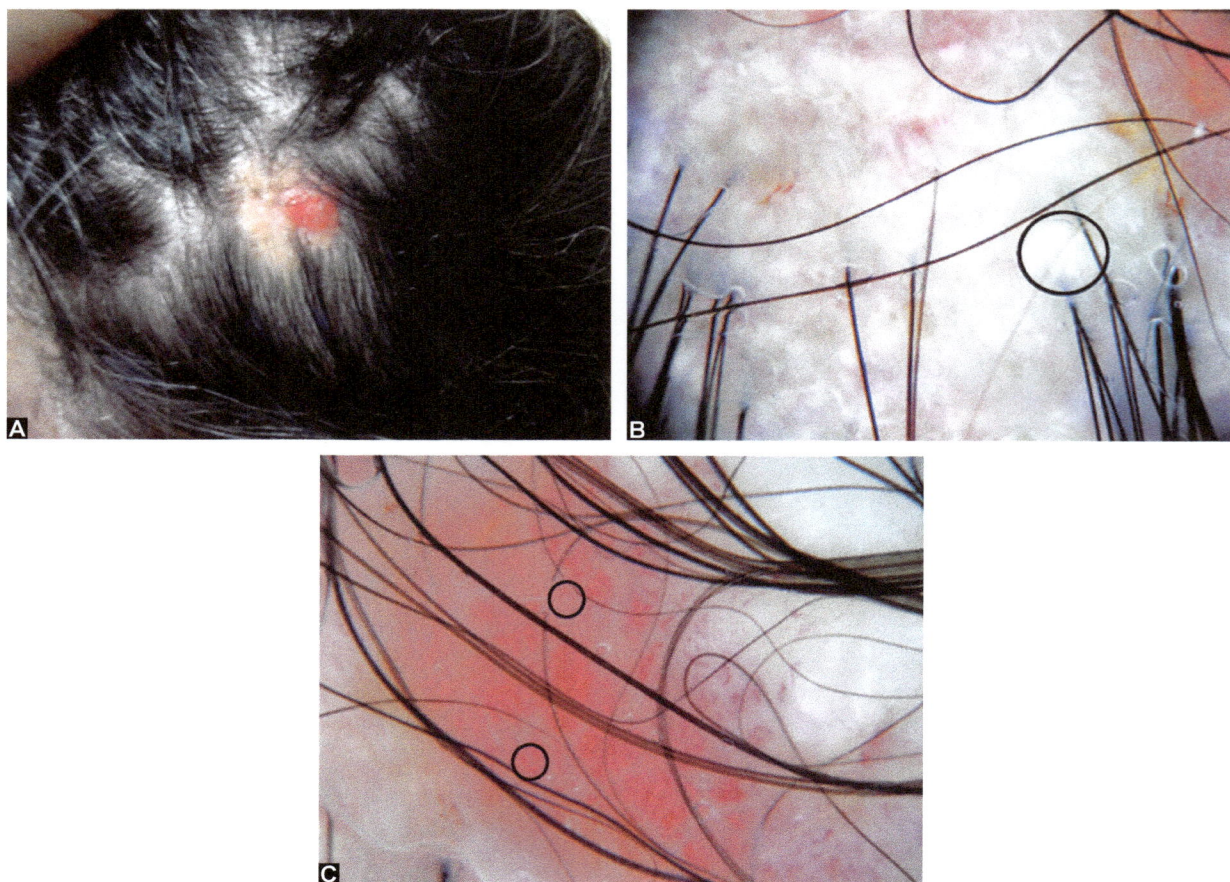

Figs. 15.8A to C: (A) Papular, yellowish-orange plaque and a lobular, exophytic lesion with a moist appearance. (B) Dermoscopy of the sebaceous nevus shows round-shaped or oval, yellowish-white structures (circled). (C) Dermoscopy of the exophytic lesion shows an erythematous background divided by whitish linear structures that demarcate lobules of different sizes. Note vascular structures of different forms: irregularly linear vessels, glomerular vessels and some vessels arranged in a horseshoe-shaped pattern (circled).
Source: Dr Carolina Barbosa Bruno.

Syringocystadenoma Papilliferum

It is a rare benign adnexal neoplasm often located on the scalp and face, with variable clinical appearance, that may arise independently or in association with an SN. Histology shows epidermal invaginations with papillary projections. Dermoscopy findings erythematous background, whitish linear structures that demarcate variable-sized lobules and multiple vascular structures (Figs. 15.8A to C).

> **Take-Home Message**
> - Syringocystadenoma papilliferum is a rare benign adnexal neoplasm that may arise independently or in association with a SN.
> - Dermoscopy shows whitish linear structures, polymorphic vessels, peripheral hairpin-like vessels; vessels arranged in a horseshoe-shaped pattern have already been described.

Trichoblastoma

It is a rare benign skin neoplasm of rudimentary hair follicles. Clinically, it presents as a solitary flesh-colored to brown or bluish-black papule/nodule mostly located on the scalp. It may arise independently or in association with an SN. Histology reveals aggregations of basaloid cells with a peripheral palisading and several rudimentary follicular papillae. Nonspecific dermoscopy findings, sometimes mimicking malignant tumors, such as yellow plates, whitish regions, and "tree-like" telangiectasias have been reported in the literature (Figs. 15.9A and B).

> **Take-Home Message**
> - Trichoblastomas are a rare benign neoplasm of rudimentary hair follicles.
> - They may arise independently or in association with a SN.
> - Dermoscopic structures mimicking malignant neoplasms such as "tree-like telangiectasias" have been described.

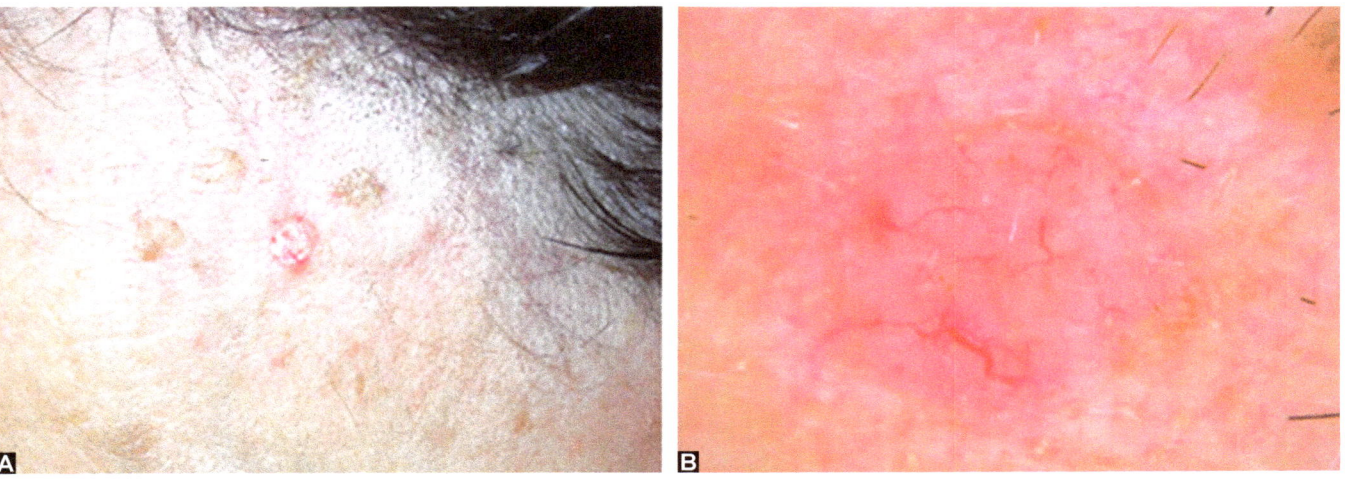

Figs. 15.9A and B: Trichoblastoma. (A) Translucent papule on the front. (B) Note typical arborizing vessels.
Source: Dr Giuseppe Argenziano.

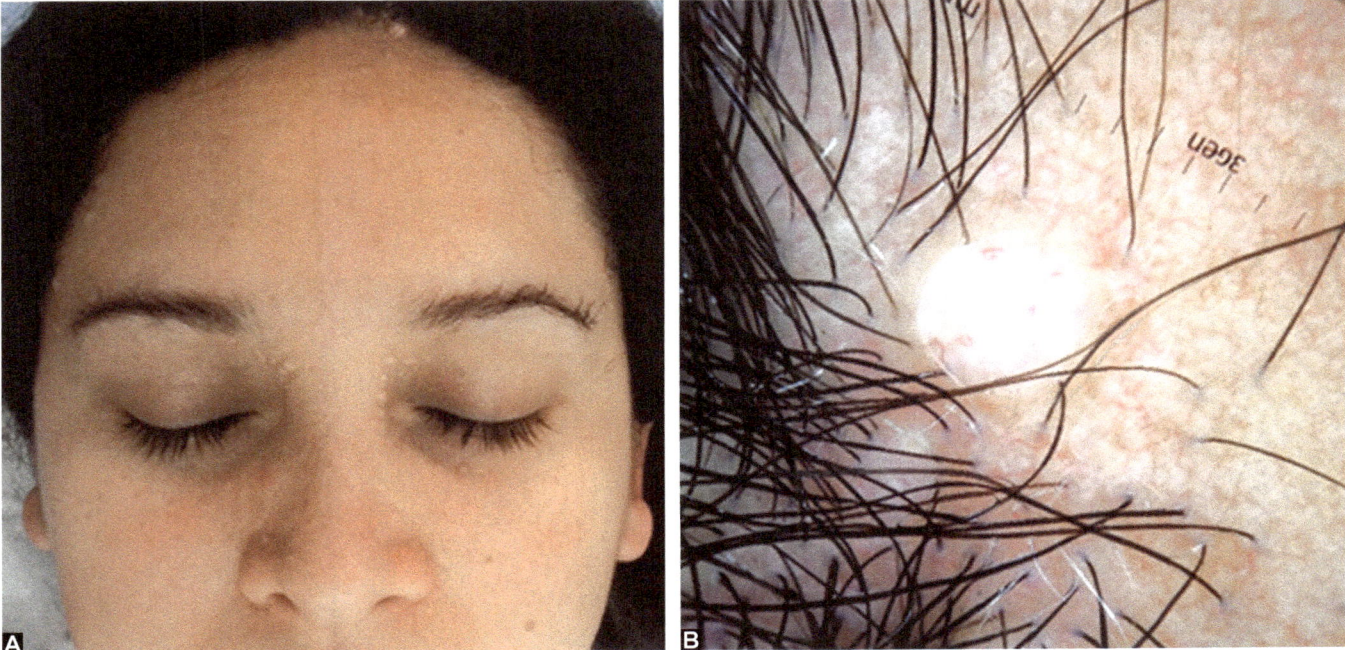

Figs. 15.10A and B: Multiple familial trichoepitheliomas. (A) Clinical presentation shows small white-yellowish papules around the eyes. (B) Dermoscopy shows in-focus arborizing vessels, multiple milia-like cysts and rosettes amidst a whitish background. (Contact nonpolarized light view, x10).
Source: Dr Cristián Navarrete-Dechent.

Trichoepithelioma

It is a rare benign adnexal neoplasm originating from the hair follicle. It presents as a solitary lesion, but multiple familial trichoepitheliomas on the face and sometimes on the scalp represent an autosomal dominant disease. Dermoscopy findings include arborizing vessels, milia-like lesions and white shiny structures (Figs. 15.10A and B and 15.11A and B).

> **Take-Home Message**
> - Trichoepitheliomas are benign hair follicle neoplasms that might occur as a solitary lesion or as multiple familial lesions in an autosomal dominant inheritance.
> - Dermoscopic findings are arborizing vessels, milia-like cysts and rosettes on a whitish background.

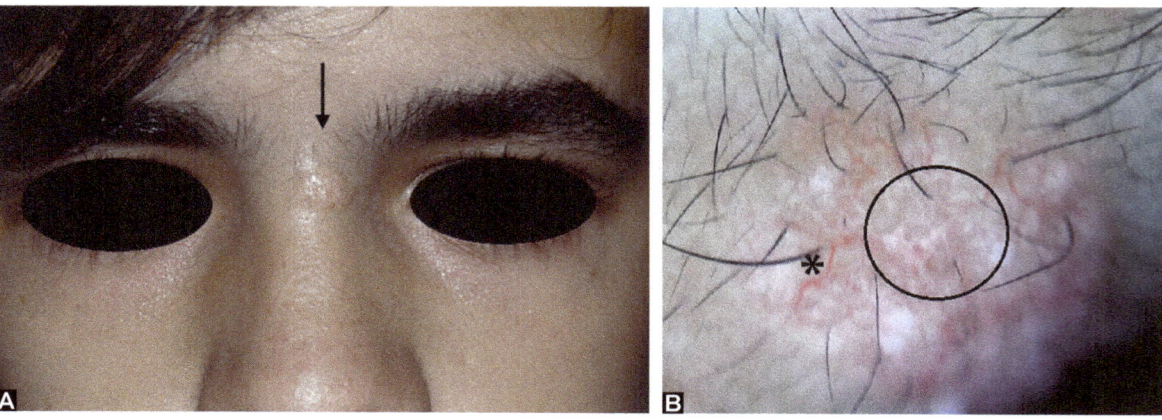

Figs. 15.11A and B: Trichoepithelioma: (A) An isolated flesh-colored papule on the front of a 14-year-old boy. (B) Dermoscopy shows in-focus arborizing vessels (*) and white shiny streaks, knows also as chrysalis (circled).

Cylindroma

It is a benign adnexal tumor that can occur as a solitary, sporadic, slow-growing, asymptomatic or painful skin-colored, bluish or reddish papule, nodule or tumor on the head and neck, or as multiple lesions mostly on the scalp, sometimes covering the entire area ("Turban tumors") in the autosomal dominant Brooke–Spiegler syndrome. Histology shows a well circumscribed lesion with islands or cords of basaloid cells in a puzzle pattern. Dermoscopy shows arborizing telangiectasia, mostly on the center of the lesion, and scattered white globules on a milky to salmon-pink background (Figs. 15.12 to 15.13).

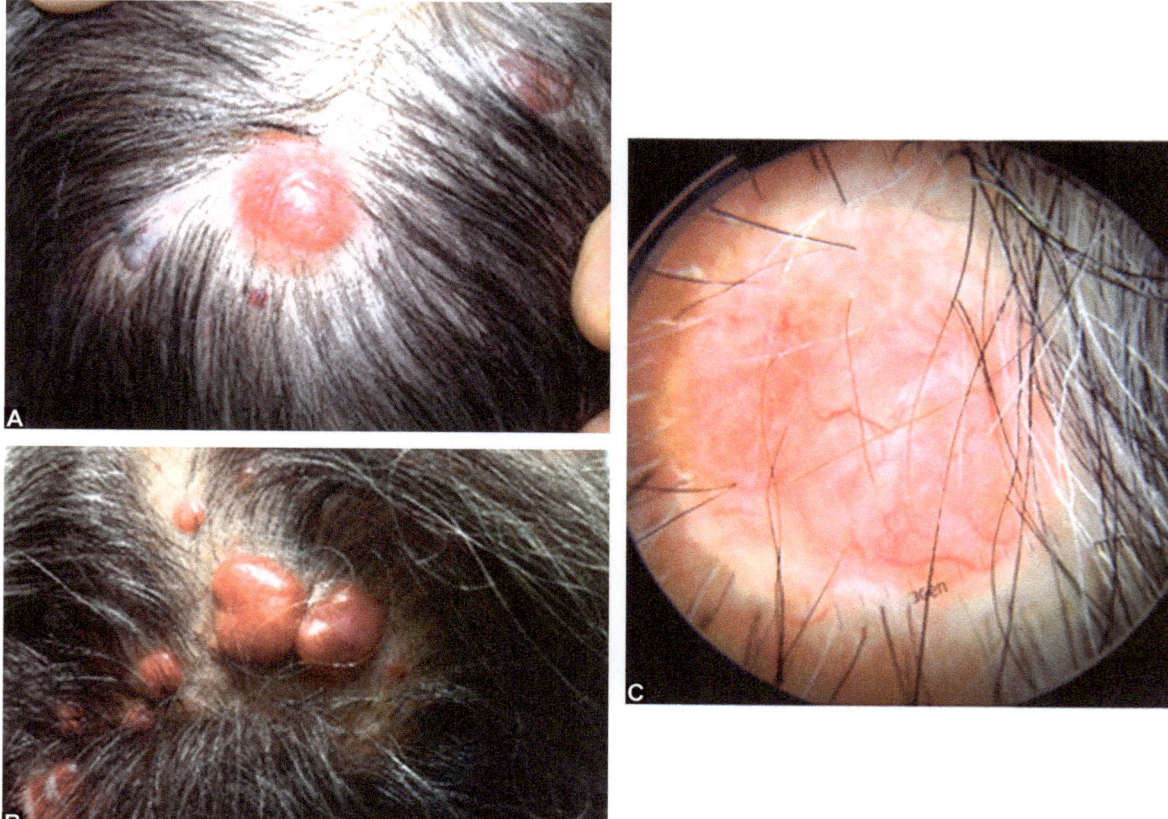

Figs. 15.12A to C: Scalp lesions. (A and B) Confluent erythematous telangiectatic nodules and papules on the scalp, consistent with spiradenocylindromas and cylindromas. (C) Dermoscopy shows arborizing telangiectasia and scattered white globules on a milky to salmon–pink background.

Source: Dr André Castro Pinho.

Nonmelanocytic Scalp Tumors

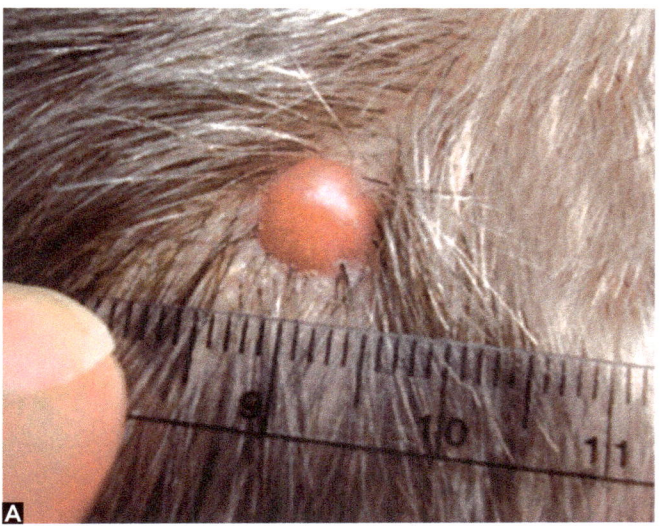
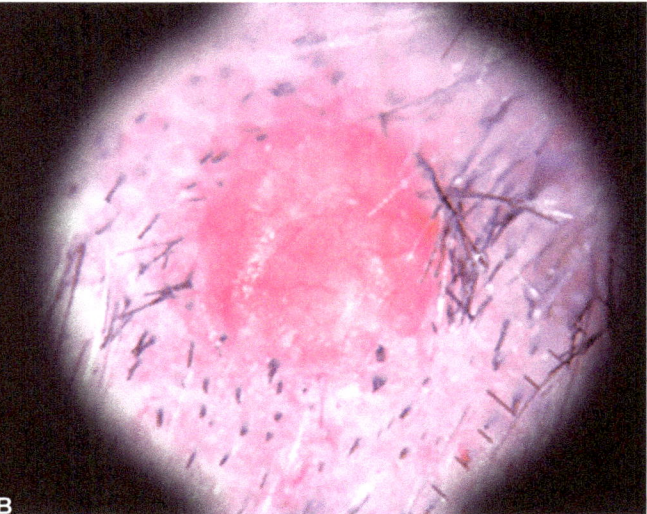

Figs. 15.13A and B: (A) Clinical view of the cylindroma on the left parietal scalp. (B) Dermoscopy shows several scattered white globules and arborizing telangiectasia on a white to salmon-pink background. The vascular branches are more pronounced at the periphery and they extend from the periphery towards the center of the lesion.

Source: Cohen YK, Elpern DJ. Dermatoscopic pattern of a cylindroma. Dermatol Pract Concept. 2014;4(1):67-8.

> **Take-Home Message**
> - Cylindroma is a benign adnexal tumor characterized by papule, nodule or tumor on the head and neck.
> - It can occur as a solitary, sporadic lesion or as multiple lesions mostly on the scalp ("Turban tumors") in Brooke–Spiegler syndrome.
> - Dermoscopic descriptions include white globules and arborizing telangiectasia on a white to salmon-pink background.

Eccrine Poroma

It is a rare adnexal tumor composed of cells similar to those of the acrosyringium. It occurs as a solitary, slow-growing, pedunculated or sessile papule or nodule, most frequently on the palms and soles. Histology reveals aggregations of uniform basaloid cells that radiate from the basal layer to the dermis. A rare description of a lesion on the scalp with its dermoscopy features is shown on Figure 15.14.

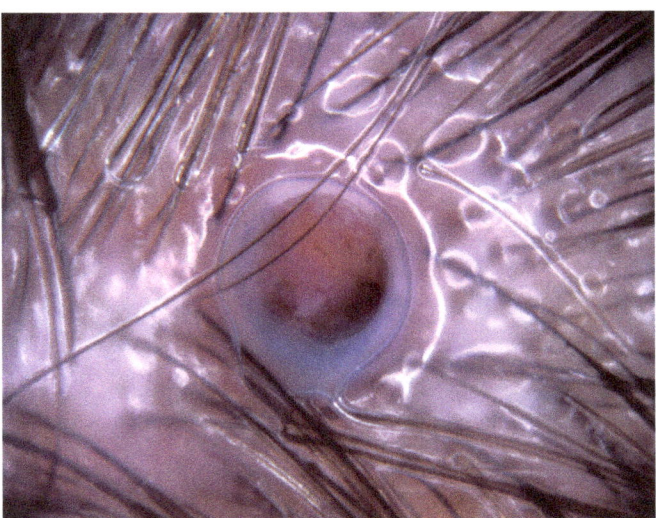

Fig. 15.14: Eccrine poroma on the scalp. Dermoscopy shows a peripheral blue–white homogeneous color with central polymorphic "out of focus" vessels.

Source: Dr Paula Ferreira (case sent for publication)

> **Take-Home Message**
> - Eccrine poroma is a rare adnexal tumor most frequently occurring on the palms and soles.
> - A rare case of a scalp lesion with a peripheral blue–white homogeneous color with central polymorphic "out of focus" vessels is described.

cystic, skin-colored or pigmented nodules, mainly located on the head and neck region and the upper extremities. Some dermoscopic findings reported in the literature are described in Figures 15.15A to C.

Pilomatrixoma

It is a benign adnexal tumor, also known as Malherbe's calcified epithelioma. It is derived from immature matrix cells and manifests most frequently as single, solid or

> **Take-Home Message**
> - Pilomatrixoma is a benign adnexal tumor most frequently located on the head and neck or upper extremities.
> - Dermoscopy shows yellowish lobules surrounded by crown-like vessels, fishing net-like streaks and polymorphous vessels.

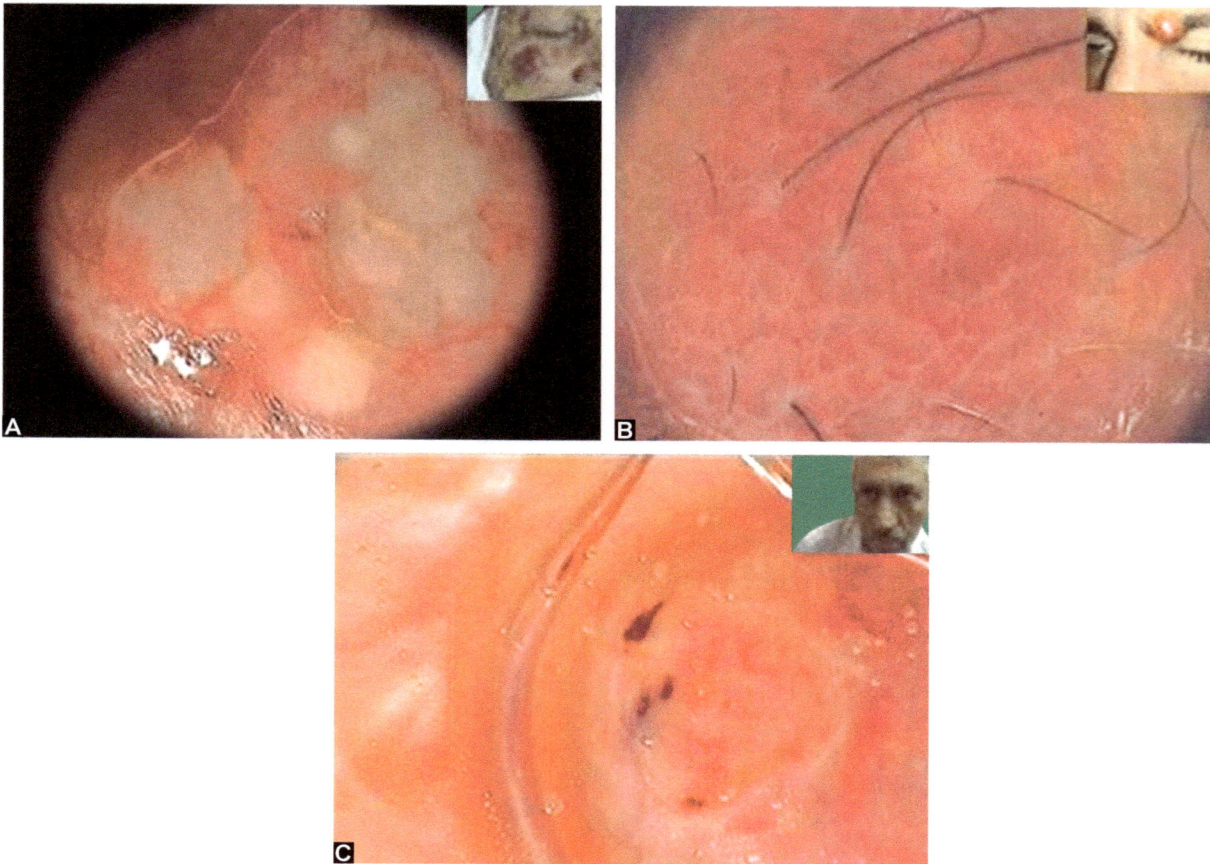

Figs. 15.15A to C: Pilomatrixoma. (A) Dermoscopy shows yellowish lobules surrounded by crown-like vessels (gross tumor is seen in the right-upper corner of the image, 10X). (B) Bluish-white fishing net-like streaks is seen in the entire image (inset of gross tumor in the right-upper corner of image, 10X). (C) Polymorphous vessels (predominated linear irregular vessels), bluish areas (left-middle side of the image) and ulcerations (inset of gross tumor in the right-upper corner of image, 10X).
Source: Ayhan E, Ertugay O, Gundogdu R. Three different dermoscopic view of three new cases with pilomatrixoma. Int J Trichology. 2014;6(1):21-2.

Epidermal Cysts

They are the most common cutaneous cysts, classically presenting as dermal or subcutaneous mobile nodules, with a central punctum (the orifice of an obstructed hair follicle), filled with keratin. Sometimes, black dots may be found surrounding the cyst (Fig. 15.16). In cases where the central punctum is not visible, dermoscopy might be a helpful tool.

VASCULAR TUMORS

Angiosarcoma

It is a rare, aggressive, malignant tumor of vascular origin that can occur in three variants—classical angiosarcoma (AS) (elderly, head and neck areas); Stewart–Treves syndrome (in areas of chronic lymphedema); and post-radiation AS. It presents as single or multiple "bruise-like"

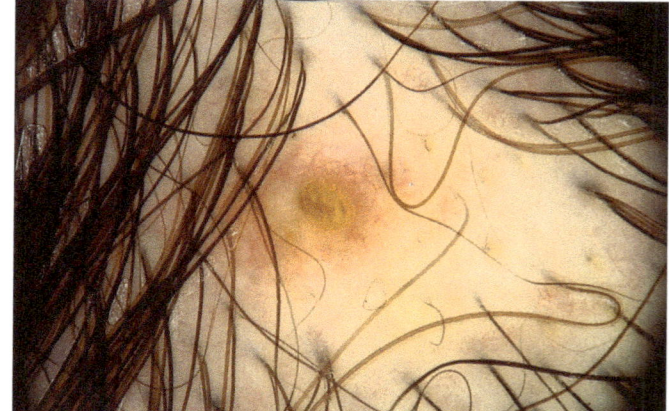

Fig. 15.16: Scalp cyst. Note the central orifice filled with keratin. Note also some black dots, yellow dots and telangiectatic vessels surrounding the lesion.
Source: Dr Isabella Doche.

patches, that become more violaceous and ill-defined with nodular areas.

On dermoscopy, the already described findings were structureless areas (without vessels or lacunae) of various colors gradations (red—light and dark, purple, blue), intermingled with white to skin-colored perifollicular areas, with white lines or white veil (on the nodular areas) (Figs. 15.17A and B).

> **Take-Home Message**
> - Angiosarcoma is a rare, aggressive, malignant vascular tumor with poor prognosis.
> - The classical variant usually presents as "bruise-like" patches or violaceous nodules on the scalp of elderly people.
> - Previous dermoscopy descriptions include structureless areas of various color gradations, intermingled with white perifollicular areas.

OTHER TUMORS

Merkel Cell Carcinoma

It is a malignant neuroendocrine carcinoma of the skin, which affects elderly people with frequent recurrences, regional and distant metastases and a high mortality rate. Lesions can have a cyst-like appearance, or a nontender rapidly growing nodule or tumor. Differential diagnosis includes cysts, BCC, amelanotic melanoma, cutaneous lymphoma and adnexal tumors. The main features in dermoscopy are irregular linear vessels, some of them long and curved (horseshoe-like structures) over a homogeneous pinkish background, or poorly and sharply focused vessels, milky-red areas, and globules with shiny white areas (Figs. 15.18A and B).

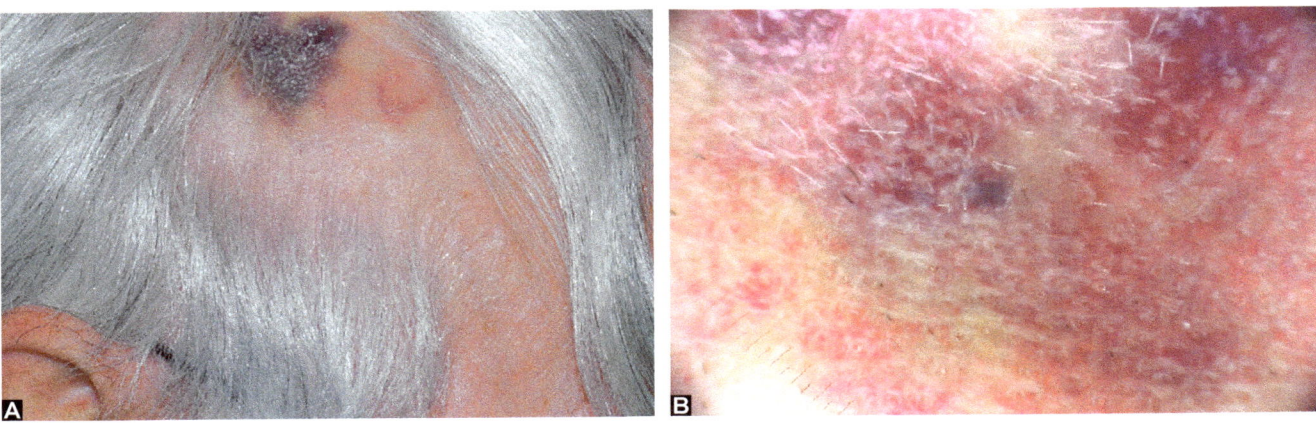

Figs. 15.17A and B: (A) Angiosarcoma on the scalp with a bruise-like appearance. (B) Dermoscopy shows structureless red-purple areas intermingled with white to yellow roundish appearing follicular openings.
Source: Dr Iris Zalaudek.

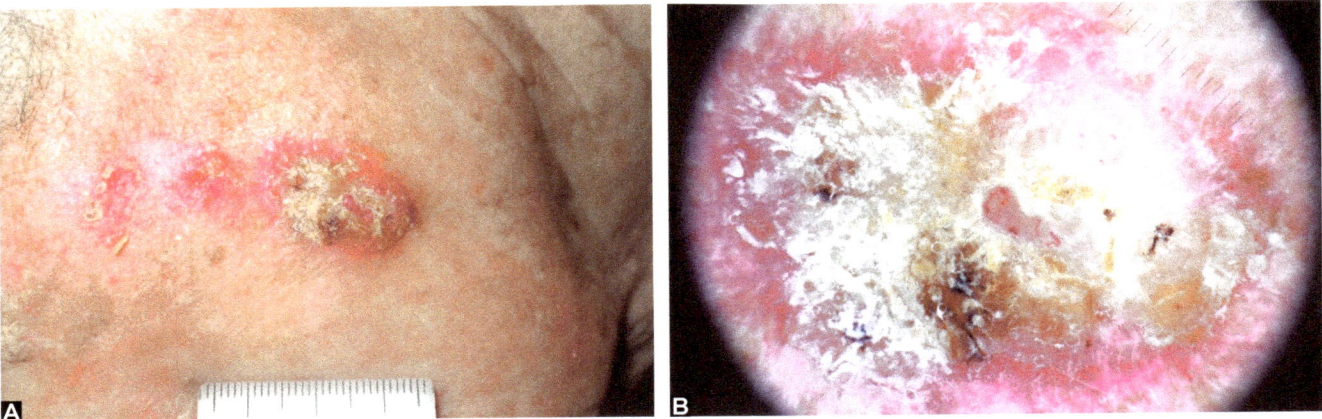

Figs. 15.18A and B: Merkel cell carcinoma. (A) Fast-growing, asymptomatic, shiny and violaceous nodule. (B) Linear irregular and polymorphous vessels, poorly focused vessels, milky-red areas, white areas, structureless areas and architectural disorder. Pigmented structures are absent. Note yellow crusts. (20X).
Source: Dr Giuseppe Argenziano.

Take-Home Message

- Merkel cell carcinoma (MCC) is a malignant neuroendocrine carcinoma of the skin with a high mortality rate.
- Dermoscopy shows irregular linear vessels, milky-red areas, and no pigmented structures.

LYMPHOPROLIFERATIVE DISORDERS

Cutaneous lymphomas represent 3.9% of all non-Hodgkin lymphomas, with mycosis fungoides (MF) representing the majority of cases. It is an indolent T-cell lymphoma that usually manifests as patches, plaques, or tumors on doubled covered areas of the body. The folliculotropic variant usually affects the face and scalp, with the development of infiltrated plaques and tumors and areas of alopecia. There is as yet no description in the literature of the findings from the dermoscopy of such lesions on the scalp, only rare reports on patches at other body areas. Clinical and dermoscopic aspects are shown on Figures 15.19 and 15.20.

Besides folliculotropic MF, another lymphoproliferative disorder, less frequent, but that usually affects the scalp, is the follicle center B-cell lymphoma. It presents as solitary or grouped erythematous plaques, nodules, and tumors, preferentially located on the scalp or forehead or on the trunk. It is also an indolent disease with rare extracutaneous dissemination. Clinically, the lesions are quite similar to secondary skin infiltration of systemic B-cell lymphomas (Figs. 15.21A and B).

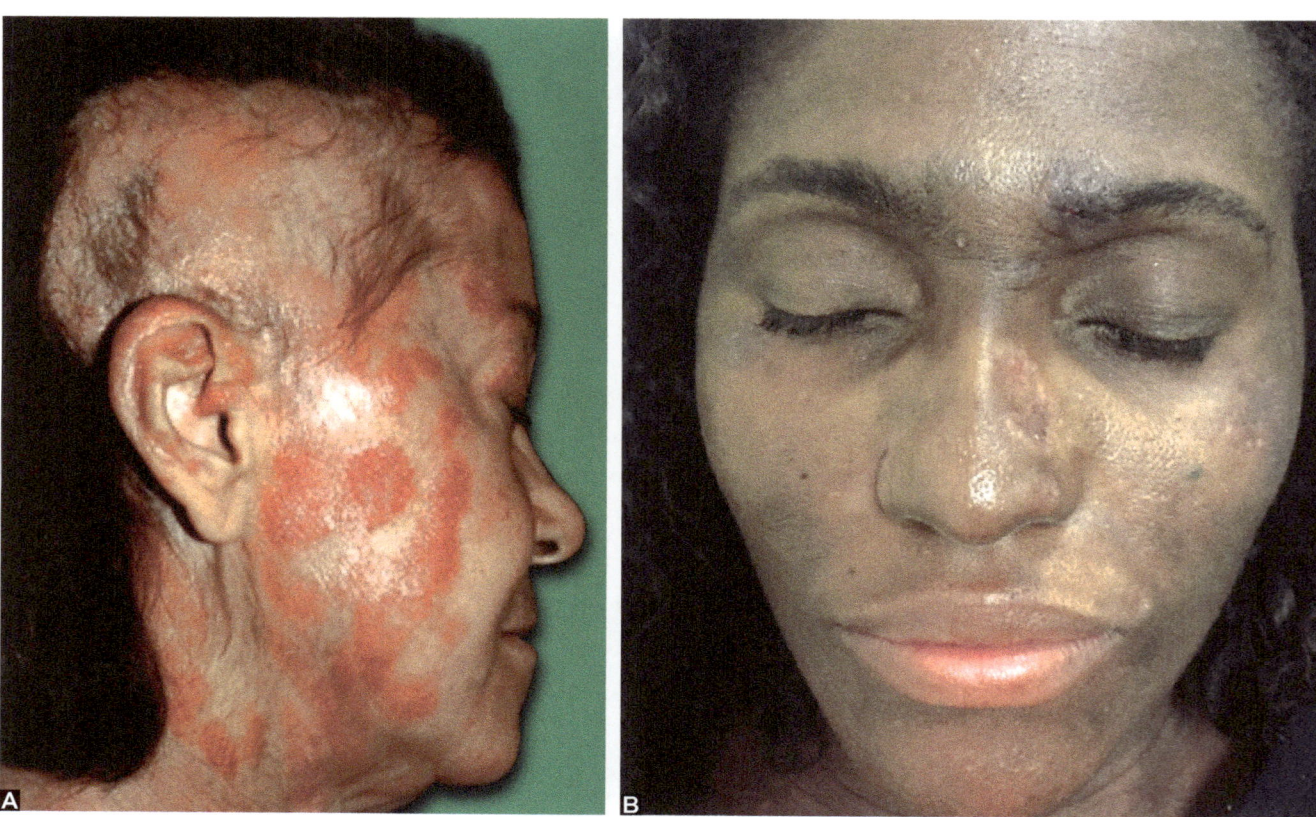

Figs. 15.19A and B: Folliculotropic mycosis fungoides. Note infiltrated plaques on the face, neck and scalp, with areas of alopecia.

Nonmelanocytic Scalp Tumors

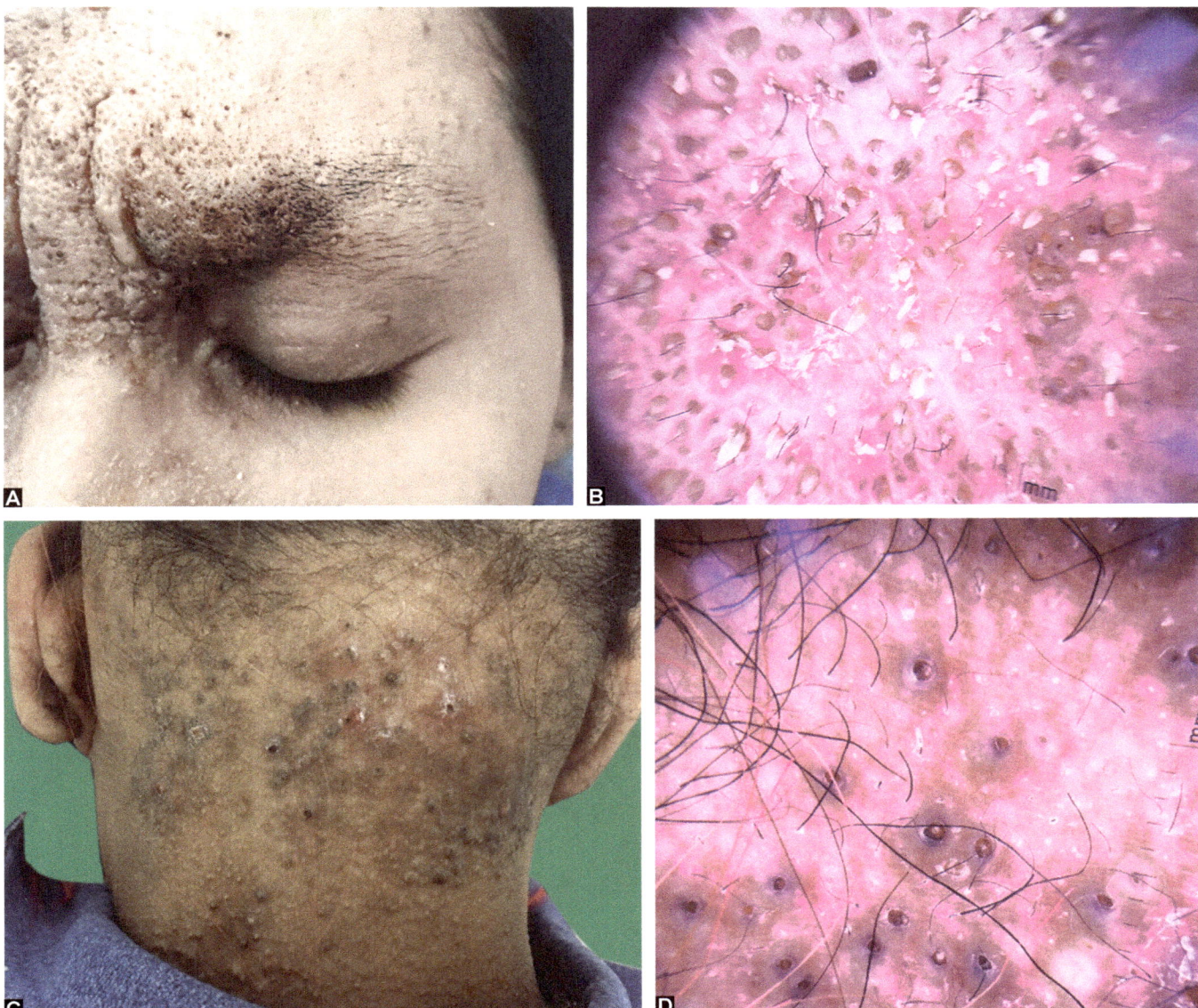

Figs. 15.20A to D: (A and C) Folliculotropic mycosis fungoides with infiltrated, follicular, and cystic lesions on the glabella and occipital area with alopecia and loss of the eyebrows. (B and D) Dermoscopy shows follicles are filled with keratin, multiple milia-like cysts and comedo-like openings.

Take-Home Message
- Mycosis fungoides is an indolent T-cell lymphoma and represents the most common form of cutaneous lymphoma.
- The folliculotropic variant usually affects the head and neck areas. Dermoscopy shows follicles filled with keratin, milia-like cysts and comedo openings and are here described.
- Cutaneous B-cell lymphoma is less frequent, but follicle center B-cell lymphoma has a predilection for the scalp, presenting as erythematous or violaceous nodules or tumors.
- Systemic lymphoproliferative diseases might also secondarily affect the skin.

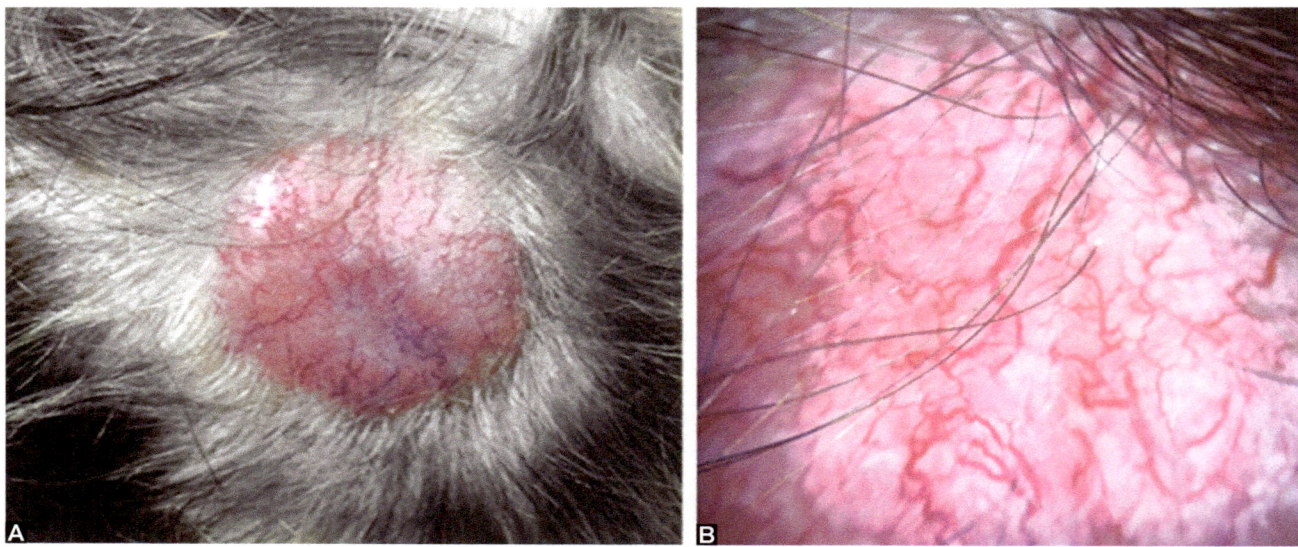

Figs. 15.21A and B: Systemic B-cell follicular lymphoma infiltrating the skin. (A) Clinically, a slow-growing erythematous tumor on the scalp. (B) Dermoscopy shows multiple arborizing telangiectasias.

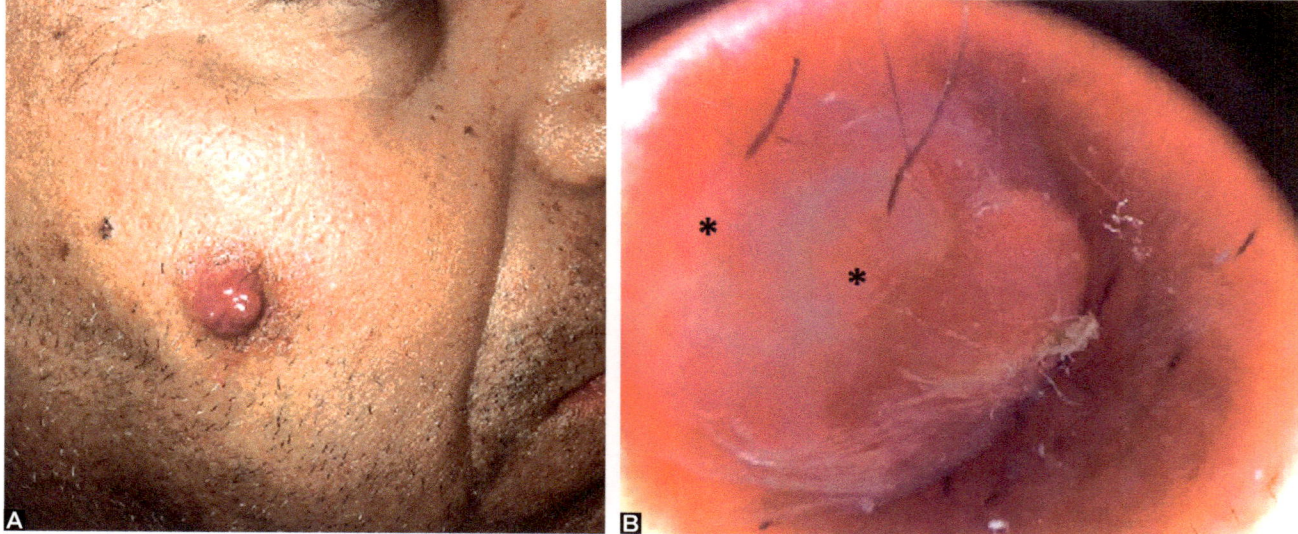

Figs. 15.22A and B: Clear cell renal carcinoma—cutaneous metastasis. (A) Clinically, a rapidly enlarging purple-red nodule on the cheek. (B) Dermoscopy shows a whitish-red color with some linear vessels (*).

CUTANEOUS METASTASIS

Cutaneous metastases are rare, occurring in 0.7–9% of solid neoplasms, with the most common primary tumor being of breast cancer, in the lung, gastrointestinal tract, uterus, and kidneys. The scalp accounts for 4–6.9% of all cutaneous metastases. They can arise by contiguity, iatrogenically or via lymphatic or hematogenic dissemination.

The clinical aspect is variable and may appear as single or multiple firm nodules, papules or plaques, usually painless. They may occur before, concurrently with or after the diagnosis of the primary neoplasia. Histologically they resemble the tumor of origin and are related to a worse prognosis. Rare dermoscopic descriptions of cutaneous metastases are available, and no specific pattern has been described so far. One example is shown in Figures 15.22A and B.

Take-Home Message
- Skin metastases from solid tumors are rare, but the scalp accounts for 4–6.9% of all cutaneous metastases.
- The clinical aspect is variable and may appear as single or multiple firm nodules, papules or plaques, usually painless.
- Dermoscopy is not specific.

SUGGESTED READING

1. Ayhan E, Ertugay O, Gundogdu R. Three different dermoscopic view of three new cases with pilomatrixoma. Int J Trichology. 2014;6(1):21-2.
2. Bruno CB, Cordeiro FN, Soares Fdo E, et al. Dermoscopic aspects of syringocystadenoma papilliferum associated with nevus sebaceus. An Bras Dermatol. 2011;86(6):1213-6.
3. Ciudad C, Avilés JA, Alfageme F, et al. Spontaneous regression in merkel cell carcinoma: report of two cases with a description of dermoscopic features and review of the literature. Dermatol Surg. 2010;36(5):687-93.
4. Cohen YK, Elpern DJ. Dermatoscopic pattern of a cylindroma. Dermatol Pract Concept. 2014;4(1):67-8.
5. Donati A, Cavelier-Balloy B, Reygagne P. Histologic correlation of dermoscopy findings in a sebaceous nevus. Cutis. 2015;96(6):E8-9.
6. Duman N, Ersoy-Evans S, Erkin Özaygen G, et al. Syringocystadenoma papilliferum arising on naevus sebaceus: a 6-year-old child case described with dermoscopic features. Australas J Dermatol. 2015;56(2):e53-4.
7. Ghigliotti G, De Col E, parodi A, Bombonato C, et al. Trichoblastoma: is a clinical or dermoscopic diagnosis possible? J Eur Acad Dermatol Venereol. 2016;30(11):1978-80.
8. Laureano A, Cunha D, Pernandes C, et al. Dermoscopy in Merkel cell carcinoma: a case report. Dermatol Online J. 2014;20(2):21543.
9. Lin MJ, Pan Y, Jalilian C, et al. Dermoscopic characteristics of nodular squamous cell carcinoma and keratoacanthoma. Dermatol Pract Concept. 2014;4(2):2.
10. Minagawa A, Koga H, Okuyama R. Vascular structure absence under dermoscopy in two cases of angiosarcoma on the scalp. Int J Dermatol. 2014;53(7):e350-2.
11. Mun JH, Park SM, Kim TW, et al. Importance of keen observation for the diagnosis of epidermal cysts: dermoscopy can be a useful adjuvant tool. J Am Acad Dermatol. 2014;71(4):e138-40.
12. Navarrete-Dechent C, Bajaj S, Marghoob AA, et al. Multiple familial trichoepithelioma: confirmation via dermoscopy. Dermatol Pract Concept. 2016;6(3):51-4.
13. Neri I, Savoia F, Giacomini F, et al. Usefulness of dermatoscopy for the early diagnosis of sebaceous naevus and differentiation from aplasia cutis congenita. Clin Exp Dermatol. 2009;34(5):e50-2.
14. Oiso N, Matsuda H, Kawada A. Various colour gradations as a dermatoscopic feature of cutaneous angiosarcoma of the scalp. Australas J Dermatol. 2013;54(1):36-8.
15. Pinho AC, Gouveia MJ, Gameiro AR, et al. Brooke-Spiegler syndrome—an underrecognized cause of multiple familial scalp tumors: report of a new germline mutation. J Dermatol Case Rep. 2015;9(3):67-70.
16. Picard A, Tsilika K, Cardot-Leccia N, et al. Trichoblastoma with dermoscopic features of a malignant tumor: three cases. J Am Acad Dermatol. 2014;71(3):e63-4.
17. Richmond HM, Duvic M, Macfarlane DF. Primary and metastatic malignant tumors of the scalp: an update. Am J Clin Dermatol. 2010;11(4):233-46.
18. Salemis NS, Veloudis G, Spiliopoulos K, et al. Scalp metastasis as the first sign of small-cell lung cancer: management and literature review. Int Surg. 2014;99(4):325-9.
19. Stanganelli I, Argenziano G, Sera F, et al. Dermoscopy of scalp tumours: a multi-centre study conducted by the international Dermoscopy society. J Eur Acad Dermatol Venereol. 2012;26(8):953-63.
20. Soares GH, Lallas A, Lombardi M, et al. Cutaneous metastasis of renal carcinoma. J Am Acad Dermatol. 2015;72(1 Suppl):S45-6.
21. Suppa M, Micantonio T, Di Stefani A, et al. Dermoscopic variability of basal cell carcinoma according to clinical type and anatomic location. J Eur Acad Dermatol Venereol. 2015;29(9):1732-41.
22. Warszawik-Hendzel O, Olszewska M, Maj M, et al. Non-invasive diagnostic techniques in the diagnosis of squamous cell carcinoma. J Dermatol Case Rep. 2015;9(4):89-97.
23. Zalaudek I, Gomez-Moyano E, Landi C, et al. Clinical, dermoscopic and histopathological features of spontaneous scalp or face and radiotherapy-induced angiosarcoma. Australas J Dermatol. 2013;54(3):201-7.

CHAPTER 16

Melanocytic Scalp Tumors

Maximilian Uranitsch, Roberta Giuffrida, Iris Zalaudek

MELANOMA

Maximilian Uranitsch, Roberta Giuffrida, Iris Zalaudek

PRIMARY SCALP MELANOMA

Primary scalp melanoma is referred to as the "invisible killer" because of its unnoticed growth and poorer prognosis compared with thickness-matched melanomas of the trunk. Advanced age, male sex, and scalp subsite all portend poor prognosis in patients with cutaneous head and neck melanoma.

Although scalp melanoma is a rare condition, it is mandatory that dermatologists perform scalp inspections during dermatological examinations, in order to detect lesions early. Dermoscopy should be considered standard of care in the diagnosis and management of scalp tumors.

Breslow thickness, mitotic rate, ulceration, satellitosis, and regional nodal status are recognized as important prognostic features that guide management algorithms. Recent evidence supports the clinical observation that primary melanoma occurring in the head and neck is associated with worse rates of locoregional disease control and overall survival.

The prevailing dermoscopic patterns of scalp melanoma depend on the tumor type, growth rate, and thickness. Atypical pseudonetwork or (atypical) network pattern of brown to black color and regression is predictive for thin scalp melanomas (Figs. 16.1A and B). Thin scalp melanoma often also shows an area of regression or diffuse hypopigmentation. Thick, fast-growing, nodular melanoma often lacks specific dermoscopic patterns; yet, its diagnosis relies mostly on a history of rapid growth and the dermoscopic presence of different shades of blue and black (Figs. 16.2A and B).

It is recommended to follow a very low biopsy threshold for thick scalp melanoma, as they can mimic a wide range of benign skin tumors. Thin scalp melanoma may have similar details to regressing seborrheic keratosis and pigmented actinic keratosis. Therefore, a biopsy of all flat scalp tumors showing regression (even in the absence of melanoma specific criteria) is recommended in order not to overlook any melanomas. Early detection and prompt treatment are the best options for improving the survival of scalp melanoma. It always must be considered when performing a regular examination that higher age and male sex raise the probability of melanoma.

Melanocytic Scalp Tumors

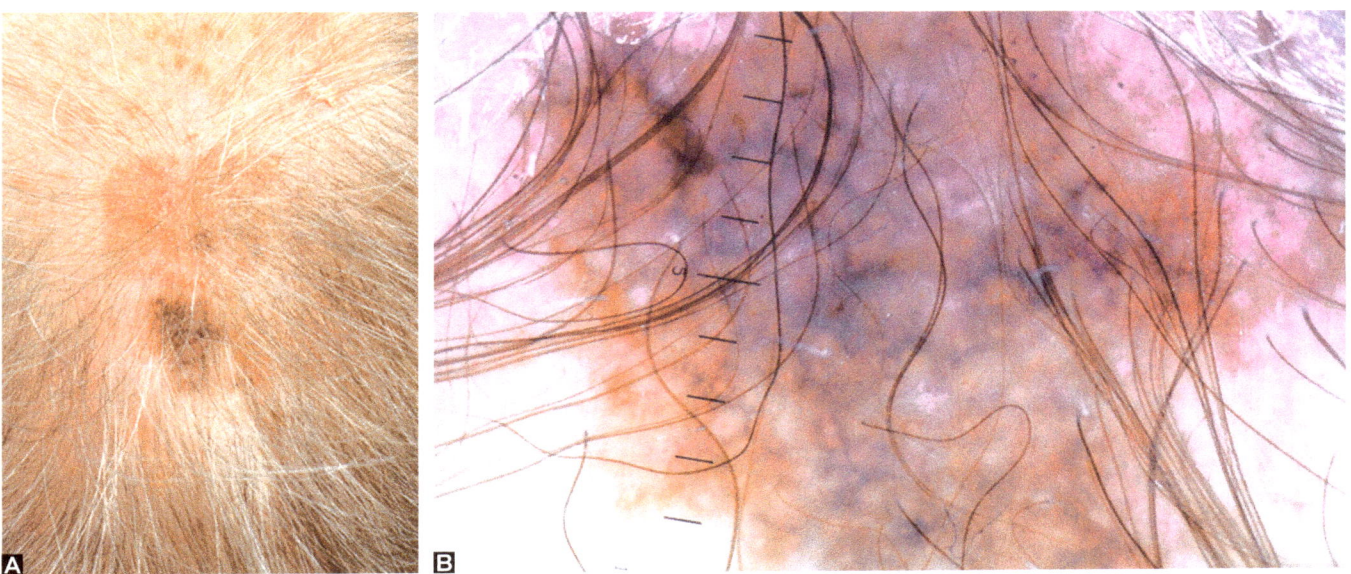

Figs. 16.1A and B: (A) Minimal invasive scalp melanoma (tumor thickness 0.5 mm). (B) Dermoscopy shows structureless brown pattern and extensive areas of regression seen as white and gray areas.

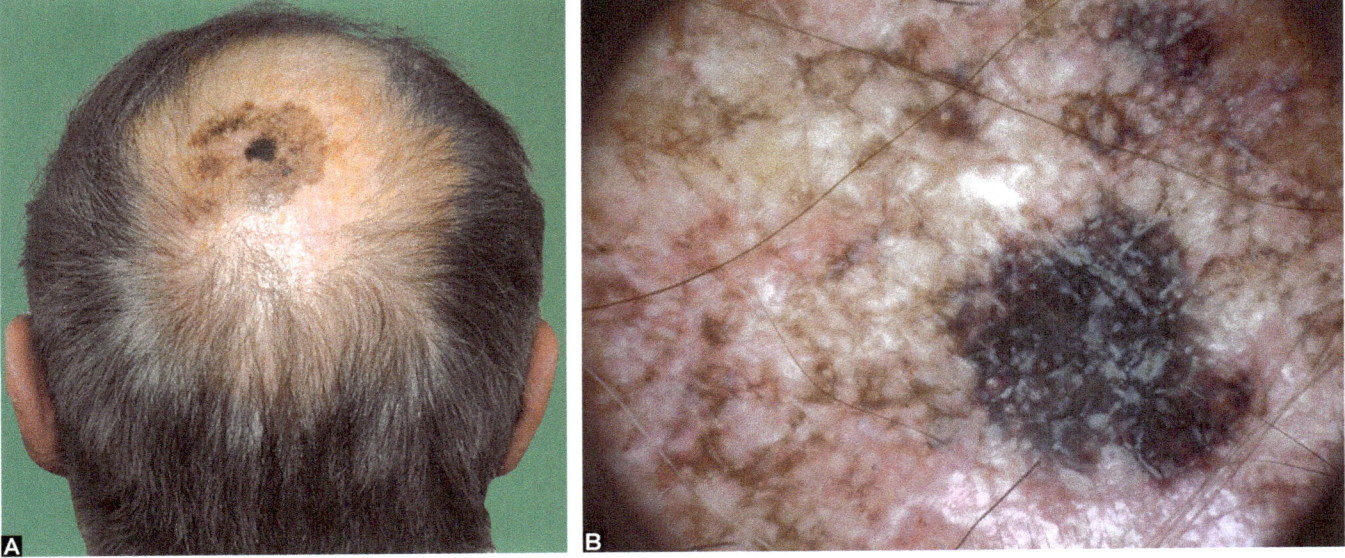

Figs. 16.2A and B: (A) Invasive melanoma (tumor thickness >2 mm). (B) Dermoscopy of the invasive area (corresponding to central blue hyperpigmentation in Figs. 16.1A and B) reveals structureless blue areas with white thick lines (seen only under polarized dermoscopy) whereas the more superficial areas show structureless brown and gray patterns.

Take-Home Message
- Primary melanoma occurring in the head and neck is associated with worst prognosis.
- Atypical pseudonetwork or atypical network pattern of brown to black color and regression is predictive for thin scalp melanomas.
- Thin scalp melanoma often also shows an area of regression or diffuse hypopigmentation.
- Thick, fast-growing, nodular melanoma often lacks specific dermoscopic patterns; yet, its diagnosis relies mostly on a history of rapid growth and the dermoscopic presence of different shades of blue and black.

BENIGN TUMORS

Maximilian Uranitsch, Roberta Giuffrida, Iris Zalaudek

The scalp is a site with predilection for benign lesions, but histologically, atypical nevi demonstrate varying levels of architectural disorder. For this reason, scalp nevi are also commonly referred to as nevi with site-related atypia. Importantly, the histopathological atypia does not translate into a higher risk of malignant transformation as the great majority of scalp nevi have a completely benign course.

Scalp nevi also appear to be indicators for an above average total nevus count and are often seen in so-called "moly" children. Scalp nevi are significantly associated with younger age, male sex, and the presence of atypical nevi elsewhere on the body. Based on specific clinical and dermoscopic patterns, scalp nevi can be classified into six main groups—(1) common, (2) papillomatous, (3) eclipse, (4) congenital, (5) blue, and (6) unclassifiable (atypical) nevus.

Common nevi present clinically flat, slightly elevated or nodular, dome-shaped nevus with an overall symmetric appearance and textured or smooth surface. Dermoscopically if flat, they are characterized by a structureless brown pattern or a reticular pattern. Sometimes, hypopigmented hair follicles may cause some clinical border irregularity (Figs. 16.3A and B). If raised, their dermoscopic aspect is that of a nonpigmented skin-colored nodule without any specific patterns.

Papillomatous nevi are raised to nodular tumors with a papillomatous surface. Upon dermoscopy, a clod (cobblestone) pattern with color variegations from brown to gray can be seen. In cases of hypopigmented tumors, curved (comma) vessels can be often seen within the papilla (Figs. 16.4A and B). Sometimes, these nevi can also show marked hyperkeratosis (Figs. 16.5A and B).

Eclipse nevi are composed by a hypopigmented center and surrounded by a pigmented brown rim, which may exhibit a reticular or structureless brown pattern under dermoscopy (Figs. 16.6A and B).

Congenital nevi are defined as present since birth or development within the first 2 years of postnatal life (Figs. 16.7A and B). They are often large (>6 mm) and exhibit dermoscopically a brown clod (globular) pattern with a uniform or central hyperpigmented pigment distribution.

Blue nevi may be challenging because of color variegations of structureless blue, white, and brown colors (Figs. 16.8A and B). Moreover, elongated or dotted vessels may be additionally seen. They are important simulators for melanoma and the threshold for biopsy should be particularly lowered if there is a missing convincing, subjective history of a long-standing and unmodified presence.

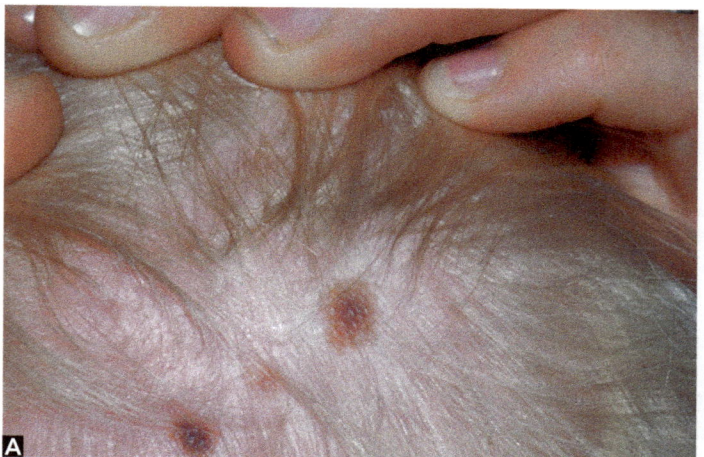 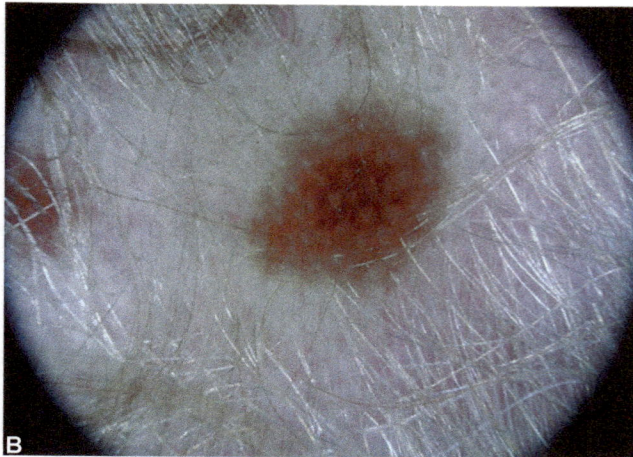

Figs. 16.3A and B: (A) Common nevus. (B) Dermoscopy shows a regular network and perifollicular hypopigmentation.

If a nevus shows none of the above-mentioned patterns of benign nevi, they are referred to as atypical or unclassifiable nevi (Figs. 16.9A and B). They may show asymmetry in shape, border irregularity, often more than three colors, or a diameter greater than 6 mm. Dermoscopically, these nevi exhibit asymmetry of colors and structures. Such lesions should be excised to rule out melanoma.

Scalp nevi show some age-related differences. They are commonly flat and pigmented in children, while being raised and nonpigmented in adults. This observation is important as it implies that any flat, pigmented macule on the scalp in an adult should raise the index of suspicion for melanoma even in the absence of other melanoma-specific features (Figs. 16.10A and B).

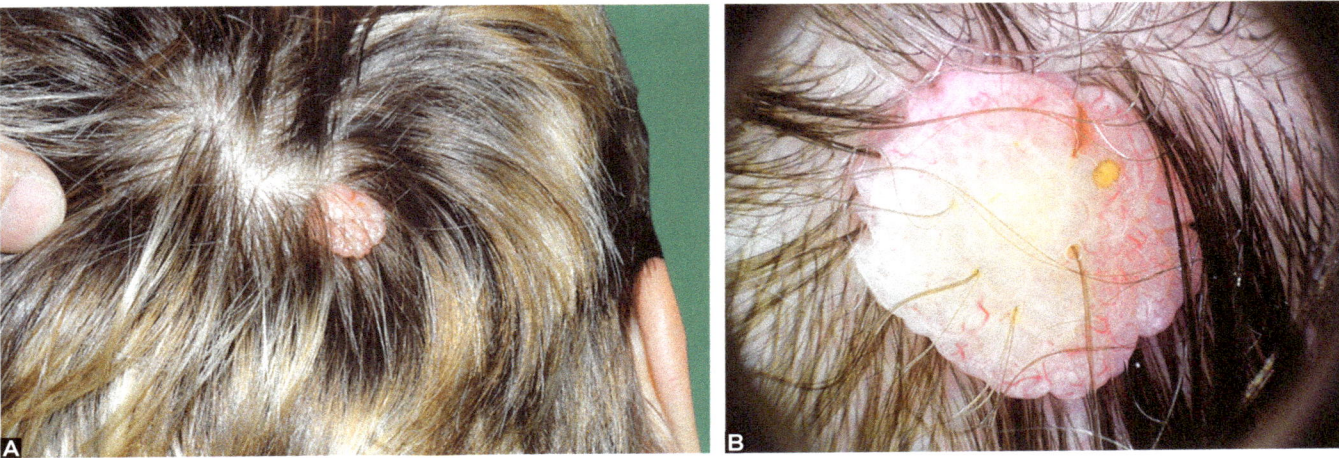

Figs. 16.4A and B: (A) Hypopigmented papillomatous nevus. (B) Dermoscopy shows monomorphous curved (comma-shaped) vessels that vary in size and diameter but not in their morphology.

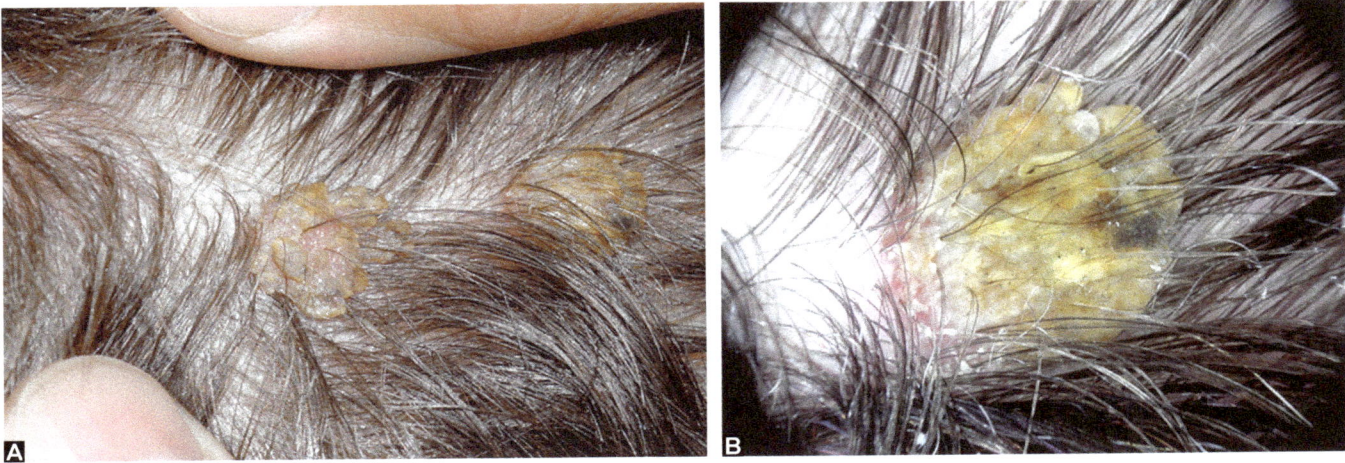

Figs. 16.5A and B: (A) Hypopigmented papillomatous nevus showing marked hyperkeratosis. (B) Dermoscopy shows structureless amorphous areas.

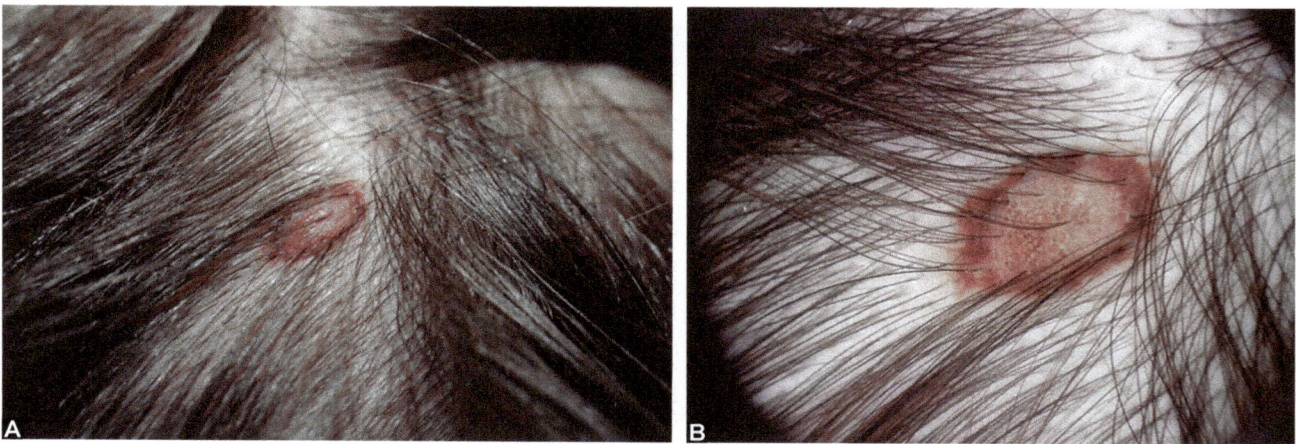

Figs. 16.6A and B: (A) Eclipse nevus. (B) Dermoscopy reveals a central elevated and hypopigmented are surrounded by rim of brown pigmentation with brown lines.

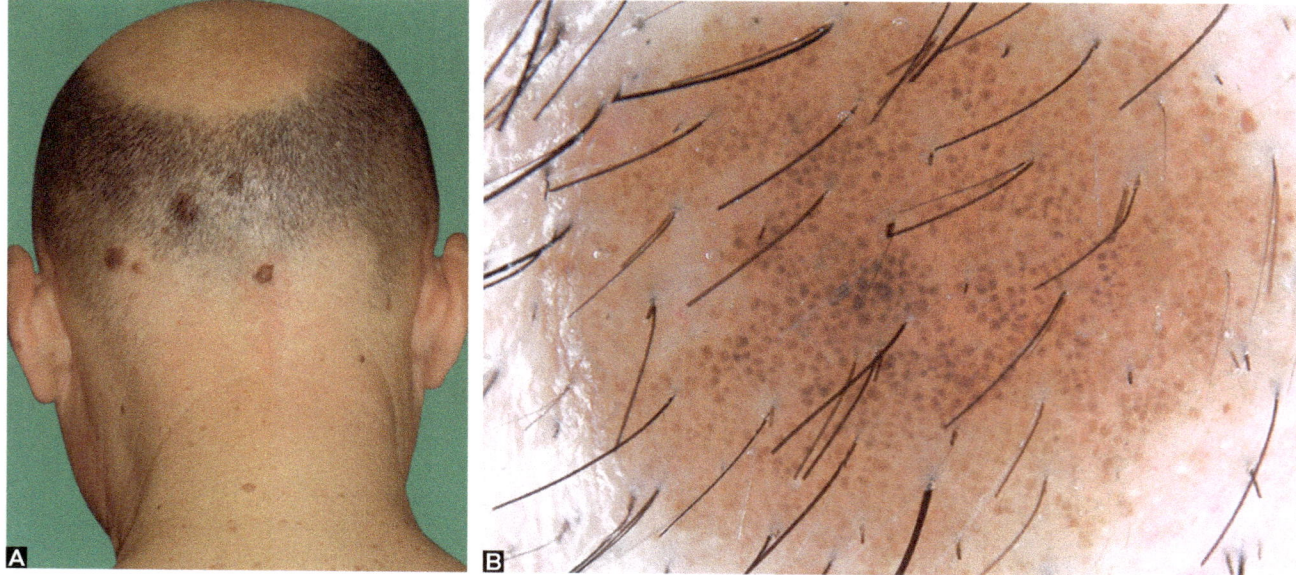

Figs. 16.7A and B: (A) Congenital nevus. (B) Dermoscopy shows regular brown clods (globules).

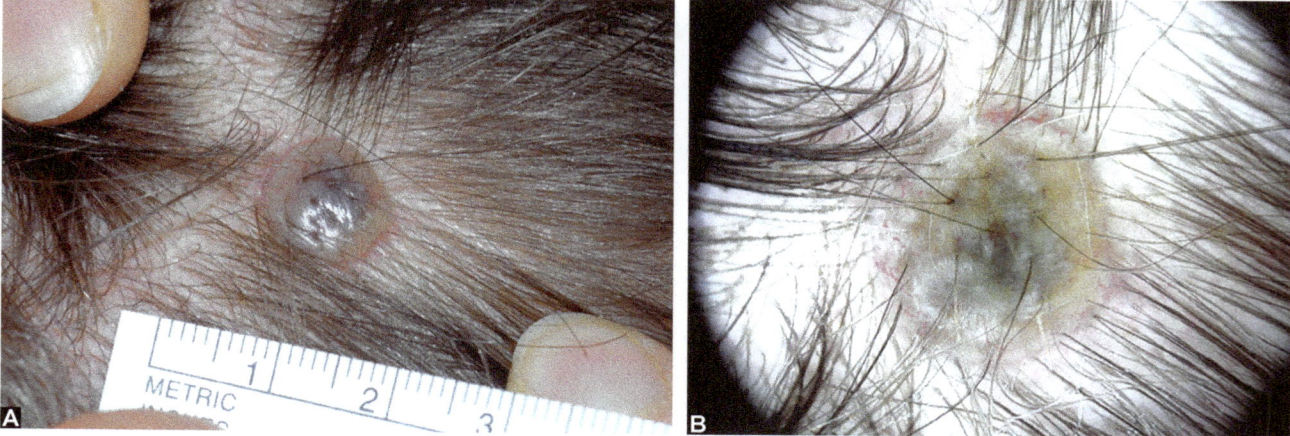

Figs. 16.8A and B: (A) Blue nevus. (B) Dermoscopy of a blue nevus showing color variegations and polymorphic vessels.

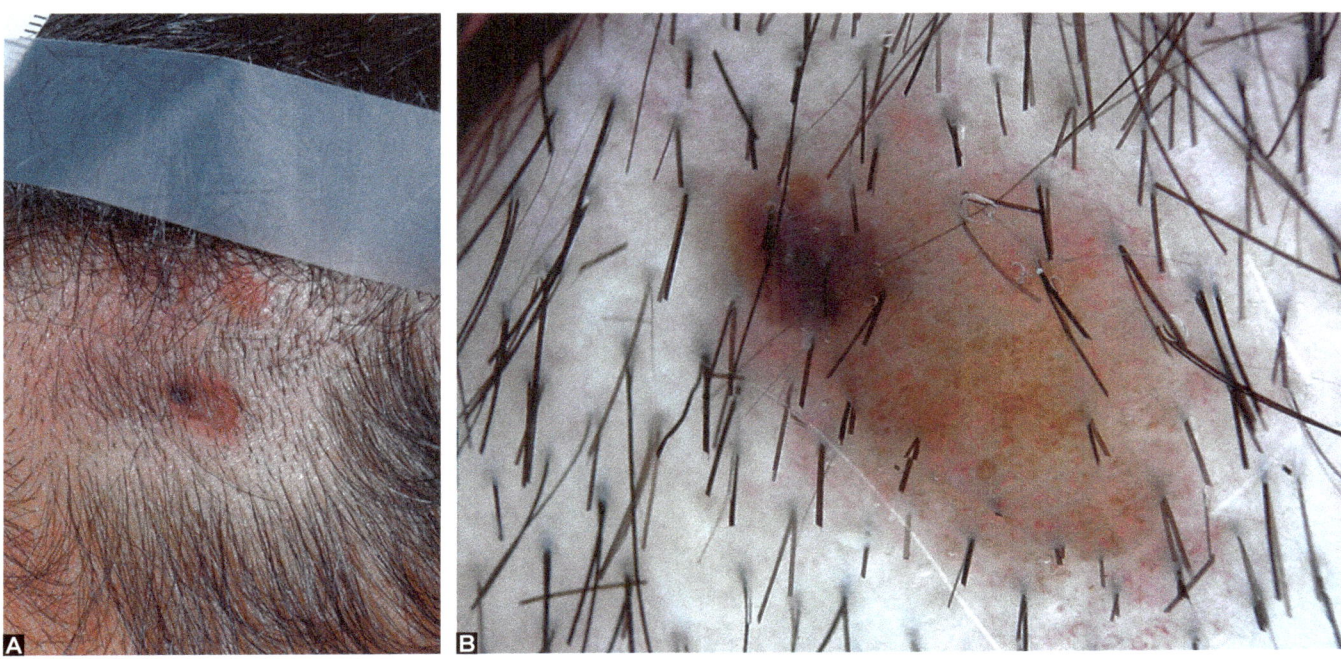

Figs. 16.9A and B: (A) Unclassified nevus. (B) Dermoscopic patterns of the nevus do not fit with any of the other benign nevus patterns.

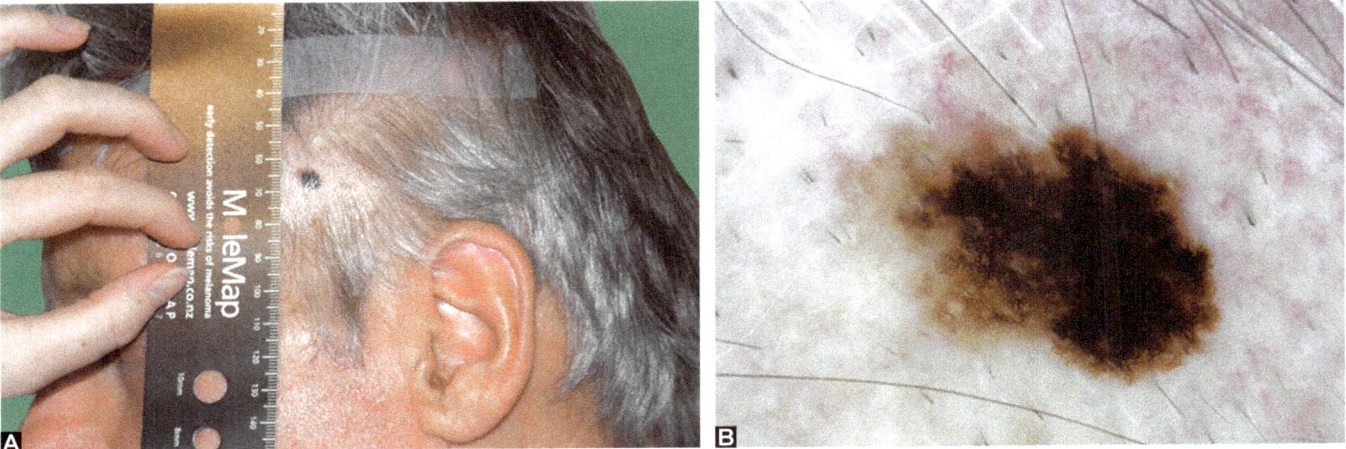

Figs. 16.10A and B: (A) In situ melanoma presenting as pigmented flat macule on the scalp of an adult. (B) Dermoscopy exhibits a more or less typical network and some irregular brown-black pigmentation. The clue to the diagnosis in this case is that a heavily pigmented macule on the scalp in this age is a highly unusual finding.

Take-Home Message

- Benign lesions may show varying levels of architectural disorder even on histopathology.
- Types: Common, papillomatous, eclipse, congenital, blue, and unclassifiable (atypical) nevus.
- Scalp nevi are commonly flat and pigmented in children, while being raised and nonpigmented in adults.

SUGGESTED READING

1. Argenziano G, Longo C, Cameron A, et al. Blue-black rule: a simple dermoscopic clue to recognize pigmented nodular melanoma. Br J Dermatol. 2011;165(6):1251-5.
2. Balch CM, Gershenwald JE, Soong SJ, et al. Final version of 2009 AJCC melanoma staging and classification. J Clin Oncol. 2009;27(36):6199-206.

3. Benmeir P, Baruchin A, Lusthaus S, et al. Melanoma of the scalp: the invisible killer. Plast Reconstr Surg. 1995;95(3):496-500.
4. De Giorgi V, Sestini S, Grazzini M, et al. Prevalence and distribution of melanocytic naevi on the scalp: a prospective study. Br J Dermatol. 2010;162:345-9.
5. Gandini S, Sera F, Cattaruzza MS, et al. Meta-analysis of risk factors for cutaneous melanoma: common and atypical naevi. Eur J Cancer. 2005;41(1):28-44.
6. Ferrara G, Soyer HP, Malvehy J, et al. The many faces of blue nevus: a clinicopathologic study. J Cutan Pathol. 2007;34(7):543-51.
7. Hosler GA, Moresi JM, Barrett TL. Nevi with site-related atypia: a review of melanocytic nevi with atypical histologic features based on anatomic site. J Cutan Pathol. 2008;35(10):889-98.
8. Kadakia S, Chan D, Mourad M, et al. The prognostic value of age, sex, and subsite in cutaneous head and neck melanoma: a clinical review of recent literature. Iran J Cancer Prev. 2016;9(3):e5079.
9. Lachiewicz AM, Berwick M, Wiggins CL, et al. Survival differences between patients with scalp or neck melanoma and those with melanoma of other sites in the surveillance, epidemiology, and end results (SEER) program. Arch Dermatol. 2008;144:515-21.
10. Stanganelli I, Argenziano G, Sera F, et al. Dermoscopy of scalp tumours: a multi-centre study conducted by the international dermoscopy society. J Eur Acad Dermatol Venereol. 2012:26(8):953-63.
11. Torres F, Fabbrocini G, Hirata SH, et al. Dermoscopy of scalp melanoma: report of three cases. Cancers. 2010;2(3):1597-601.
12. Tosti A, Pazzaglia M, Piraccini BM. Scalp tumors. In: Blume-Peytavi U, Tosti A, Whiting DA (Eds). Hair Growth and Disorders. Berlin: Springer; 2008. pp. 380-7.
13. Zalaudek I, Argenziano G, Ferrara G, et al. Clinically equivocal melanocytic skin lesions with features of regression: a dermoscopic-pathological study. Br J Dermatol. 2004;150(1):64-71.
14. Zalaudek I, Leinweber B, Sawyer HP, et al. Dermoscopic features of melanoma on the scalp. J Am Acad Dermatol. 2004;51:S88-90.
15. Zalaudek I, Schmid K, Niederkorn, et al. Proposal for a clinical–dermoscopic classification of scalp naevi. Br J Dermatol. 2014;170:1065-72.

CHAPTER 17

Pearls and Pitfalls

Isabella Doche, Giselle Martins, Patricia Damasco

INTRODUCTION

Trichoscopy may be tricky sometimes. Some cosmetics, contact gels, and artifacts may mimic similar structures and lead to a misdiagnosis. In this chapter, we will review the main pitfalls in trichoscopy and discuss some pearls to enhance the visualization of typical findings and features.

STEROID DEPOSITS AND MILIA

The steroid deposits and multiple milia are shown in Figures 17.1A and B.

MOLLUSCUM CONTAGIOSUM AND SEBACEOUS HYPERPLASIA

Molluscum contagiosum and sebaceous hyperplasia are shown in Figures 17.2A and B.

HAIR FIBERS (CAMOUFLAGE PRODUCTS) AND BROKEN HAIRS

The hair fibers (camouflage products) and broken hairs are shown in Figures 17.3A and B.

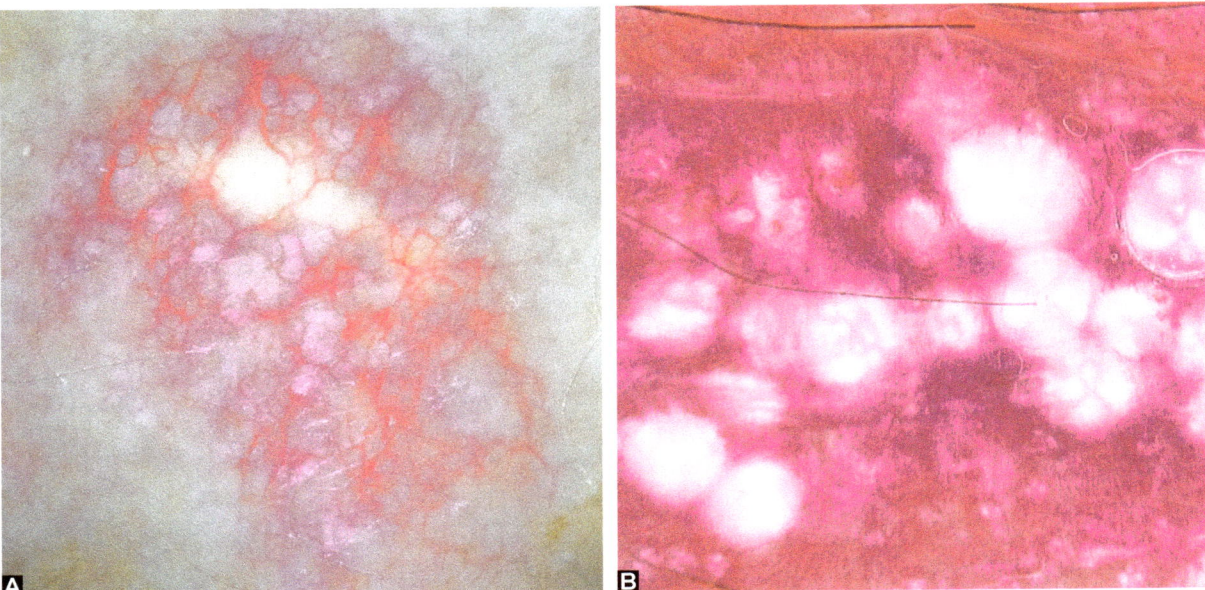

Figs. 17.1A and B: (A) Yellowish deposits in an atrophic skin after steroid injections. Note the multiple telangiectasia. (B) Multiple milia lesions in a patient with acquired epidermolysis bullosa. Note the whitish round structures.
Source: Division of Dermatology, Hospital das Clínicas, University of São Paulo Medical School.

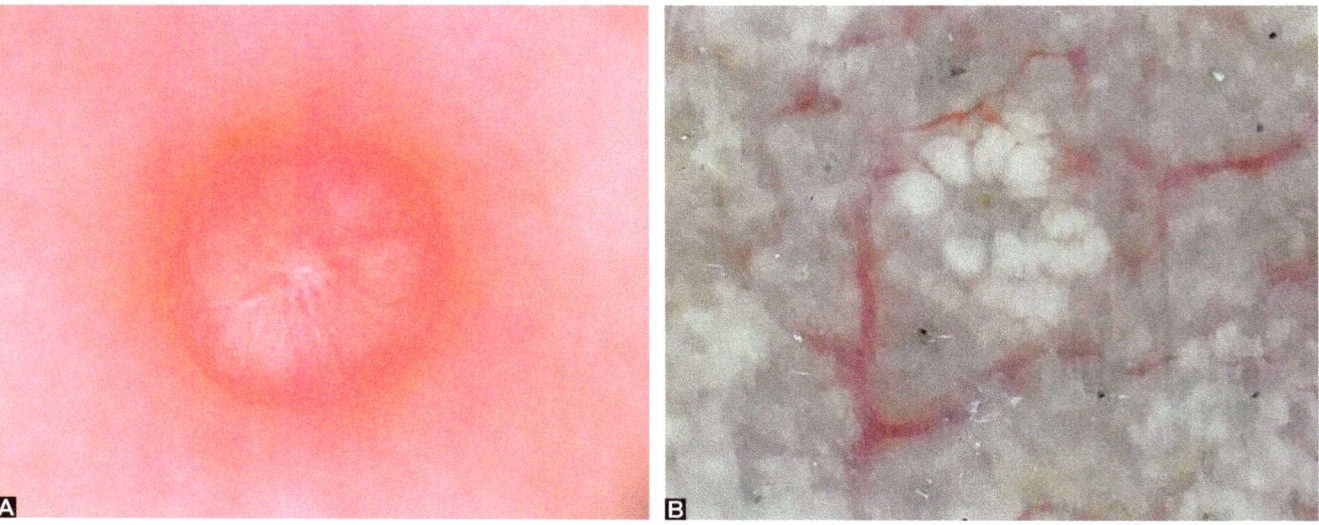

Figs. 17.2A and B: (A) Molluscum contagiosum. Peripheral crown vessels with a radial distribution and some amorphous white-yellowish polylobular structures in the center of the lesion. (B) Sebaceous hyperplasia. Crown vessels, telangiectasias with central polylobulated white-yellowish areas that do not cross the center of the lesion, where the ostium of the gland is seen as a small crater.
Source: (A) Marina Lino Vieira.

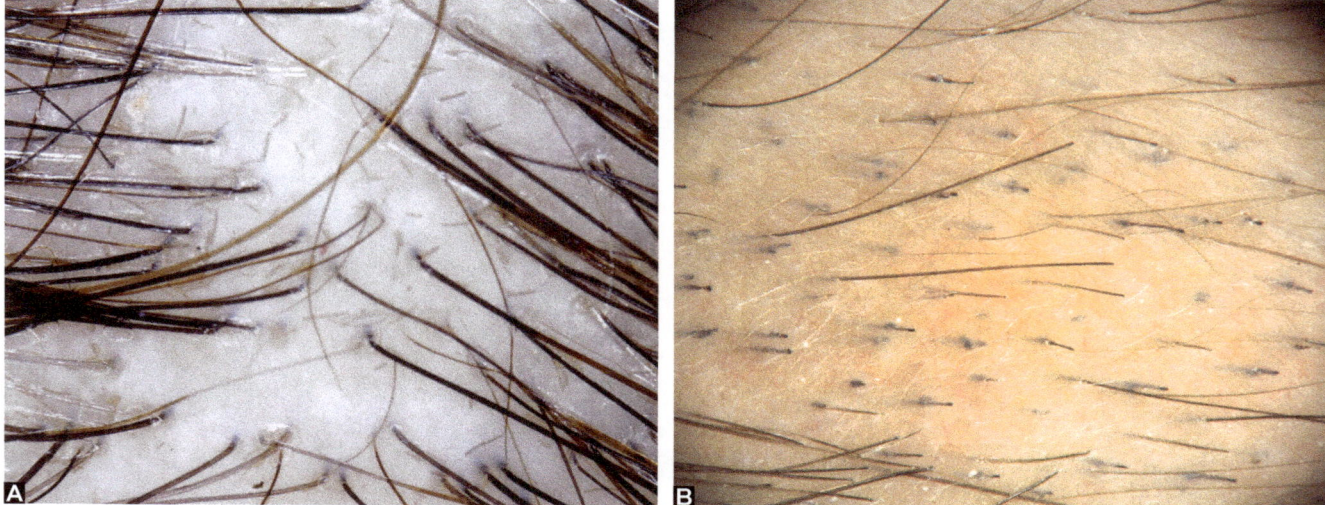

Figs. 17.3A and B: (A) Hair fibers. Note monomorphous residues of camouflage product over the scalp. No black dots are seen. (B) Multiple broken hairs in a patient with trichotillomania. Note broken hairs at variable lengths and black dots.

HAIR POWDER (CAMOUFLAGE PRODUCTS) AND GRAIN-LIKE STRUCTURES IN CHEMOTHERAPY-INDUCED ALOPECIA

Hair powder (camouflage products) and grain-like structures in chemotherapy-induced alopecia are shown in Figures 17.4A and B.

PERIPILAR SIGN AND HAIR DYE

The peripilar sign and hair dye are shown in Figures 17.5A and B.

SCATTERED BROWN SKIN IN SCARRING ALOPECIAS AND HAIR DYE

The scattered brown skin in scarring alopecias and hair dye are shown in Figures 17.6A and B.

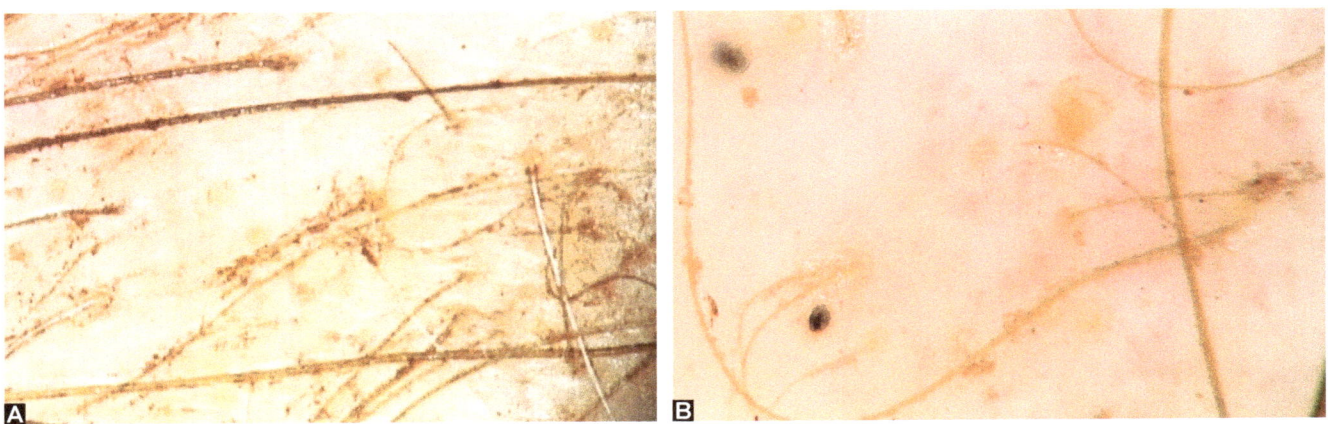

Figs. 17.4A and B: (A) Multiple residues of hair powder can be seen attached to the hair shafts and to the scalp. (B) In chemotherapy-induced alopecia, some grain-like structures can be found surrounding defective regrowing hair shafts.

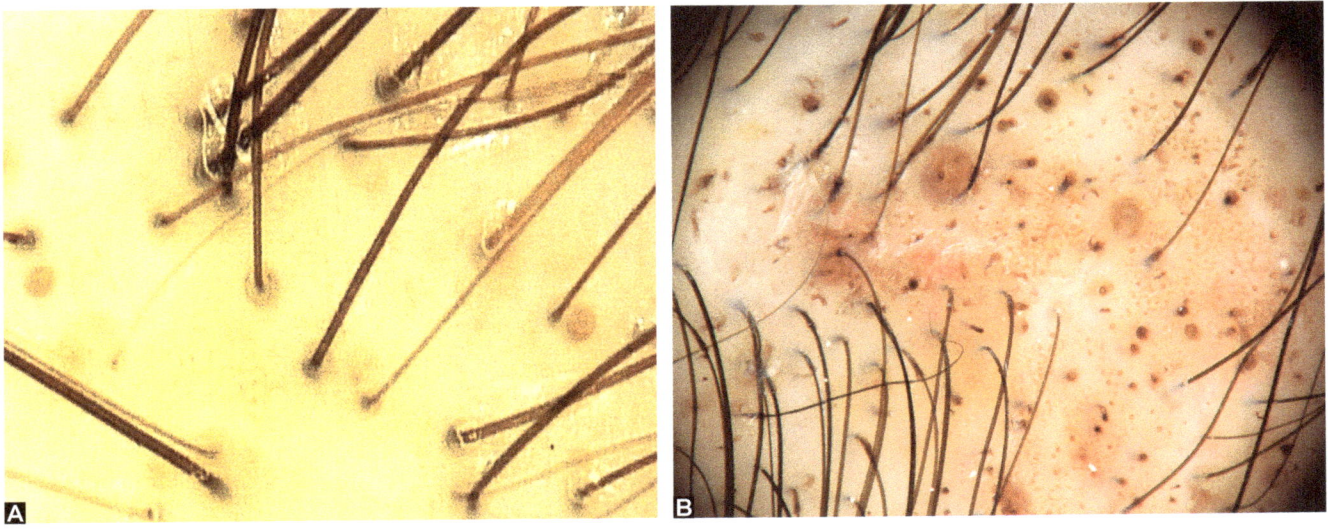

Figs. 17.5A and B: (A) Peripilar sign appears as a large brown homogeneous peripilar halo mostly around terminal or intermediate hairs of patients with early androgenetic alopecia. Note increased hair diameter variability, vellus hairs and the honeycomb pattern due to sun exposure. (B) The remains of hair dye can adhere mostly to empty follicles, and to scalp skin in an irregular distribution.

Source: (B) Division of Dermatology, Hospital das Clínicas, University of São Paulo Medical School.

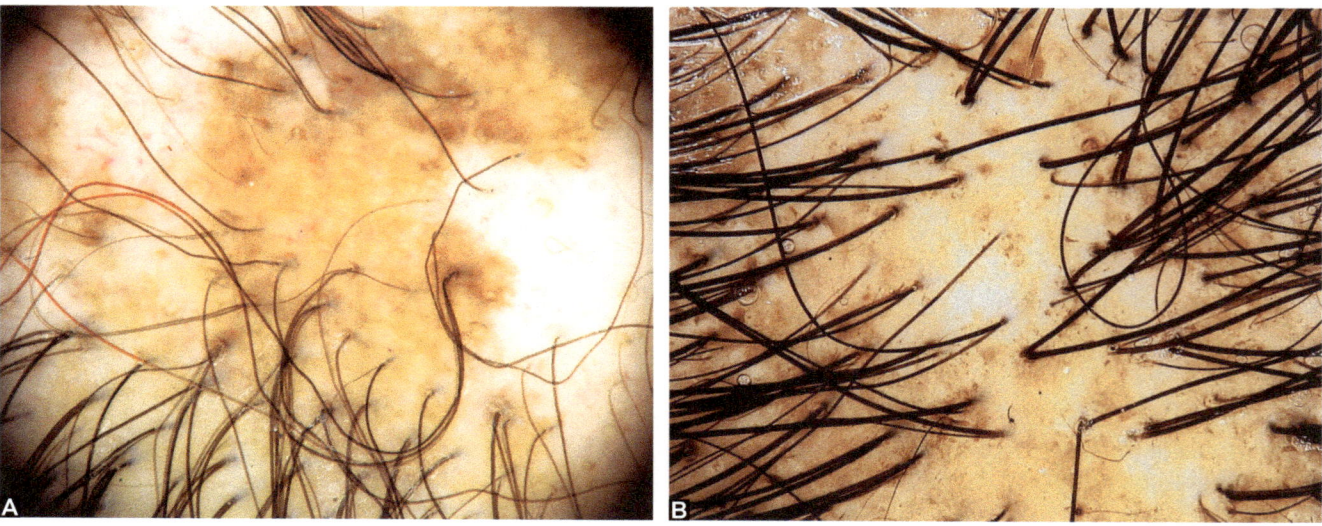

Figs. 17.6A and B: (A) Scattered brown skin areas can occur mostly in discoid lupus erythematosus due to interfollicular inflammation. Note the white scarring areas, small keratin plugs and the thick arborizing vessels. (B) The remains of hair dye can adhere to interfollicular skin and to empty follicles in an irregular distribution. Note the absence of scarring features.

Source: (A) Division of Dermatology, Hospital das Clínicas, University of São Paulo Medical School.

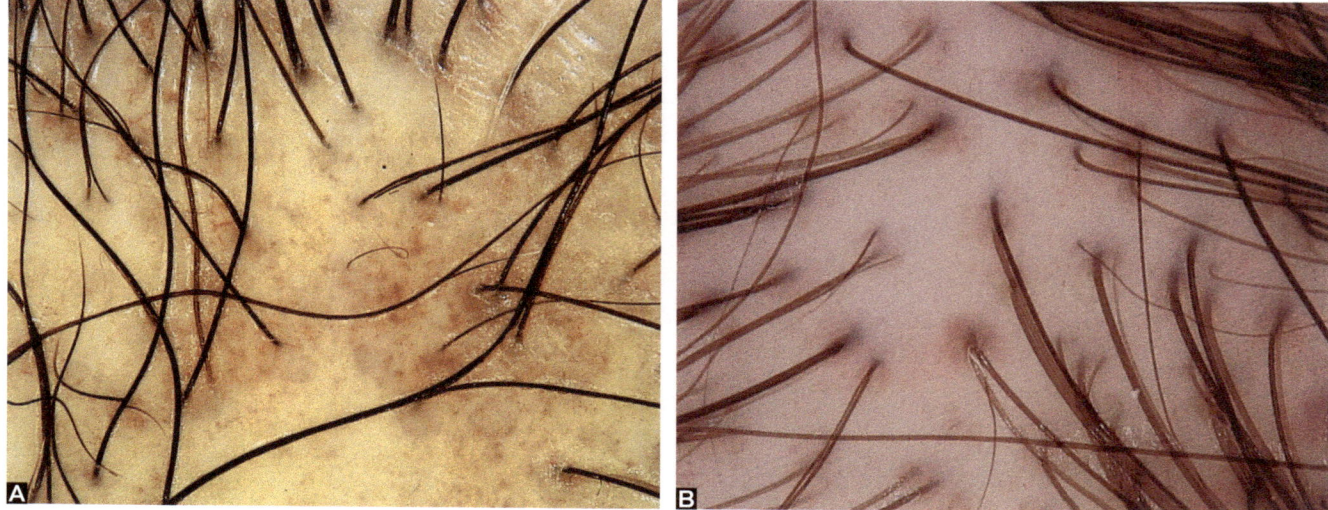

Figs. 17.7A and B: (A) Brown-gray areas indicate pigment incontinence and appear as large heterogeneous peripilar halos with blunt borders, mostly in scarring disorders, such as lichen planopilaris. Note scarring areas with absence of follicular openings and scalp scattered discoloration. (B) Peripilar sign is usually seen in early androgenetic alopecia, as large brown homogeneous peripilar halos. Note the increased hair diameter variability and vellus hairs.

BROWN-GRAY PERIPILAR PIGMENTATION AND PERIPILAR SIGN

Brown-gray peripilar pigmentation and peripilar sign are shown in Figures 17.7A and B.

ANTHRALIN DYE AND BLACK DOTS

Anthralin dye and black dots are shown in Figures 17.8A and B.

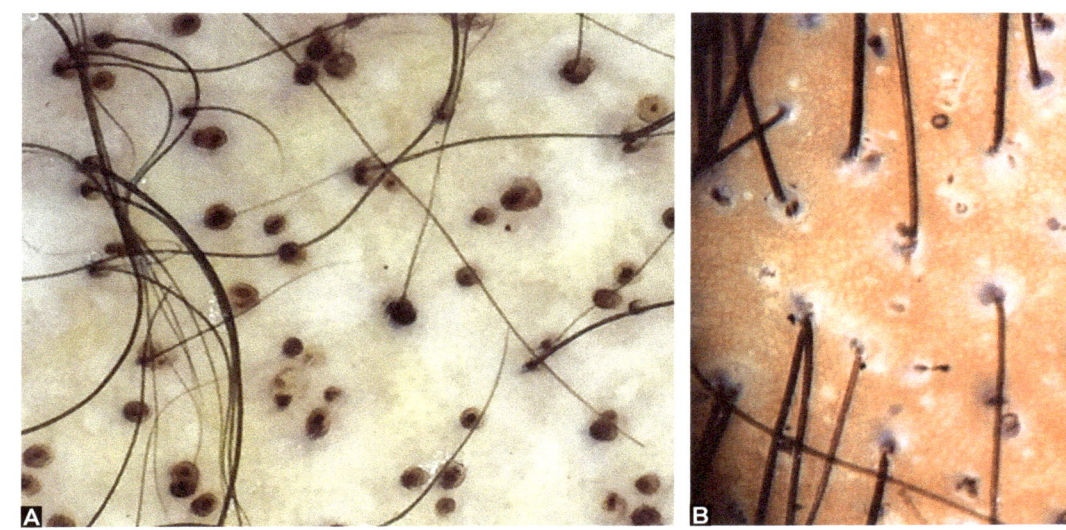

Figs. 17.8A and B: (A) Sometimes anthralin dye may adhere to empty follicles and mimic black dots in low magnifications. (B) Black dots in a severe case of monilethrix. Note some cadaverized hairs broken at the level of scalp emergence and some broken hairs with different lengths.

Source: (B) Division of Dermatology, Hospital das Clínicas, University of São Paulo Medical School.

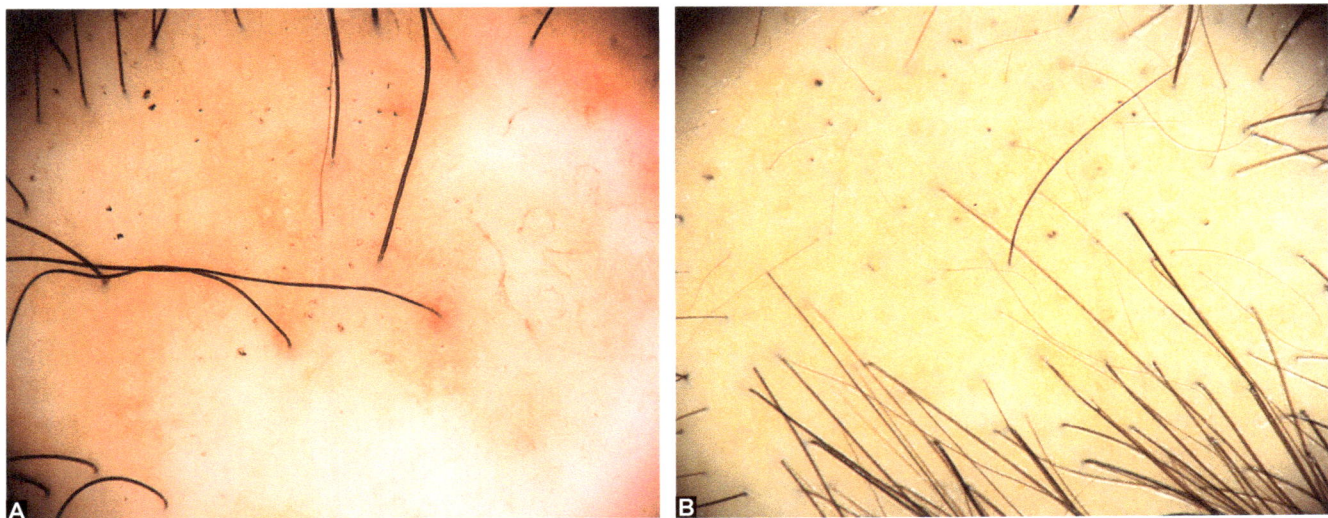

Figs. 17.9A and B: (A) Dirty dots are very common in children and elderly people. They appear as heterogeneous black structures unrelated to follicular openings that can be easily removed after shampooing. (B) Black dots are hairs broken at the level of scalp emergence and can be present mostly in active alopecia areata. They indicate disease activity and cannot be removed after shampooing.

Source: (A and B) Division of Dermatology, Hospital das Clínicas, University of São Paulo Medical School

DIRTY DOTS AND BLACK DOTS

Dirty dots and black dots are shown in Figures 17.9A and B.

SHORT REGROWING HAIRS AND PLUCKED HAIRS IN THE EYEBROWS

Short regrowing hairs and plucked hairs in the eyebrows are shown in Figures 17.10A and B.

TRICHOSTASIS SPINULOSA AND BLACK DOTS

Trichostasis spinulosa and black dots are shown in Figures 17.11A and B.

BROOM HAIRS AND TRICHOSTASIS SPINULOSA

Broom hairs and trichostasis spinulosa are shown in Figures 17.12A and B.

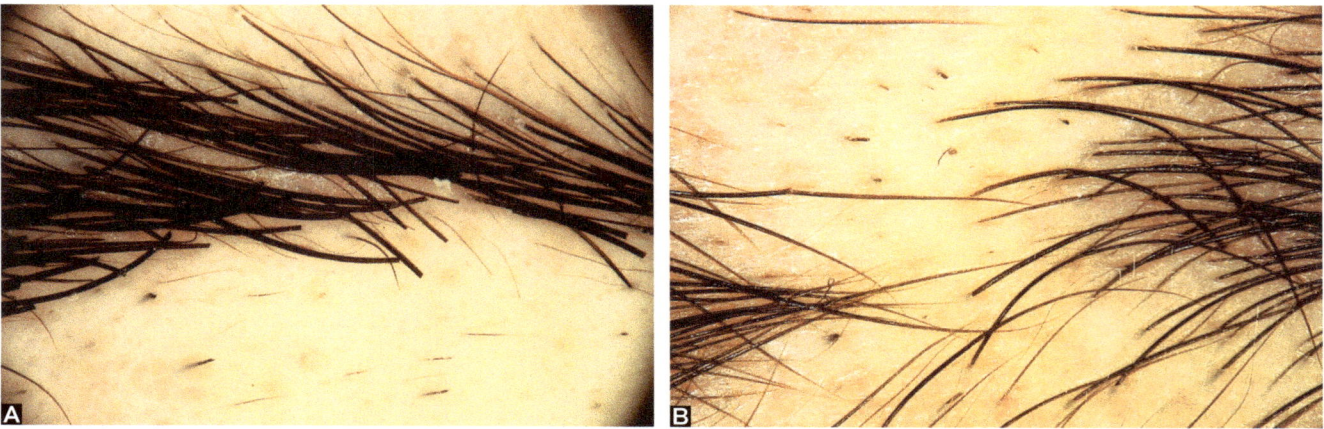

Figs. 17.10A and B: (A) Note some short hairs and black dots in the lower part of the eyebrow from a healthy patient. They correspond to short regrowing hairs after hair plucking. (B) Broken hairs and black dots in a patient with alopecia areata in the scalp and in the eyebrow. Note partial madarosis.

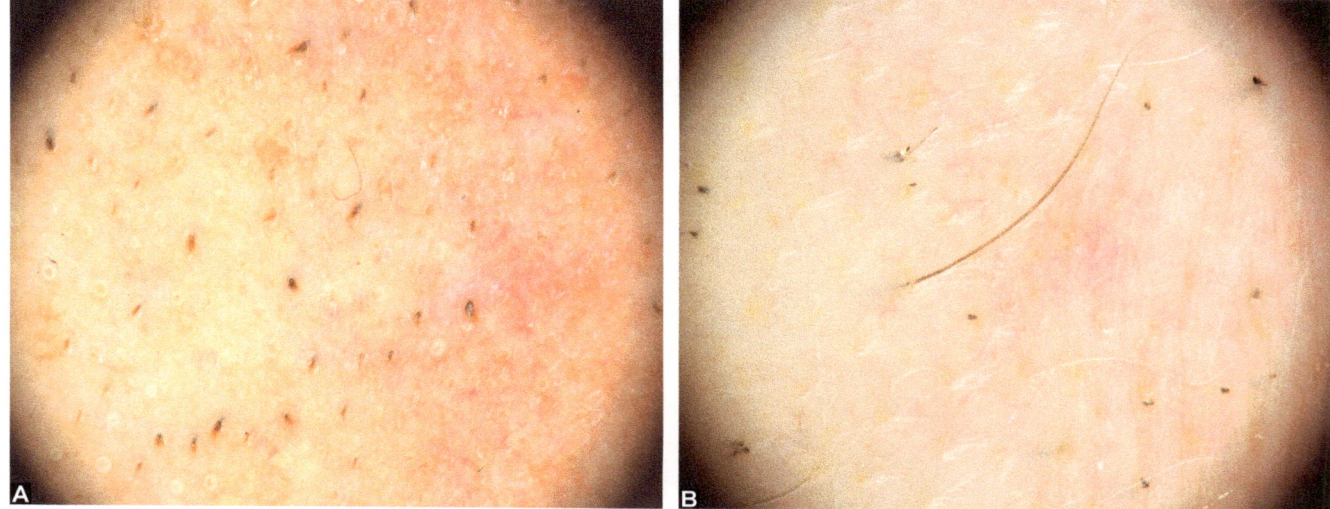

Figs. 17.11A and B: (A) In low magnifications, trichostasis spinulosa (many vellus hairs in the same follicular openings) may mimic black dots. Note the presence of small keratin plugs and the absence of broken hairs. (B) Black dots, multiple broken hairs and yellow dots in a patient with alopecia areata.
Source: (A and B) Division of Dermatology, Hospital das Clínicas, University of São Paulo Medical School

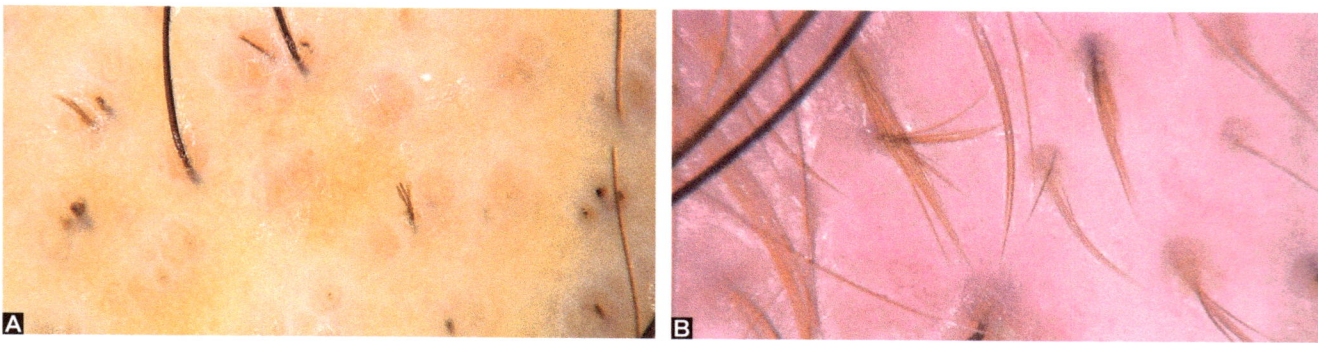

Figs. 17.12A and B: (A) "Broom-like hairs" or "brush hairs" can be found in nonscarring and scarring alopecias. They correspond to multiple thin and short hair shafts emerging from the same follicular opening. (B) Trichostasis spinulosa are clusters of vellus hairs embedded within hair follicles, resulting in dark, spiny papules on the face or trunk. Usually it is an accidental finding, and often is misdiagnosed as comedo structures or keratosis pilaris.

CLOTHING FIBERS, BROKEN HAIRS, AND PILI TORTI

Clothing fibers, broken hairs, and pili torti are shown in Figures 17.13A to D.

PROXIMAL TRICHORRHEXIS NODOSA, TRICHOTEMNOMANIA, AND HAIR TUFTING

Proximal trichorrhexis nodosa, trichotemnomania, and hair tufting are shown in Figures 17.14A to C.

DOLL-LIKE IMPLANTED HAIRS AND HAIR TUFTS

"Doll-like implanted hairs" and hair tufts are shown in Figures 17.15A and B.

CIRCLE HAIRS, COMMA AND CORKSCREW HAIRS

Circle hairs, comma and corkscrew hairs are shown in Figures 17.16A and B.

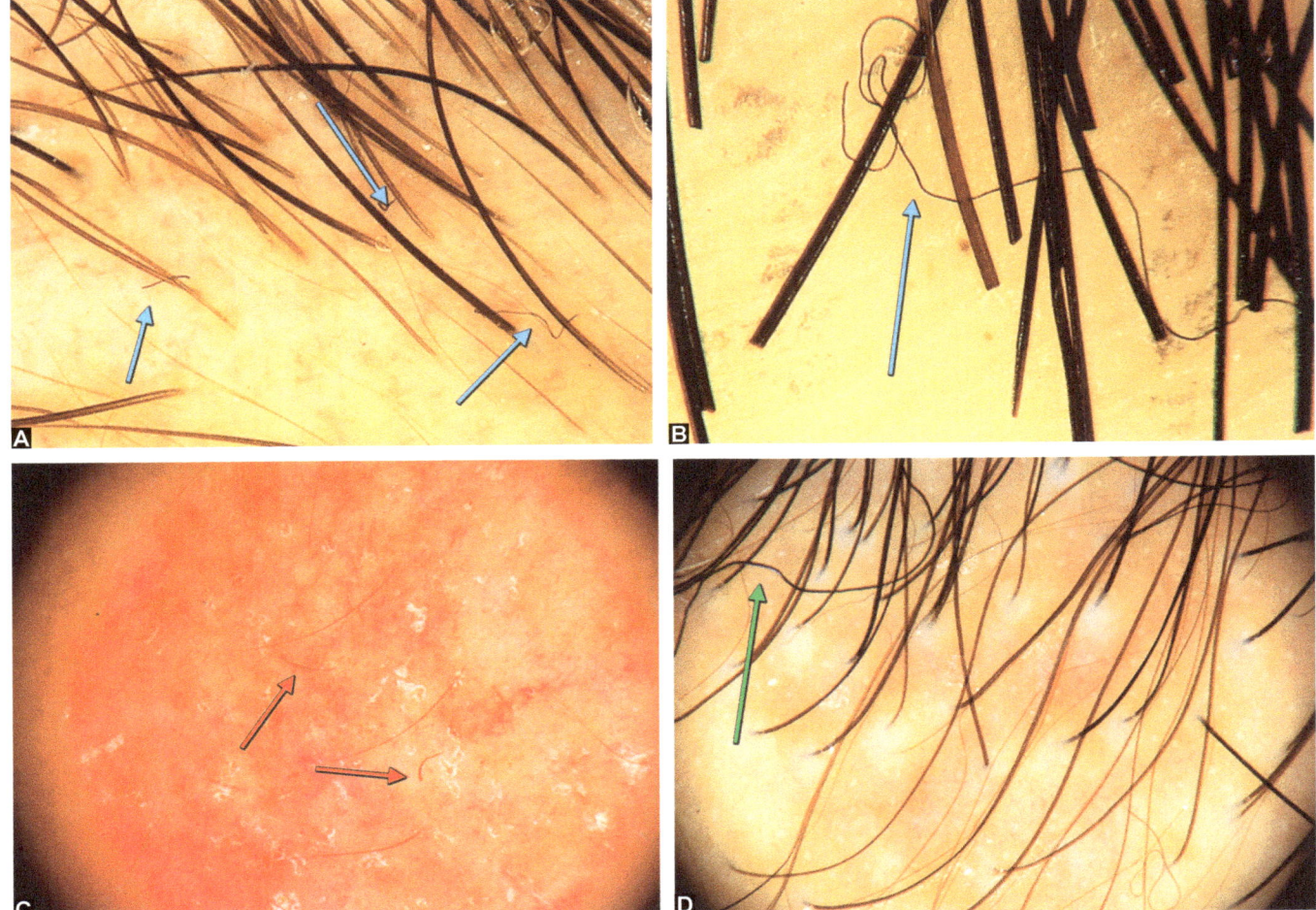

Figs. 17.13A to D: (A and B) Note some clothing fibers within hair shafts. Note that the fibers are thinner and curlier compared to the normal shafts (blue arrows). (C) Broken hairs (red arrows). (D) Pili torti (green arrow).

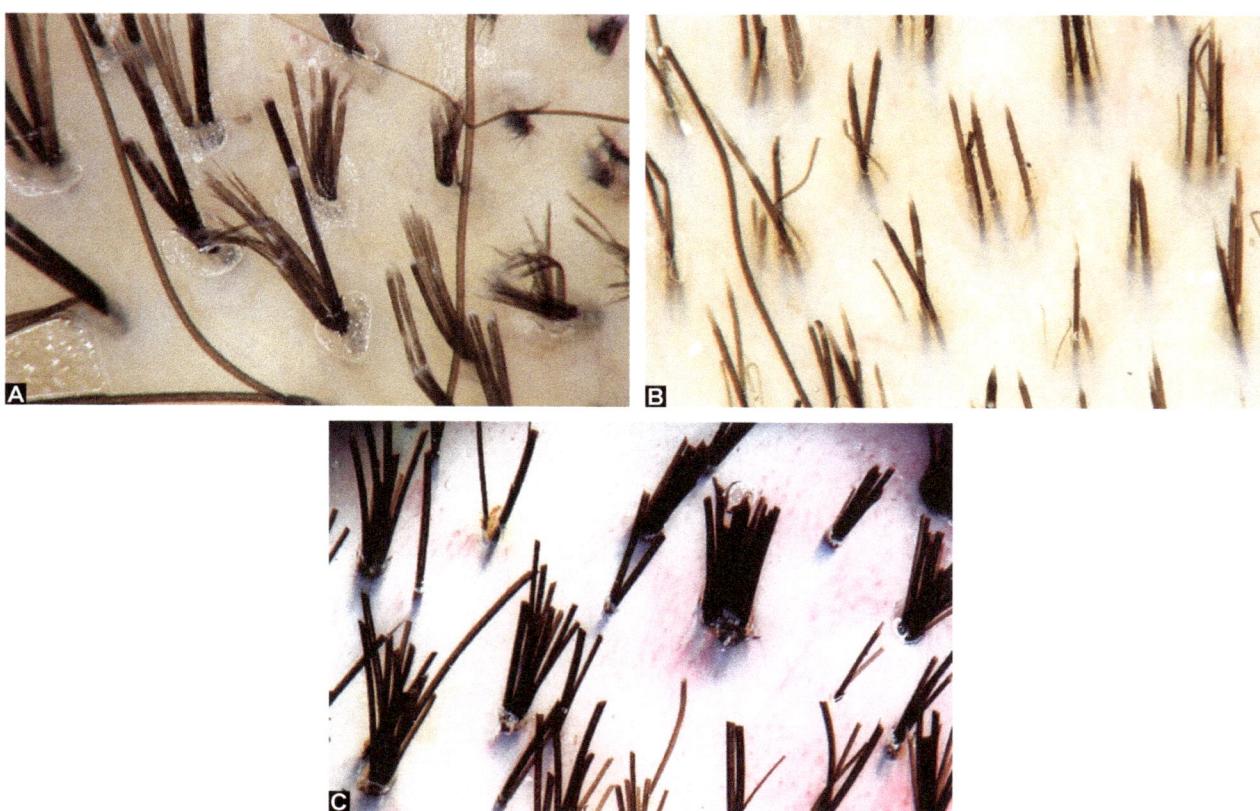

Figs. 17.14A to C: (A) Proximal trichorrhexis nodosa usually occurs in cases of pruritus in the scalp, also known as trichoteiromania. Note the multiple broken hairs at variable lengths. (B) Trichotemnomania is an obsessive-compulsive habit of cutting or shaving the hair. Note regular follicular units containing one to three hair shafts. Note all tips are cut in the same length. (C) Hair tufting in folliculitis decalvans. Note several hair shafts emerging from the same follicular opening. In this case the diagnosis may be tough due to the short haircut.
Source: (B) Division of Dermatology, Hospital das Clínicas, University of São Paulo Medical School.

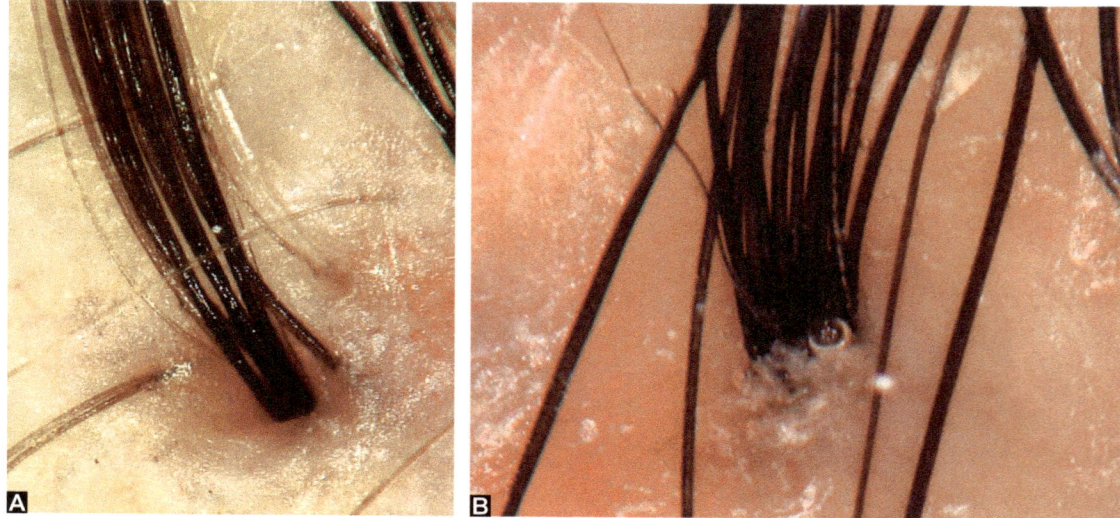

Figs. 17.15A and B: Hair plugs correspond to multiple hairs in the same follicular opening. (A) Old hair transplantation techniques used to implant multiple follicular units in the same skin opening, leading to a doll-like appearance. Note the deep and reddish surface surrounding the hair implant. (B) Multiple hair tufts with more than 10 hair shafts are usually seen in folliculitis decalvans associated with thick peripilar scales and absence of follicular openings.

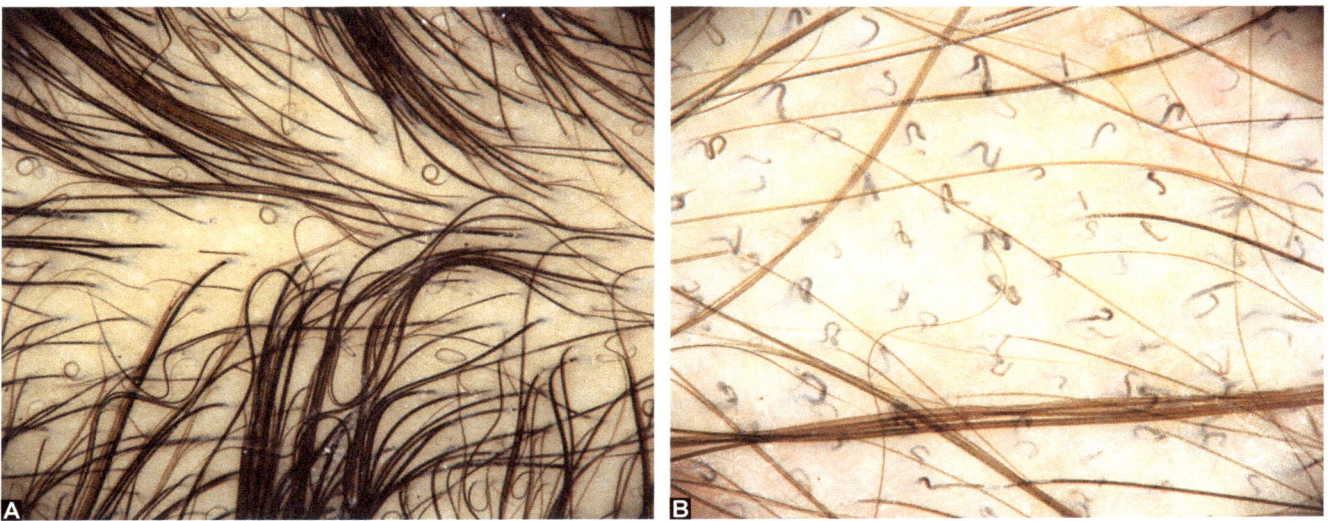

Figs. 17.16A and B: (A) Circle hairs or pigtail hairs are short and twisted regrowing hairs. They can occur in androgenetic alopecia and alopecia areata. A few isolated circle hairs can be seen in androgenetic alopecia. Multiple circle hairs (more than six) usually indicate alopecia areata. In this case, circle hairs may be the unique finding of the disease. (B) Comma and corkscrew hairs are pathognomonic features of tinea capitis. Comma hairs are shorter and less curling than corkscrew hairs and both can coexist.

Source: (B) Division of Dermatology, Hospital das Clínicas, University of São Paulo Medical School.

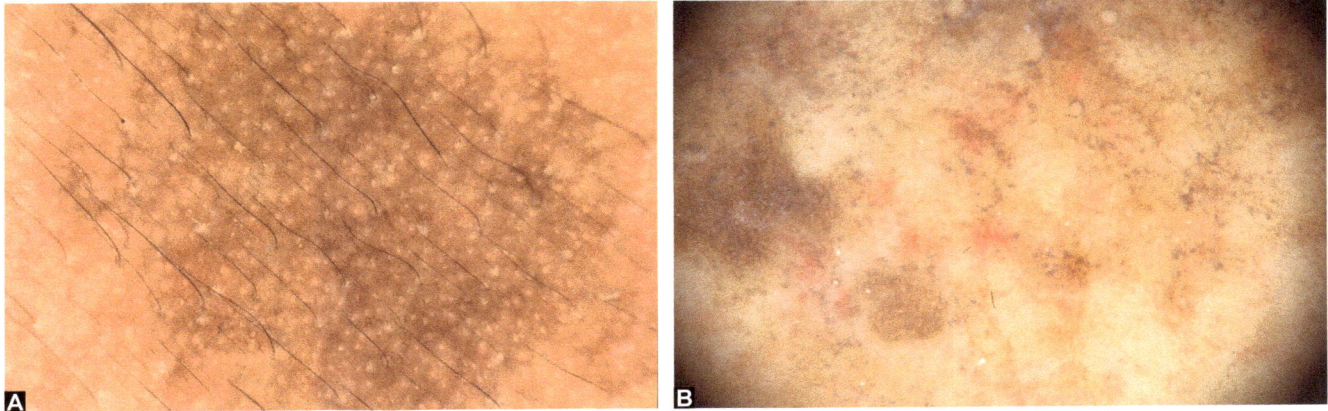

Figs. 17.17A and B: (A) Melasma is very common in dark-skinned patients. Although a mild erythema can be seen in patients using containing-acids products, there is no telangiectatic vessels in dermoscopy. Note multiple facial vellus hairs and a light and homogenous skin pigmentation. (B) Lichen planus pigmentosum is usually associated with frontal fibrosing alopecia in dark-skinned patients. Note telangiectasia and heterogeneous skin pigmentation. In some cases, target lesions can be present as well.

Source: Division of Dermatology, Hospital das Clínicas, University of São Paulo Medical School.

MELASMA AND LICHEN PLANUS PIGMENTOSUM

Melasma and lichen planus pigmentosum are shown in Figures 17.17A and B.

YELLOW DOTS AND YELLOWISH HUE

Yellow dots and yellowish hue are shown in Figures 17.18A and B.

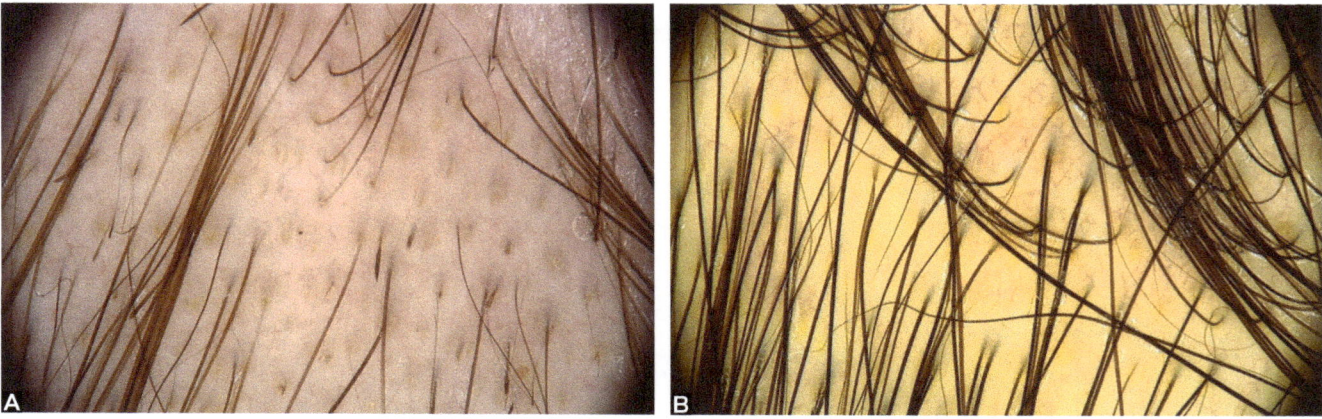

Figs. 17.18A and B: (A) True yellow dots are homogenous small structures in place of follicular openings. Some may contain black dots, dystrophic hairs, and vellus hairs and can be present in many types of hair loss, including alopecia areata, and androgenetic alopecia. Note that some may have a double margin filled with a central keratin plug. (B) A large yellowish hue can be seen surrounding terminal or intermediate hair shafts in an oily scalp. They are not necessarily associated with hair miniaturization. In this case, the patient had seborrheic dermatitis and short regrowing hairs due to a telogen effluvium and has not washed the hair for the last 3 days. These halos can be mostly removed after shampooing.

HAIR CASTS AND PSEUDOCASTS

Hair casts and pseudocasts are shown in Figures 17.19A and B.

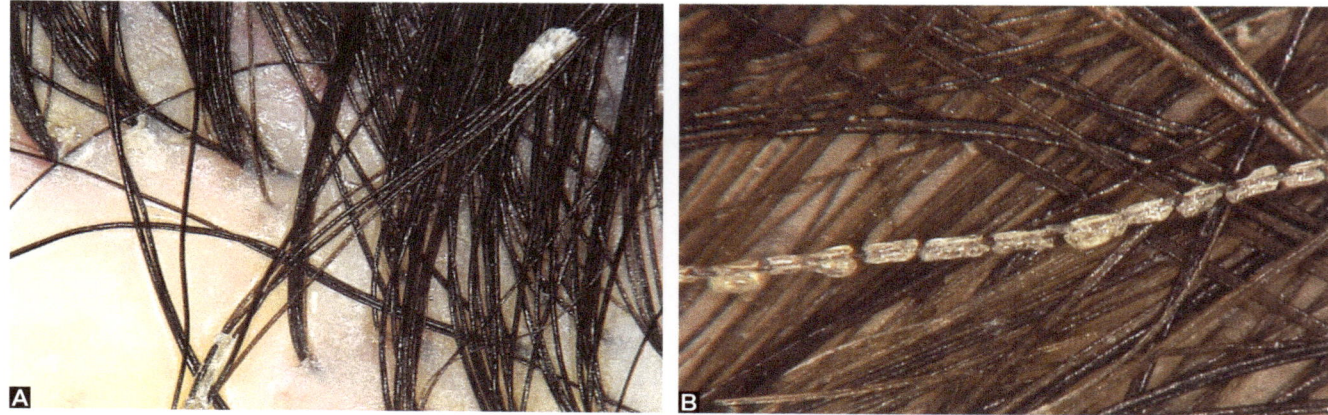

Figs. 17.19A and B: (A) True hair casts are tubular movable structures formed by keratin cells from the outer root sheath. They can be seen surrounding the hair shafts from patients with many inflammatory hair disorders, such as lichen planopilaris, seborrheic dermatitis and folliculitis decalvans. (B) Pseudocasts appear as irregularly shaped concretions with variable length, thickness, and surface, irregularly attached to the hair shafts. They can be seen after the use of hair spray, deodorants, and dry shampoos.

Source: (A and B) Dr Antonella Tosti.

TRICHORRHEXIS NODOSA, WHITE PIEDRA, AND DRY SHAMPOOS

Trichorrhexis nodosa, white piedra, and dry shampoos are shown in Figures 17.20A to C.

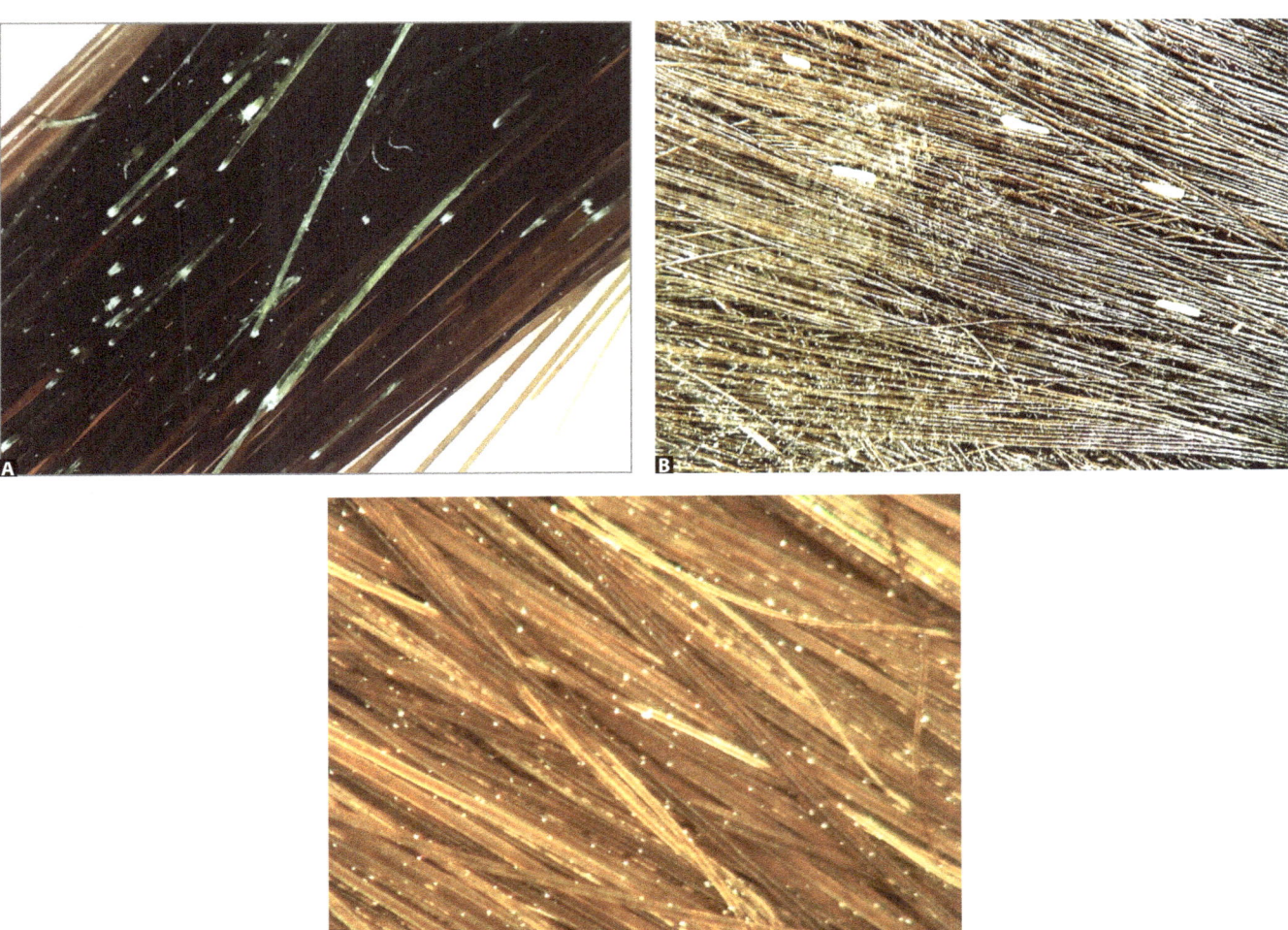

Figs. 17.20A to C: (A) In low magnifications, the knots from trichorrhexis nodosa may mimic fungal infections, nits, casts, and pseudocasts caused by the use of some cosmetics. (B) White piedra can be seen as small masses of fungal structures attached to the hair shafts. (C) The use of some cosmetics as dry shampoos may lead to small irregular concentrations that attach to the hair shaft. In this case, it is very import to perform dermoscopy in high magnifications (70 ×) to make the correct diagnosis.

SUGGESTED READING

1. Alfaro-Castellón P, Mejía-Rodríguez AS, Valencia-Herrera A, et al. Dermoscopy distiction of eruptive vellus hair cysts with molluscum contagiosum and acne lesions. Pediatric Dermatol. 2012:29(6):772-3.
2. Angra K, LaSenna CE, Nichols AJ, et al. Hair dye: a trichoscopic pitfall. J Am Acad Dermatol. 2015;72(4):e101-2.
3. Chagas FS, Donati A, Soares II, et al. Trichostasis spinulosa of the scalp mimicking alopecia areata black dots. An Bras Dermatol. 2014;89(4):685-7.
4. Doche I, Vincenzi C, Tosti A. Casts and pseudocasts. J Am Acad Dermatol. 2016;75(4):e147-8.
5. Elghblawi E. Tinea capitis children and trichoscopic criteria. Int J Trichology. 2017;9(2):47-9.
6. Gallouj S, Rabhi S, Baybay H, et al. Trichotemnomania associated to trichotillomania: a case report with emphasis on the diagnostic value of dermoscopy. Ann Dermatol Venereol. 2011;138(2):140-1.
7. Ianhez M, Cestari Sda C, Enokihara MY, et al. Dermoscopic patterns of molluscum contagiosum: a study of 211

lesions confirmed by histopathology. An Bras Dermatol. 2011;86(1):74-9.
8. Inui S. Trichoscopy for common hair loss diseases: algorithmic method for diagnosis. J Dermatol. 2011;38(1):71-5.
9. Kawaguchi M, Suzuki T. Dermoscopy is useful for the diagnosis of milia-like idiopathic calcinosis cutis. Australas J Dermatol. 2018;59(1):63-4.
10. Kim NH, Zell DS, Kolm I, et al. The dermoscopic differential diagnosis of yellow lobularlike structures. Arch Dermatol. 2008;144(7):962.
11. Kowalska-Oledzka E, Slowinska M, Rakowska A, et al. 'Black dots' seen under trichoscopy are not specific for alopecia areata. Clin Exp Dermatol. 2012;37(6):615-9.
12. Ku SH, Cho EB, Park EJ, et al. Dermoscopic features of molluscum contagiosum based on white structures and their correlation with histopathological findings. Clin Exp Dermatol. 2015;40(2):208-10.
13. Lacarrubba F, Misciali C, Gibilisco R, et al. Circle hairs: clinical, trichoscopic and histopathologic findings. Int J Trichology. 2013;5(4):211-3.
14. Lacarrunna F, Verzì AE, Dinotta F, et al. Dermoscopy in inflammatory and infectious skin disorders. G Ital Dermatol Venereol. 2015;150(5):521-31.
15. Lam M, Crutchfield CE III, Lewis EJ. Hair casts: a case of pseudonits. Cutis. 1997;60(5):251-2.
16. Miteva M, Lima M, Tosti A. Dirty dots as a normal trichoscopic finding in the elderly scalp. JAMA Dermatol. 2016;152(4):474-6.
17. Pirmez R, Abraham LS, Duque-Estrada B, et al. Trichoscopy of steroid-induced atrophy. Skin Appendage Disord. 2017;3:171-4.
18. Pirmez R, Duque-Estrada B, Donati A, et al. Clinical and dermoscopic features of lichen planus pigmentosum in 37 patients with frontal fibrosing alopecia. Br J Dermatol. 2016;175(6):1387-90.
19. Rakowska A, Slowinska M, Kowalska-Oledzka E, et al. Trichoscopy of cicatricial alopecia. J Drugs Dermatol. 2012;11(6):753-8.
20. Zaballos P, Ara M, Puig S, et al. dermoscopy of sebaceous hyperplasia. Arch Dermatol. 2005;141(6):808.

Index

Page numbers followed by *b* refer to box, *f* refer to figure, and *t* refer to table.

A

Acne 100*f*
   keloidalis 67
      nuchae 97, 100, 106, 106*f*, 107, 107*f*
   necrotica 67
Adalimumab 100
Adnexal tumor 212
   benign 216
African hair 1
   shafts, normal 4*f*
African scalp, normal 1, 3*f*
African vertex scalp, normal 3*f*
Alopecia 138, 144, 150, 221*f*
   active traction 12*f*
   chemotherapy-induced 28, 56, 56*f*, 57*f*, 58, 232
   cicatricial 59, 91, 95*f*
   complete 163
   congenital triangular 141, 144, 144*f*, 145*f*
   diffuse 138*f*, 154*f*
      nonscarring 121*f*
   during childhood 141
   early
      androgenetic 233*f*
      frontal fibrosing 75*f*
      scarring 108*f*
   fibrosing 80, 80*f*, 81*f*, 82, 82*f*
   frontal fibrosing 10*f*, 67, 74*f*-78*f*, 167*f*, 191, 195*f*
   frontotemporal 74*f*
   hot comb 91
   late stage of traction 9*f*
   linear patch of 62*f*
   mild androgenetic 22*f*
   mimicking traction 74*f*
   neutrophilic primary scarring 100
   nonscarring 33, 236*f*
      patchy 121*f*
      pattern of 120*f*
   of scalp, progressive scarring 97
   patchy moth-eaten 138
   permanent 56*f*, 58
      diffuse 60*f*
   pressure 66*f*
   pressure-induced 65, 65*t*, 66
   primary scarring 67*t*
   psoriatic scarring 114*f*, 115*f*
   radiation-induced 59
   radiotherapy-induced 59, 59*f*, 60*f*
   scarring 236*f*
      patch of 100*f*
   secondary cicatricial 151
   senescent 40, 40*f*
   senile 40, 41
   severe androgenetic 9*f*
   temporal scarring 75*f*
   totalis 44*f*, 47
   type of 156
   universalis 44
Alopecia areata 8*f*, 9*f*, 10*f*, 15, 26*f*, 28, 28*f*, 31*f*, 44*f*-47*f*, 49, 52, 54, 66, 66*f*, 93*f*, 95*f*, 96, 144, 146, 166, 167*f*, 190, 191, 239*f*
   diagnosis of 45*f*
   incognito 49*f*, 50*f*
   mimicking 75*f*
   of eyebrows 193*f*
   of eyelashes 194*f*
Alopecia mucinosa 67, 95, 95*f*, 96*f*
   trichoscopy of 95
Alopecic patch 62*f*
   diffuse scarring 68*f*
   multiple scarring 104*f*
   unique 44*f*
Amorphous hair residues 51
Amyloidosis 132
   type of 132
Anagen 30
   effluvium 56*f*, 57*f*, 60*f*, 191
   hair 176*f*
      dye 30*f*
Androgenetic alopecia 13*f*, 19*f*, 33, 40, 43*f*, 80, 239*f*
   mild male-pattern 22*f*
Angiosarcoma 218, 219
   on scalp 219*f*
Anhidrotic ectodermal dysplasia 191
Anhidrotic type 152
Anisotrichosis 22*f*
Anthralin 47*f*
   dye 234
Anti-androgens drugs 38
Anticoagulants 191
Antithyroid drugs 191
Aplasia cutis 213
   congenita 44, 141, 141*f*, 142*f*, 144
Apocrine 210, 212
Arborizing capillaries, diffuse thin 18*f*
Arborizing vessels 117*f*
Areata alopecia 198
Argininosuccinic aciduria 183
Asian female's eyelashes 190
Asian scalp, normal 4, 4*f*
Atopy 97
Atrichia congenital 191
Atrophic scarring patch 93*f*
Autoimmune bullous disorders 156
Autoimmune skin disorders 156
Axillary alopecia 97
Axillary hairs shafts 207*f*
Azathioprine 85, 161

B

Bacterial folliculitis 54*f*
Bacterial infections, frequent 171
Bamboo appearance 196
Bamboo hair 171, 197*f*
Barre syndrome 166
Basal cell carcinoma 191, 210
   on scalp
      nonpigmented 211*f*
      pigmented 211*f*
Bazex-Dupré-Christol syndrome 166, 183
B-cell lymphomas 220
Biotin 183
Björnstad syndrome 166
Blaschko´s lines 127
Blepharitis, infective 191
Blood vessels, prominent frontal 74*f*
Brown skin, scattered 234*f*
Brownish halo 13*f*
Bullous pemphigoid 161

C

Calcineurin inhibitors, topical 81
Camouflage 199
   products 199
Carvajal syndrome 173
Caucasian blond-haired girls 148
Caucasian hair shaft, normal 2*f*, 3
Caucasian scalp, normal 1, 2
Caucasian temporal scalp, normal 3*f*

Caucasian vertex scalp, normal 2f, 3f
Central centrifugal cicatricial alopecia, active 12f
Centrifugal cicatricial alopecia, central 12f, 67, 91, 91f, 92, 92f
Chediak-Higashi syndrome 180, 180f, 181f
Chemotherapy 132
Cholinergics 191
Christmas-tree pattern 37f
Cicatricial alopecias, primary 67
Cicatricial scalp patch
    with crusts 136f
    with pustules 136f
Cicatricial surface, smooth 93f
Cisplatin 56
Clear cell renal carcinoma 222f
Clofazimine 85
Clothing fibers 237
Compulsive disorder 52
Cone rod dystrophy 198
Confluent erythematous telangiectatic nodules 216f
Congenital syndromes 198
Corneal dystrophy 97
Cornelia de Lange syndrome 198
Corticosteroids 81
Corynebacterium tenuis 136
Cosmetic 190
    and camouflage products 190
    hair
        products 199
        sprays 206
Costello syndrome 173
Crawling snake 173, 174f
Crusted scabies 134
Cutaneous cleft 104
Cutaneous cysts, common 218
Cutaneous lichen planus 69f
Cutaneous lupus erythematosus, chronic 67
Cutaneous lymphomas 220
Cutaneous metastasis 222
Cutaneous T-cell lymphoma 95, 191
Cyclophosphamide 161, 191
Cylindroma 216, 217
    on left parietal scalp 217f
Cysts 219

D

Dapsone 85, 100
Deafness 97
Dental abnormalities 153f
Deodorant spray, irregular residues of 207f
Deodorants 206
Dermatitis
    contact 117
    herpetiformis 160
Dermatobia hominis 137
    larva 137f

Dermatomyositis 124, 124f, 125f, 127, 198
Dermis 210
Dermoscope 5
    digital 6
    manual 8
Dermoscopy 5, 33, 42, 122, 132, 137, 144, 146, 152, 160, 178, 186, 187, 199, 219, 226f
    in androgenetic alopecia 118f
    of acute lesions 65, 66
    of anagen effluvium 56
    of early-onset scleroderma 127
    of eyebrows 190
    of eyelashes 190
    of facial lesions 119
    of hair 1
        loss 138
    of initial alopecic patches 53
    of nonscarring alopecia 124
    of scalp 1
Dimethylaminocinnamaldehyde 30f
Discoid erythematous lesions, multiple 84f
Discoid lupus
    diagnosis of 85f
    erythematosus 11f, 13f, 18, 74f, 84, 85f, 86f, 130, 167f, 192, 195f
    in eyebrow 196f
Dissecting cellulitis 53, 53f, 54f, 67, 104, 105f
    initial stage 53, 53f, 54f
    late stage 104, 104f
Doxorubicin 191
Doxycycline 74
Dry dermoscopy 14f, 17, 71f, 76f, 81f, 101f, 109f, 112f, 125f
Dry shampoos 206, 241
Dutasteride 74
Dyproterone 38
Dyschromia 195f
    scales 123f
Dysplasia, oculovertebral 191
Dystrophic epidermolysis bullosa 154f, 155f

E

Eccrine 210, 212
    poroma 217
        on scalp 217f
Ectodermal dysplasia 152, 152f, 153f, 183
Ectoderm-derived structures 152
Eczema 109
Eczematous lesions 117, 138
Ehlers-Danlos syndrome 191
Elejalde disease 180, 181f
Endocrine disease 191
Envelope trichogram 30f
Epidermal cysts 218
Epidermis 210
Epidermolysis bullosa 191
    congenital 154

Epiluminescence, digital 5
Erosive pustular dermatosis 67
    of scalp 108, 108f, 109f
Erythema 108f, 109f, 195f
    diffuse 120f, 151f
    mild 3f, 80f, 82f, 92f, 142f
Erythematous plaques 220
Erythematous skin 114f
Etoposide 56
Exogen substances 8, 15, 20
Eyebrows 52, 97, 98, 138f, 166, 171, 178
    alopecia 47, 194f
    disorder 190
    hair
        loss 204f
        shafts 206f
        shedding 56f
    loss of 221f
    makeup 192f
    micropigmentation 204f
    monilethrix in 196f
    red dots in 194f
    tattoo 191, 191f, 195f, 204f
    trichotillomania 194f
Eyelashes 97, 171, 178, 190
    disorder 190
    makeup 192f
    perifollicular scaling on 195f
    scarring alopecia 98
    trichomegaly 196, 197f, 198t
Eyelid tattoo 191f

F

Facial papules, extensive 75f
Facial rosacea 119f, 120f
Facial ulerythema ophryogenes 97
Fallot tetralogy 198
Familial trichoepitheliomas, multiple 215f
Familial trichomegaly 198
Fertility, decreased 178
Fibrotic scarring patches 86f
Finasteride 38, 74
Flaky yellowish interfollicular scales 16f
Floppy sock appearance 146
Focal atrichia 38f
Follicular epidermis 84
Follicular hair and scalp patterns 8b
Follicular keratosis lesions 163
Follicular keratotic plugging 109f
Follicular mucinosis 95, 191
Follicular occlusion tetrad 53
Follicular openings 8, 8f, 20f, 81f, 85f
    absence of 18, 71f, 82f, 94f, 98f, 106f, 109f
    atrophic patch with loss of 142f
    loss of 86f, 89f
Follicular ostia 74
    absence of 71f, 76f
Follicular papules 119

Follicular patterns 8
Follicular pustules 102f
Follicular units, single 38f
Folliculitis 67
    decalvans 16, 20f, 29f, 67, 100, 100f, 101f, 102, 102f, 106f, 109, 167f, 191
        lesions 100f
    dissecting 191
    keloidalis 67, 106
        nuchae 100, 100f
    necrotica 67
    superficial 54f
Folliculotropic mycosis fungoides 95, 95f, 96f, 220f, 221f
Folliculotropism 95
Friar tuck sign 51
Friction alopecia from scratching 117f
Fried egg sign 156, 159f
Fringe sign 62f, 88, 89
Frontotemporal scalp 144
Fungal infection 109, 191

G

Genetic skin diseases 150
Genetic syndromes 166
Glue-in technique 201f
Goldstein Hutt syndrome 198
Golf-tee
    hairs 171
    sign 197f
Goltz syndrome 166
Graham-Little syndrome 12f, 67, 70f
Gray-white halos 8, 12, 12f
Griscelli-Prunieras syndrome 180-182f

H

Hair 152
    additions 201
    at birth, normal 163
    body 176f
    breakage 150
    brittle 178
    broken 21, 24, 26, 26f, 47, 47f, 136f, 138, 199, 231, 235, 237
    broom-like 236f
        structures 46
    brush 236f
    bubble 186, 186f
    bulbs 109f
    cadaverized 60f
    caucasian 1, 4f
    circle 237, 239f
    club 43f
    coiled 47
    collar sign 141, 142f
    comma 135f, 237, 239f
    concretions 21
    corkscrew 28f, 135f, 237
    curly 28f
    cutaneous cleft containing multiple 102f
    damaged 186
    dermoscopy 5, 6, 8
    diameter variability 21, 22, 22f, 37
    disorders, inflammatory 240f
    doll-like implanted 237
    dystrophic 21, 24, 26f, 45f, 47f, 60f, 144, 190
        anagen 31f
    exclamation mark 66f
    extension 201, 201f, 202
    fibers 199f, 200f, 231, 232f
    flame 28, 28f, 47, 60f
    folliculitis, tufted 97, 156
    fracturing, brush-like 184f
    grooming practices 169
    implant 238f
    in eyebrows, plucked 235
    isolated coiled 28
    length 148
    morse code 136f
    multiple
        broken 26f
        circle 28f, 239f
        vellus 60f
    plugs 238f
    regrowing 54f, 57f, 72f, 199
    regrowth 44f, 47f
    short 21, 23
        regrowing 23f, 235
        vellus 23f
    silvery blond 180f
    single terminal 74f
    spray 200f, 206
    structures, compound 82
    terminal 35
    tuftings 21, 29, 29f, 237
    tulip 26f
    twisted regrowing 239f
    units, multiple single 40f
Hair and scalp
    dermoscopy, devices for 5
    patterns 8
        interfollicular 15b
Hair casts 30, 63f, 156, 194f, 240
    true 240f
Hair density 3, 21, 22f, 38f, 40f, 60f
    decreased 138, 139f, 146, 155f
Hair dye 232
    irregular residues of 15f
    scattered brown skin in 232
Hair follicle 21f, 38f, 54f, 84, 190, 210, 212
    base of 14f
    hypopigmented 226
    obstructed 218
Hair loss 65, 75f
    chronic 42
    female-pattern 37, 37f, 38
        mild 38f
        moderate 38f
        severe 38f
    male-pattern 33, 34f, 37
        early 34f, 35f
        moderate 35f
        severe 35f
    partial 80f
    permanent and diffuse 59f
    severe 80f
Hair matting 208
    acute 208, 208f, 209f
Hair powder 51, 200f, 232
    multiple residues of 233f
Hair pull
    disorder 51
    test 42
Hair roots 8, 30, 141
    anagen 30
    dystrophic 30
    elongated 142f
    patterns of 30b
    pigmented 142f
    telogen 30
Hair shaft 8, 21, 152, 181f
    abnormalities, treatment for congenital 171
    defective regrowing 233f
    disorder 163, 171
        acquired 187, 191
        congenital 146
    fractured 208
    hypopigmented 57f
    in scalp hairs, triangular-like 176f
    irregular 176f
    medullated 190
    normal 1
    on light microscopy 179f
    pigmentation, diverse 152
    proximal 206
    resembling 174f
    single 152
Hair thinning 82f
    mild frontal 37f
    moderate 37f
Hair transplant
    techniques, old 238f
    with strip harvesting 203f
Hairless plaque, congenital 213f
Hairline
    recession, extensive 74f
    unusual retention of 74f
Hairpin perifollicular vessels 18f
Hamilton-Norwood classification 33
Handheld dermoscopes 5t
Hebra lines 134
Hepatitis C 138
Hermansky-Pudlak syndrome 198

Herpes simplex 191
Herpes zoster 191
Honeycomb pattern 19f, 20, 34f, 35f, 76f
Honeycomb-pigmented network 3f
Horseshoe-like structures 219
Human immunodeficiency virus 138
    infection 191, 198
Hydrochloric acid 30f
Hydroxychloroquine 74, 81
Hyperparathyroidism 191
Hyperpigmented perifollicular halo 92f
Hyperpigmented peripilar halos 78f
Hyperthyroidism 191
Hypohidrotic ectodermal dysplasia 146
Hypoparathyroidism 191
Hypopigmented papillomatous nevus 227f
Hypopituitarism 191, 183, 191
Hypotrichosis, congenital 148
Hypoxia 137

I

Ichthyosiform erythroderma 171, 178
    congenital 151, 151f
    multiple 171f
Ichthyosis 150, 150f, 151f, 173, 178, 183, 191
    types of 150
    vulgaris 150
Immunossupressive drugs 132
In situ melanoma 229f
Infection, sign of lice 30f, 206
Infectious disease 191
Inflammatory disease, chronic 106
Infliximab 100
Intelligence impairment 178
Interfollicular epidermis 95
Interfollicular scales
    intense 16f
    mild 16f
    moderate 16f
Interfollicular simple red loops 3f
Interfollicular telangiectasia 120f
Interfollicular white flaky scales 111f
Interfollicular white scale 101f
Invasive melanoma 225f
Invasive squamous cell carcinoma 212f
Iron deficiency 183
Isotretinoin 74, 85

K

Kabuki syndrome 183
Keloid lesions 104
Keratin cells 63f
Keratin plugs
    multiple small 13f
    small and multiple 13
Keratosis follicularis spinulosa 97, 98
    decalvans 67, 97, 97f, 98f

Keratosis pilaris 70f, 98
    diffuse 97
    lesions of 97f
Keratotic plugs 8, 13
Kerion celsi 136, 136f
    treatment of 136
Kindler syndrome 154

L

LA hairs 146
Lamellar ichthyosis 150f, 151
Laron syndrome 183
Leprosy 191, 196
    madarosis in 197f
Lichen planopilaris 12f, 14f, 16, 16f, 20f, 26, 29f, 30f, 67, 68, 68f-73f, 80, 82, 102, 167f, 234f
    classic 67
    diagnosis of 69f
    lesions 85f
Lichen planus pigmentosum 75f, 77f, 239
Lid coloboma 191
Loose anagen syndrome 44, 146, 146f, 147f
Lung cancer 56
Lupus erythematosus 109
Lupus vulgaris 191
Lymphocytic scarring alopecia
    chronic 68, 84
    progressive 68
Lymphoproliferative disorders 220

M

Madarosis
    diseases with 191t
    partial 194f
Malherbe's calcified epithelioma 217
Malnutrition 166
Marie Unna syndrome 175
Melanin granules, larger 181f
Melanocytic scalp tumors 224
Melanoma 224, 227
    malignant 191
    primary 224
    probability of 224
Melasma 239
Meningioma radiation therapy 59f
Menkes disease 183
Menkes syndrome 166, 167f
Mental retardation 178
Merkel cell carcinoma 219, 219f, 220
Methotrexate 85
Microsporum canis 136
Milia 231
    lesions in knee 154f
Minoxidil, topical 33
Miotics 191
Molluscum contagiosum 231, 232f

Monilethrix 163, 163f, 164f, 187, 192
    like congenital hypotrichosis 183
    like hairs 44, 46f
Morphea 127
    types of 127
Multibacillary leprosy 196
Mycofenolate mofetil 85, 161
Mycosis fungoides 221
Myelogenous leukemia, acute 56
Myiasis 137, 137f

N

N-acetylcysteine 52
Nail 152
    fold capillaroscopy 127
    lichen planus 69f
Nail-patella syndrome 146
Natural hair, amount of 201
Naxos disease 173
Neck melanoma 224
Netherton syndrome 171f
Neuroendocrine carcinoma, malignant 219
Neurofibromatosis 146
Neutropenia 178
Nevus
    blue 228f
    common 226f
    congenital 226, 228f
    unclassified 229f
Nodular lesions, diagnoses of 133
Nonmelanocytic scalp tumors 210
Noonan syndrome 146, 173
North American Hair Research Society 91
    classification 104
    workshop on cicatricial alopecia 67

O

Oculomandibular dysostosis 191
Oliver McFarlane syndrome 198
Onychotrichodysplasia 178
Ophiasis pattern 44f
Oral doxycycline 81
Oral finasteride 33, 81
Oral griseofulvin 135
Oral lichen planus 69f
Oral retinoid 171
    treatment 166
Oral steroids 136
Oral vitamin E 85

P

Pale-to-orange discoloration 130f
Palmoplantar keratoderma 97
Papillomatous nevus 226
Papulosquamous skin lesions 138
Paracoccidioidomycosis 191

Patches
    alopecia over, acute nonscarring
        irregular 59*f*
    irregular small 135
    white irregular 20*f*
    with scales, irregular 135*f*
Patchy hair loss 146
Pediculosis 133, 133*f*, 134*f*
Pediculus capitis 133
Pemphigoid 161
Pemphigus 156
    foliaceus 109, 156, 158*f*, 160*f*
    remains 156
    subtypes of 156
    types of 156
Pemphigus vulgaris 156, 158*f*, 160*f*
    and foliaceus, blood extravasation in 157*f*
Penicillin 138
Perifollicular
    erythema 62*f*, 63*f*
    hyperpigmentation 63*f*
    hyperpigmented halos 47*f*
    pustules, large 54*f*
    scale 16*f*, 71*f*, 85*f*, 92*f*
    seborrheic scales 201*f*
    thick concentric scale 101*f*
    tubular whitish scaling 159*f*
Perifolliculitis abscedens et suffodiens 67
Periorbital heliotropic rash 124
    discoloration 107*f*
    erythema 74, 74*f*
    pigmentation, brown-gray 234
    scale 8, 14, 14*f*, 16*f*, 29*f*, 35*f*, 72*f*, 74, 76*f*, 78*f*, 81*f*, 82*f*, 85*f*, 106*f*, 107*f*, 123*f*
    sign 8, 13, 13*f*, 22*f*, 38*f*, 232, 233*f*, 234
Peripilar whitish halos 94*f*
Photophobia 97
Phthirus pubis 133
Phylloid hypomelanosis 198
Physical retardation 178
Piedra 136
    black 136*f*
    white 136*f*, 241
Piedraia hortae 136
Pigment 15, 19
    botches 203
    incontinence 73*f*
Pigtail hairs 28*f*, 35*f*, 57*f*, 239*f*
Pili annulati 169, 169*f*, 170*f*
    canaliculi 152
    torti 72*f*, 76*f*, 78*f*, 86*f*, 109*f*, 152, 166, 166*f*, 167*f*, 187
    acquired 104*f*
        diseases with 166*t*
    congenital diseases with 166*t*
    on eyelashes 195*f*
    trianguli 175
    et canaliculi 175, 175*f*-177*f*

Pilomatrixoma 217, 218*f*
Pinpoint white dots 8, 9
Pituitary necrosis syndrome 191
Pityriasis amiantacea 16*f*, 111, 112*f*, 113
Pohl-Pinkus constrictions 26*f*
Pollitt syndrome 183
Polycyclic yellow dots 49
Polytrichia 100, 100*f*
    severe 100*f*
Potassium hydroxide 135
Progeria 191
Pseudocasts 30*f*, 206*f*, 207*f*, 240
Pseudofringe sign 74*f*, 88, 89
Pseudomonilethrix hairs 26, 44, 46*f*, 47
Pseudopelade 44
    of Brocq 93, 93*f*, 94, 94*f*
        classic 67
Pseudotinea amiantacea 111
Psoriasis 18*f*, 114, 191
Pubic hair loss 70*f*
Pull test 49, 51, 148*f*
Pustular psoriasis 109

R

Rapp-Hodgkin syndrome 166
Renal metastatic adenocarcinoma 198
Retinopatic ichthyosis 151
Rituximab 161
Ronchese syndrome 166
Rosacea 119
Rosacea-like dermatosis of scalp 119, 119*f*, 120*f*
Rothmund-Thomson syndrome 191

S

Sarcoidosis 130, 130*f*, 131*f*
Sarcoptes scabiei var hominis 134
Scabies 134, 135*f*
    mite 134*f*
Scalp 208
    atrophy 74*f*, 98*f*
    central 98
    cicatricial alopecia 154*f*
    contact dermatitis 117*f*, 118*f*
    cyst 218*f*
    dermoscopy 73
    disorders, inflammatory 111
    erythema, intense 98*f*
    infections of 133
    infestations of 133
    inflammatory disorders 203
    involvement 124
    mycosis fungoides of 96
    nevus 226
    nodules, differential diagnosis for 210
    noninflammatory infection of 135
    normal 1

    normal-appearing 73, 73*f*, 106, 107
    patch with pustules and crusts, inflammatory 136*f*
    pruritic infestation of 133
    pruritus, conditions with 183
    psoriasis 16*f*, 54*f*, 101*f*, 114, 114*f*, 115*f*
    sarcoidosis 130
    scale 150
        over central region of 80*f*
    surface, white-porcelain 69*f*
    tattoo 204*f*
    vessels, normal 1, 3
Scalp alopecia 59, 69*f*
    parietal 138*f*
Scalp hairs
    affected 175
    unruly and frizzy 175*f*
Scalp lesions 216*f*
    in bullous pemphigoid 162*f*
    in dermatitis herpetiformis 161*f*
    in pemphigus
        foliaceus 157*f*
        vulgaris 156*f*, 157*f*
    therapy-resistant 156
Scalp melanoma 224
    minimal invasive 225*f*
    primary 224
Scalp micropigmentation
    after 203*f*
    before 203*f*
Scalp tumors 210
    diagnosis of 224
    management of 224
Scaly skin 150
Scarring alopecia 17, 26*f*, 29*f*, 45*f*, 67, 73*f*, 104*f*, 109*f*
    occipital patches of 74*f*
    of central scalp 97*f*
    scattered brown skin in 232
Scarring patches over scalp, multiple oval-shaped 86
Scleroderma 127, 128, 191
    linear 127, 148
    localized 127, 127*f*, 128*f*
    types of 127
Sebaceous gland carcinoma 191
Sebaceous hyperplasia 231, 232*f*
Sebaceous nevus 141, 213
Seborrheic blepharitis 191
Seborrheic dermatitis 16*f*, 18*f*, 111, 111*f*, 112*f*, 113, 139*f*, 190, 191
    mild 18*f*
    of eyebrow 193*f*
    of eyelashes 192*f*
Seborrheic keratosis 213
Shampoo residues 207*f*
Short anagen syndrome 148, 148*f*
Silvery hair 180
    syndromes 180
        differences in 180*t*

Skin
- absence of 141
- and mucosa 156
- atrophy 108f, 109f
  - intense 29f
- cancer
  - treatment 108f
  - type of 210
- disease 191

Spacious follicular openings 96
Spironolactone 38
Squamous cell carcinoma 109, 191, 210, 212
Staphylococcal blepharitis 191
Staphylococcus aureus 100
Starburst hair follicles 141, 142f
Starburst sign 101f
Stem-cell transplant 132
Sterile pustules, multiple 108f
Steroid 132
- deposits 231
- injections, atrophic skin after 231f
- topical 74

Stevens-Johnson syndrome 191
Stewart-Treves syndrome 218
Strawberry ice cream pattern 72f
Sun exposure, chronic 35f
Sweat glands 152
Swiss-cheese appearance 186
Syphilic alopecia 138
Syphilis
- infections 138
- secondary 191
- tertiary 191

Syphilitic alopecia 138, 138f, 139f
- types of secondary 138

Syringocystadenoma papilliferum 213, 214
Systemic amyloidosis 132, 132f
Systemic B-cell follicular lymphoma infiltrating skin 222f
Systemic corticosteroids 130, 161
Systemic diseases 121
Systemic infectious diseases 138
Systemic lupus erythematosus 84, 121, 121f-123f, 127
Systemic sclerosis 127

T

Tacrolimus, topical 74
Tattoo 190, 203
Tay syndrome 183
T-cell lymphoma 220
Teeth 152

Telangiectasia 130, 141
- marked 142f
- prominent 131f

Telogen 30
Telogen effluvium 23f, 42, 43, 43f, 191
- acute 43f
- chronic 42, 42f, 43f

Telogen hairs
- positive with multiple 148f
- retained 208

Telogen roots entrapped 202f
Thiouracil 191
Tiger tail
- hairs 178, 179f
- pattern 178

Tinea capitis 16f, 17, 28f, 28f, 44, 135, 135f, 136f, 239f
- inflammatory 136
- microsporic 135f

Tissue disorders, connective 198
Tonsure trichotillomania 51
Traction alopecia 28f, 30, 30f, 44, 52, 62, 62f, 63f, 64, 88, 89, 89f, 91f, 144
- early stage of 9f
- initial stage 62f
- late stage 88f, 89f

Trauma 191
Trichoblastoma 213, 214, 215f
Trichodental syndrome 148
Trichodynia 42
Trichodysplasia-xeroderma 166
Trichoepithelioma 215, 216f
Trichogram, modified 30f, 31f
Trichomycosis 136, 137f
Trichonodosis 187, 189, 189f
Trichophytic tinea capitis 135f
Trichophyton mentagrophytes 136
Trichoptilosis 187, 187f
- central 187, 187f

Trichorhinophalangeal syndrome 146
Trichorrhexis invaginata 171, 171f, 187, 196
- in eyebrow 171f, 197f

Trichorrhexis nodosa 152, 178, 183, 183f, 184f, 187, 208, 241
- conditions with 183t
- proximal 118f, 237, 238f

Trichoschisis 178, 179f
Trichoscopy 1, 5, 8, 43, 51f, 52f, 96f, 231
- patterns 8

Trichosporon spp 136
Trichostasis spinulosa 235, 236f
Trichotemnomania 237

Trichothiodystrophy 166, 178, 178f, 179f, 183, 187
- signs of 178
- symptoms of 178
- syndromes with 178b

Trichotilloma 28
Trichotillomania 26f, 28f, 47, 51, 51f, 52f, 144, 146, 190
- treatment of 52
- trichoscopy of 51

Tumors
- benign 226
- vascular 218

Turban tumors 216

U

Ungual dysplasia 178

V

Vascular abnormalities 161
Vellus hairs 4f, 35f, 40f, 43f, 45f, 54f, 57f, 60f, 63f, 74, 75f, 76f, 89f, 233f, 236f
- absence of 71f

Vessels 15, 17
Videodermoscope 8
- devices 5

Violaceous keloid-like papules, small 106f
Violaceous peripilar halo 72f
Vogt-Koyanagi-Harada syndrome 191

W

White scarring
- dots 130f
- patches 72f

Woolly hair 146, 173
- diffuse partial 173f
- familial recessive 173
- hereditary dominant 173
- nevus 173, 173f
- sporadic recessive 173
- syndrome 174f, 175
- treatment for 173

X

Xeroderma pigmentosum 178

Z

Zigzag hairs 26, 26f
Zinc deficiency 183

EU GSPR Authorised Reprsentative
Logos Europe, 9 rue Nicolas Poussin
1700, La Rochelle, France
Phone: +33 (0) 6 67 93 73 78
E-mail: contact@logoseurope.eu